REFERENCE MANUAL
ROSENOW ET AL

✳✳✳

"MEDICAL GUIDE OF THE FUTURE" [JAMA 1938]: MICROBIAL INFECTION, VARIATION, LOCALIZATION

Narratives,
compilations &
annotations
by

S. Hale Shakman
INSTITUTE OF SCIENCE
www.InstituteOfScience.com

INSTITUTE OF SCIENCE
InstituteOfScience.com
mail@InstituteOfScience.com
First Printed 1998
Reprinted 2010
Reprinted 2016 with new "Preface to the Second Edition"

Warning and Disclaimer: Although every possible effort has been
made to assure the accuracy and correctness of information
herein, the publisher hereby: apologizes and disclaims liability
for any errors which have escaped editing; and disclaims any and
all dental, medical or legal liability in the event the contents
of this book are utilized as a direct source of any dental or
medical advice. The reader is encouraged to access original
works discussed herein to assure accuracy of information,
particularly on such critical matters as vaccine preparation,
etc., and to refer any medical questions concerning discussions
herein and related dental or medical treatment to appropriate
professionals. A proper professional assessment of all of a
person's medical conditions must always be taken into account
prior to development of a treatment plan. In this regard, as
differing professional opinions abound, a "second opinion" (or
more) is highly recommended.

The AUTOMED Project:
- *AUTOHEMOTHERAPY REFERENCE MANUAL*
- *REFERENCE MANUAL ROSENOW ET AL*
- *MEDICINE'S GRANDEST FRAUD PHD*

Printed in the United States of America

TABLE OF CONTENTS & LIST OF TABLES

(cont.)

LIST OF TABLES AND FIGURES:

ABOUT THE AUTHOR AND THIS PROJECT

S. Hale Shakman has served in program analysis, consulting, and management capacities on health, medical and related programs for several government and private organizations, including the U.S. Department of State's Agency for International Development, where he received a Meritorious Service award for his assessment of the Public Health Project Program requirements in Vietnam. He subsequently worked at the U.S. Office of Economic Opportunity (program management) and the Pathfinder Fund (population planning); and served as consultant to the U.S. Department of Health, Education & Welfare (research methodology); Maryland, Washington State and Alaska (nutrition programs); and USAID's Africa Bureau (program management). He also compiled and wrote the Summer Youth Sports Program Guide for the President's Council on Physical Fitness and Sports, and was a participant in the Scholars' Colloquium at the Library of Congress.

His writing has appeared in USA Today, Nature (London) and numerous other publications. Mr. Shakman attended Northwestern University (BA) and Georgetown University Graduate School (direct to PhD Program in History of Political Thought, earning honors), withdrawing to accept temporary assignment to Vietnam for the U.S. State Department. He resumed and completed his PhD Program requirements in History of Dentistry by special petition through the American Academy of Biological Dentistry. His PhD dissertation is published under the title, *MEDICINE'S GRANDEST FRAUD PHD*.

Over the past several years, Shakman has intensively studied the works and career of Edward C. Rosenow, M.D., (head of experimental bacteriology for the Mayo Foundation from 1915-44), and the relation of his monumental body of work to historical and contemporary medical theory and practice. Rosenow was a gifted, brilliant and thorough researcher, and his work may well mark the beginning of a new epoch in medical history.

Above all, Rosenow conclusively delineated the role of "oral foci" (infected teeth and/or tonsils) in the cause of many other diseases, including many "mysterious" disease conditions. Using organisms from oral foci of patients with various diseases, he consistently transmitted the same respective diseases to laboratory animals, demonstrating the "elective localization" of the organisms within tissues corresponding to the human diseases. His vaccines, made from these organisms, reportedly worked miracles. An accidental but inescapable postscript-hypothesis following from study of Rosenow's work is that it also encompasses, indeed provides an essential perspective for understanding, the modern nemesis known as AIDS.

This work evolved from conversations with R. Cuyugan in 1988 concerning autologous blood therapy, inspiring a research trail leading from autohemotherapy through vaccine-therapy to Rosenow. Autohemotherapy and other autologous therapies, from ancient times to current trends in cancer, vaccine, and bone-marrow-transplant research, are discussed in detail in the volume, *AUTOHEMOTHERAPY REFERENCE MANUAL*.

DISEASE CONDITIONS DISCUSSED BY ROSENOW

Alcoholism
Alkaline phosphatic
    cystitis
Allergies
Amyotrophic lateral
    sclerosis
Anemia
Angina
Appendicitis
Arthritis
Asthma
Brain tumor
Bronchiectasis
Bronchitis
Bronchopneumonia
Cancer
Cholecystitis
Chorea
Colitis
Common Cold
Compulsive
    violence
Convulsions
Coronary heart
    disease
Cystic ovaries
Cystitis
Dermatology
Diabetes
Duodenal ulcer
Embolism
Encephalitis
Encephalomyelitis
Endocarditis
Endocervitis
Epilepsy
Erythema
Ether convulsions
Eye Diseases, e.g.,
    chorioretinitis
    glaucoma
    iridocyclitis
    iritis
    uveitis
Fibrositis
Gallbladder disease
Gallstones
Gastroenteritis
Gastric ulcer
Gastroduodenal
    ulcer
Goiter
Habit spasm
Hayfever

Headache (migraine)
Herpes
    Duhring's dis.
    simplex
    zoster
Hiccup, epidemic
    & post-operative
Hodgkin's disease
Hyperpnea
    w/arrhythmia
Hypertension
Hypotension
Infertility
Influenza
Intercostal Neuralgia
Lethargy
Leukemia
Lobar pneumonia
Lupus erythematosus
Meningitis
Mental Illness
Mernier's disease
Migraine
Mononucleosis
Multiple neuritis
Multiple sclerosis
Mumps
Muscular dystrophy/
    atrophy
Myasthenia gravis
Myocardial lesions
Myoclonic
    encephalitis
Myositis
Nephritis
Nephrolithiasis
Nervous system
    diseases
Neuritis
Neuralgia
Neurofibromyositis
Neuromyositis
Osteitis deformans
Ovaritis
Paget's disease
Pancreatic disease
Parkinsonian
    encephalitis
Parotitis
Pemphigus
Periodic Ophthalmia
Pernicious anemia
Pneumonia
Pneumococcus infection

Poliomyelitis
Portal thrombosis
Prostatitis
Puerperal infection
Pulmonary diseases
Pulpitis
Pyelonephritis
Pyemia
Respiratory infect.
Rheumatic fever
Rheumatism
Scarlatinal
Scarlet fever
Schizophrenia
Sciatica
Sclerosis
Skin diseases
Sneeze, persistent
Sore throat
Spasmodic
Spasms during
    anesthesia
Splenic anemia
Stomach ulcer
Sydenham's Chorea, St.
    Vitus' dance
Thrombosis
Thyroiditis
    (exophthalmic)
Tonsillitis
Torticollis
Transverse myelitis
Trigeminal neuralgia
Ulcerative colitis
Ulcer
Urinary calculus,
    stone, tumor
Uveitis
Vagotonic neurosis
Venous thrombosis
Violent criminality
Zoster, Herpes

PREFACE TO THE SECOND EDITION - 2016

THE BOTTOM LINE:

The **mind-boggling essential finding** of E.C.Rosenow's five-decade-plus career - including three decades as head of Experimental Bacteriology at the Mayo Foundation, as exhaustively documented in 300-plus articles in the medical literature -

TO WIT -- **A _single fastidious and insidious strain_ of a very common micro-organism is fundamentally and specifically implicated in a vast bulk of chronic disease identities that plague human-kind.** The "mother" family of this organism is commonly found in the mouths and elsewhere in humans in a harmless streptococcal form, along with other, usually-innocuous, microbial residents.

Through several decades of efforts to identify the microbial cause(s) of a range of chronic diseases, which from an early stage gravitated towards exploring and unraveling the nature of this particularly dastardly enemy, Rosenow was able to expose, albeit with great difficulty, its uncanny ability to hide among related and non-related organisms found in oral areas in general and in infections elsewhere in body.

Usual methods did not and do not readily deliver up the culprit, insofar as co-existing other organisms tend to outgrow and crowd out the harmful strain in these usual culture methods. But using specially designed media that afford variations of oxygen gradients, in conjunction with extreme serial dilution culture methods, the specifically-implicated non-hemolytic or green-producing alpha streptococcus is and was reliably isolated and starkly exposed. Rosenow himself was astonished by the ability of these extreme dilutions to deliver up the sought entity, as noted in 1938:
>"I wish to state clearly that I am fully aware of the growth to be expected from mathematical relationship after successive tenfold dilutions. Nevertheless, growth has been observed in dilutions which cannot be explained on this basis. The significance, if any, of this growth is under investigation."

Simply stated, the resulting degree of extreme dilution makes it virtually impossible that an intact single organism could continue to exist, from which a viable colony might grow. (One possibility Rosenow mentioned was the question of whether a single unit might have adhered to the nichrome wire that been used to stir the succeeding dilutions.) Not long afterwards, in 1940, Rosenow seemingly touched on the extremes at which life itself might exist - indeed the question of the essential nature of the "flavor" that inhabits the essential properties of living beings - at least that which enables infectivity:
>"The property or tendency of these streptococci to localize and produce lesions electively has been shown to be referable to a toxic substance or substances elaborated by the organisms within themselves and free in the medium in which they grow. Filtrates of actively growing cultures of the respective streptococci, the dead bacteria and the live culture, all to tend to localize and produce symptoms and lesions specifically or electively in the tissues or organs characteristic of the disease the patient had and from whose foci the streptococci were isolated." (Appendix D5; 1940)

Moreover, as so isolated and then grown in pure culture, the strain of this microbe as derived from various respective disease conditions is virtually indistinguishable "morphologically and culturally" from this same strain derived from other respective disease conditions. At the same time, the respective entities are endowed with an uncanny affinity for their respective specific disease entities. As Rosenow had described the phenomenon as early as 1915:

> "It appears that the cells of the tissues for which a given strain shows elective affinity take the bacteria out of the circulation as if by a magnet -- adsorption." (Appendix D1)

This phenomenon was further demonstrated through a range of conclusive tests – including animal experiments, precipitation and agglutination tests, skin reactions for circulating antibody and antigen, and cataphoretic studies (e.g., see page 116). And correspondingly these microbes are endowed with uncanny specific curative powers relative to these respective specific disease entities, when incorporated in specific vaccines in conjunction with specific antibody.

Thus it may be useful, at this very early point in this volume, to focus on Rosenow's final summary article (from 1958), included within this compilation as Appendix D4. As particularly exhibited therein, Rosenow was able to obtain more than 75% favorable clinical results in a number of conditions with a combination of specific streptococcal vaccine and antibody treatment. It is further useful to be reminded that these conditions included the likes of schizophrenia and epilepsy as well as more conventional disease conditions, i.e., respiratory infections, arthritis, MS and migraine (see Table 6). And underying these clinical results, Rosenow cited agglutination and skin tests (summarized in Tables 1-5) indicating that similar results are to be expected (and to some extent had been realized in preceding work) in such far-ranging conditions as carcinoma, coronary heart disease, muscular dystrophy, infertility, alcoholism, diabetes, poliomyelitis, etc. And lest we not forget, in the above-cited 1940 article (Appendix D5), Rosenow had mentioned a disease of the "blood-building" tissues as one in which the implicated microbe was operative. As discussed in Chapter 7 of this volume, compelling arguments might be advanced that AIDS/HIV was clearly identified by Rosenow as early as 1940.

It is also notable that this last (1958) Rosenow article did not even make the slightest reference to Rosenow's decades-long exhaustive documentation of the seemingly all-important role of oral infections in the causation of chronic diseases of mankind. Indeed, in the decade+ prior to Rosenow's having first joined the Mayo Foundation in 1915, his breakthrough work documenting the role of oral focal infections provided the statistical foundation for former AMA President Frank Billing's landmark 1916 book *Focal Infection* – as well as the medical movement of the same name. And throughout Rosenow's career, as reflected in this volume, controversy over this concept was the hallmark of opposition to his monumental career and legacy. At the same time he acknowledged that elimination of these focal infections was often insufficient alone to effect a cure, insofar as secondary infections might allow for continuation of the progress of such systemic diseases.

Interestingly, Rosenow's development of thermal antibody, prominent in therapy regimens used in his later articles, had proceeded on two separate tracks. As discussed in his last two articles and relating to a range of diseases, the thermal antibody was used in conjunction with specific vaccine – usually in somewhat measured and regularly scheduled amounts. This form of usage had progressed gradually from the earlier developments of thermal antibody in the 1930s.   But in his subsequent work with Rappaport on poliomyelitis, the thermal antibody was used alone, without reference to vaccine, in massive amounts in a last ditch effort to abort already-rapidly-progressing degrees of paralysis. Prior to the Rappaport-associated effort, Rosenow had been using antibody derived from horse serum. But just before the initial attempts of treatments with Rappaport, the supply of horse serum was depleted – so thermal antibody was used in its place. The results, as summarized in Appendix D2, were most gratifying.

Thus, Rosenow's ultimate documentation of benefits of therapeutic measures involving specific vaccine and antibody, without reference to the well-documented albeit still-controversial role of inciting oral infections, speaks volumes – and points the way to a grand future for medical science.

Stuart Hale Shakman – March 8, 2016

PREFACE TO THE FIRST EDITION 1996-8

   In a 1915 article on autogenous vaccine therapy, C.H. Pierce lavishly praised an "E.C. Rosenow" for having perfected "vaccine-therapy", placing Rosenow in the company of Koch and Ehrlich; and despite several mentions of "opsonins" and "vaccine therapy", not a single mention of their originator, Sir Almroth Wright. It was this seemingly outrageous missed turn, this seemingly horrendous historical usurpation, this seemingly preposterous failed prophesy, hidden away in the history of medicine, that led to enquiry into what Rosenow was about and what happened to him.

   It must be admitted that this enquiry was initially motivated by a desire to expose Rosenow as a wrongful usurper of Wright's mantle. However, having traced Rosenow's writing career from 1902 through 1958 to his death on March 7, 1966 (this writer's birthday), accessed about 100 of his nearly 300 published articles, and searched for some fundamental flaw ... Voila! Rosenow emerges as a most viable candidate for physician of the century, perhaps millennium. He indeed appears to have successfully identified the cause of many disease conditions in constitutionally predisposed persons, and in so doing may well have scientifically redefined the very concept of disease.

   This report comprises an overview of Rosenow's work, with particular reference to his extensive demonstrations, over a period of several decades, of the phenomenon of "elective localization" of bacteria, in conjunction with studies on microbial variation, and the wide range of "mysterious" disease conditions for which he demonstrated the cause (and appropriate therapy). Also incorporated is an overview of evidence supporting the accidental and inescapable hypothesis that the disease entity known as AIDS falls within Rosenow's scope, and hence will yield to his proscribed ameliorative course of action for such conditions.

   Much of the information is presented in the form of annotated excerpts in appendices:

-- The ROSENOW FILE, APPENDIX A, is comprised of items relating to Rosenow's published writings.

-- The FOCAL INFECTION FILE, APPENDIX B, is comprised of items primarily relating to Rosenow associates and overall history of the focal infection concept.

-- The MICROBIAL VARIATION FILE, APPENDIX C, involves considerations of mutation and dissociation.

   It is noted that two distinct factors may be credited with having particularly contributed to the relative disfavor with which the totality of Rosenow's work has come to be regarded: (a) a 1928 fraudulent misrepresentation of his early research results, and (b) his long association with polio.

Notwithstanding Rosenow's still-essential contributions and striking therapeutical successes with polio, his reputation suffered near-terminally following the advent and popularization of Salk and Sabin polio vaccines. The now-recognized need for reviving the Rosenow perspective is reviewed herein.

However, this circumstance was more akin to supplementary "icing" on a pile of cakes which had already (figuratively) buried Rosenow's work in the wake of a cleverly-camouflaged, gross, and grossly successful misrepresentation of his work. This action, including its relation to the history of root-canal-therapy and dentistry, and medicine in general, is summarized herein (see 2.4) and discussed in detail in a separate report, *MEDICINE'S GRANDEST FRAUD PHD.*)

There have been and will be many volumes written on the cause of disease and disease processes, but these can never be complete without due reference to the vital body of work discussed here - Rosenow's monumental, consistent and irreproachable legacy.

There is no way in heaven or elsewhere that an individual could have lasted three decades at the Mayo Foundation, an institution of darn-near incomparably high standards, if that individual's work did not conform to the absolutely highest of technical and ethical standards. On the contrary, Rosenow was not the type to merely "conform" or "get by". Rather, his work is characterized by continual searching for alternate tests and answers to remaining questions, with each successive one of his nearly 300 articles exploring some new aspect of the problem.

Rosenow did not claim to have accessed all the answers to questions concerning the cause of disease; however, he did make great strides towards answering many of them. Thus, while he continued to search for other factors which contribute to the cause of specific diseases, he did in fact establish that: organisms taken from oral foci of persons with a diverse range of diseases, properly preserved and/or cultured using his painstakingly-conceived and exhaustingly proven techniques, tend to cause these same diverse disease conditions in laboratory animals. Further, Rosenow was able to recover the organism from the animals and pass the disease on to other animals. With these and other confirming tests, Rosenow clearly fulfilled the Koch-Henle criteria for proving the microbial cause of many diverse diseases.

In the course of documenting the relation between infected oral foci and systemic diseases, Rosenow's and other associated works extensively demonstrated that root-canal treated teeth invariably are infected, regardless of X-ray results, and as such invariably comprise harmful, infected "oral foci". Thus it is not just coincidental that root-canal "therapy" advocacy has comprised the core of opposition to proper consideration of Rosenow's work. Unfortunately for the future prospects of root-canal-therapy, its "scientific" justification rests inextricably on a clearly-

fraudulent distortion of Rosenow's early research results,
perpetrated by W.H. Holman in 1928. Beyond and largely because
of this, Holman's fraud has come to occupy a pivotal and
indispensable position within the history of medicine and
dentistry, serving to undermine the "focal infection" concept in
general" and the whole of Rosenow's legacy. Continuing impacts
on dentistry and medicine are pervasive and major.

   In summary, this report calls attention to the magnificent
works of E.C. Rosenow, associated implications for understanding
the pathogenesis of many diseases and disease processes in
general.

   Former AMA President Walter Bierring predicted in JAMA in 1938
(Vol. 111, p. 1623-7), that "perchance it is safe to assume that
[Rosenow's work] may yet become the medical guide of the future".
   Perchance Bierring's "future" has finally arrived.

Chapter 1. OVERVIEW: ROSENOW, BACTERIOLOGY AND DISEASE

       Prior to consideration of the substance of Rosenow's work,
it may be useful to contemplate its dimensions and place in time.
 We find Rosenow listed in various series of the INDEX MEDICUS
from 1902 through 1958 - the same E. C. Rosenow!
       By 1915, the year he joined the Mayo Foundation, Rosenow had
already published nearly one-fourth of his career-total of nearly
300 articles. At the time C. H. Pierce boldly proclaimed: "The
monumental works of Rosenow ... have reversed the opinions of the
highest medical authority of the world and thrown to earth the
false theories of older medicine ..." (C.H.Pierce, 1915 [*1])
This glowing assessment of Edward C. Rosenow, then age 40, was by
no means an isolated view, as he was already generally regarded
in prominent medical circles as among the most brilliant of
modern scientists. Rosenow went on to serve as head of
experimental bacteriology for the Mayo Foundation for nearly
three decades, from 1915 to 1944, after which he continued
actively working and writing until 1958. The visible and
verifiable results of his experiments were at times so dramatic
as to have been termed "often unbelievable", and his vaccines
were said to have "worked miracles". (Rowntree, 1958 [*2])

       Rosenow's consistent and well-documented published works
built upon two venerable medical concepts: (a) the concept of
oral focal infection (Chapter 2), whereby distant and/or
generalized diseases have been attributed to the dissemination of
microorganisms or their toxins through the bloodstream from an
oral "focus" or reservoir; and (b) the ability or perhaps even
tendency of microorganisms to exist in different phases as a
result of dissociation or mutation (Chapter 3), depending on
environmental conditions.
       Rosenow's investigations consistently demonstrated the
presence of specifically virulent nonhemolytic streptococci
within the oral focus, primarily in or around teeth, including
pulpless teeth, and/or tonsils (often without visible symptoms of
infection) [*3] (see 2.1); these organisms or their derivatives
were directly and clearly implicated in a wide range of diseases
[*4] - from arthritis to schizophrenia, and even including
disease of "blood- building tissues" [*5] The key to the success
of Rosenow's investigations was the use of a laboriously-
developed methodology that most significantly correctly mimicked
conditions existing within the human body, particularly involving
a range of oxygen supply (see 4.1), rather than the customary
reliance on strictly "aerobic" (as in the air) or even strictly
"anaerobic" (zero oxygen) conditions.

       The manner in which Rosenow integrated and refined these
concepts into an understanding of a wide range of diseases may
even come to be recognized as the high point of 20th century
medicine, although his legacy is currently obscure or even
maligned. Surprisingly, this has occurred despite the association
of Rosenow with some of the most prominent names in American

medical history. Early in his career, Rosenow worked closely with Frank Billings and Charles H. Mayo, both former AMA Presidents and staunch advocates of the concept of oral focal infection as a key factor in systemic disease. And another former AMA President, Walter Bierring, in a landmark article discussing the works of Billings and Rosenow in the authoritative Journal of the American Medical Association (JAMA) in 1938, cited detailed independent results that "furnished definite confirmatory proof of Rosenow's theory of elective localization" [*6] Moreover, some 38 of Rosenow's own published articles also appeared in JAMA.

(Even before Rosenow was born, an earlier AMA president, Austin Flint, had noted in 1868 that caries of the teeth are at least an occasional cause of trigeminal neuralgia [*7] - which same condition has recently been discussed as associated with cavitations in bone from which devitalized teeth have been removed. [*8]

Rosenow emphasized two primary points relative to the therapy of a wide-range of diseases:

(a) Removal of the oral focus. [*3] Rosenow demonstrated that the oral focus, usually in or around diseased or non-vital teeth [*4,*16] (see 2.2) and/or (secondarily) tonsils [*17] (See APPENDIX A - 19R6) is the primary site of replication and dissemination, and even for the acquisition of their specificity and strength [*18](SEE APPENDIX A - 27R9, 34R5). But he and others have cautioned that removal of the focus cannot be expected to always result in a cure, insofar as a secondary infection elsewhere in the body may have already become sufficiently established so as to be able to sustain the infective process even in the absence of the primary (oral) focus; and

(b) Administration of specific therapeutic antigen (vaccine) or antibody, or both, preferably autogenous (generated from organisms taken from the patient). [*19] (see 4.5) In some of his later articles, Rosenow set forth a therapeutical regimen discussing only the administration of antigen and/or antibody, without specific reference to oral foci; however, it was noted that this therapy would need to be continued indefinitely, presumably due to the continued presence of foci (reservoirs) of infection. Thus the importance of their removal in conjunction with vaccine-therapy [*3] (see 2.3), as had been consistently and strongly emphasized by Rosenow, would appear to continue to warrant primary consideration.

Rosenow's instructions relating to the isolation, cultivation and preservation, respectively, of properly-specific pathogenic organisms (streptococci) incorporate three essential technical components (see Chapter 4): use of serial dilutions [*20] (see 4.3), oxygen gradients [*21] (see 4.1), and glycerol-salt menstruum [*3] (see 4.4). These components and other details of Rosenow's instructions for production of vaccine and antibody (see 4.5) require close attention, insofar as strict compliance consistently achieved favorable results (whereas failures invariably have been associated with and apparently attributable to non-compliance).

Further major implications of the foregoing on some popular modern medical perspectives include characterization of the concept of "animal models" as intrinsically flawed, as evident in its being at variance with the venerable Koch-Henle postulates of disease causation; reaffirmation of the validity of the Koch-Henle tradition; the essential complementarian compatibility of the Rosenow perspective with modern emphases on genetics, and exposure of the concept of "autoimmune disease" as fictional and superfluous.

- Animal Models. Nowadays, much fanfare accompanies the discovery of new "animal models" in which diseases that resemble those in man can be induced and studied. These "models" by definition do not involve the identical disease processes, but rather processes which mimic the real ones. In light of Rosenow's work, it would appear that the failure of modern practitioners to replicate many human diseases in laboratory animals simply indicates that they have the wrong organism, or a wrong or degenerative phase of the correct one. In contrast, Rosenow marvelled at how similar were the tissues of persons and animals. He readily replicated a wide range of disease conditions in laboratory animals using bacteria from oral foci of patients suffering from these same diseases.

- Koch-Henle postulates of disease. Insofar as the Koch-Henle postulates require replication of diseases in laboratory animals with the suspected disease-causing agent, a revival of Rosenow's methodology brings with it a reaffirmation of these venerable postulates. Moreover, Rosenow's work went far beyond merely fulfilling the venerable Koch-Henle postulates. [*5] (see APPENDIX A - 40R3)

- The relative role of genetics. Modern perspectives generally recognize that the genetic factor is essentially a predisposition and does not itself cause disease, but that some undisclosed environmental factor triggers the actual onset of disease. Similarly, Rosenow discussed both onset and identity of disease conditions as attributable to a combination of (a) infection by microorganisms and (b) "constitutional" or inherited predisposition. Thus, Rosenow's successful therapeutic regimens would at a minimum be expected to be complementary to gene therapy, and particularly attractive in light of the acknowledged general failure of gene therapy thus far [*22] to produce beneficial results. (see 1.3)

- The concept of "autoimmune disease". In the second half of the 20th century (coincident with Rosenow's residence in semi-obscurity), "autoimmune" processes were proposed to be causing many disease conditions for which a foreign cause presumably could not be identified; however, it has since been generally recognized that this so-called "autoimmune reaction" may be a result and not the cause of a diseased state [*23], and that the onset of "autoimmune disease" may be "triggered by unknown environmental factors acting on a predisposing genetic background" [*24]. In that Rosenow's successful methodology consistently enabled identification of specific microbial pathogens in these same conditions, the very need for an "autoimmune disease" concept may well be questioned.

- Beyond considerations of "normal" diseases, such as appendicitis, arthritis, asthma, etc., it is noted that Rosenow's scope encompassed numerous other conditions including alcoholism, infertility, mental illness and even violent criminality; and he long ago had anticipated (and solved in advance) the contemporary dilemma of "post-polio syndrome" [*25] (see Chapter 6). He also probed far-ranging disease-related topics such as the role of radiant energy in seasonality of various diseases and epidemics.[*26] (see APPENDIX A - 50R3)

As to why Rosenow's work has faded from the medical limelight, this in so small part seems attributable to a clearly fraudulent misrepresentation by W. Holman in 1928 [*10] of Rosenow's early (1915) research results [*9] . Over the next couple of decades, Holman's (incorrect) 1928 portrayal came to serve as the indispensable foundational citation for a body of incestuously cross-referenced literature [*11] which confronted Rosenow's otherwise unassailable work. This body of contrary literature, the essential core of which comprises the "scientific" justification for the field of root-canal-"therapy", continues to underly and influence modern medical and dental attitudes, theory and practice (see 2.4).

Nonetheless, the concepts of focal infection [*12] (see 2.5), mutation [*13] and dissociation [*14] (see Chapter 3), and the use of reduced oxygen gradients [*15] (see 4.2) are separately being promoted in modern medical research, providing measures of independent validation of the foundations of Rosenow's prior, integrated studies and methodology.

Overall, Rosenow's monumental body of work appears to have much to offer in relation to attaining an understanding of cause, prevention and therapy of a wide range of human disease conditions. The broad scope and immediate specific impact of Rosenow's work argue for its priority re-integration into modern medical and dental education and practice.

Postscript: Insofar as Rosenow has demonstrated that the causative agent for a wide range of diseases is disseminated through the bloodstream [*21, *27] (see 8.2), the use of autohemotherapy (see Chapter 8) is suggested for consideration as an immediately-available, temporary therapeutic expedient, pending the development and general availability of Rosenow's specific vaccines. It is further noted that numerous disease conditions have been addressed in the historical literature of both autohemotherapy and Rosenow [*28] (see 8.2).

Bibliography: OVERVIEW - ROSENOW, BACTERIOLOGY AND DISEASE

  *1. C.H. Pierce, 1915 JOURNAL-LANCET, Minneap., Aug. 1, 1915, n.s., xxxv, 414-419.
  *2. Rowntree, Leonard G., 1958, Amid Masters of TWENTIETH CENTURY MEDICINE, Charles C. Thomas, Springfield Ill. 1958
  *3. Rosenow, E.C., Jour. Lab. and Clin. Med. 14:504-512, 1929, p. 506, 510
  *4. Rosenow, E.C., Streptococci in etiology of diverse diseases, including diseases of nervous system, J. Nerv. and Ment. Dis. 117: 415-428, May 1953. Provides a comprehensive listing of disease conditions and references.
  *5. Rosenow, E.C., Proceedings, Dental Centenary Celebration, Maryland State Dental Association, 1940, pp. 261-282, 1940, p. 271, 277.
  *6. Bierring, Walter L., "Focal Infection: Quarter Century Survey", JAMA 111 (Oct. 29, 1938), 1623-1627.
  *7. Flint, Austin, A Treatise on the Principles and Practice of Medicine, 3rd Ed., Henry C. Lea, Phila., 1868, p. 688
  *8. Meinig, George, D.D.S., Root Canal Coverup, 1994, Price-Pottinger Foundation, P.O. Box 2614, La Mesa, CA. 91943-2614. (1-800-FOODS-4-U)
  *9. Rosenow, E. C., J.A.M.A. LXV 1688 (1915).
  *10. Holman, W.L., Archives Path & Lab. Med. 5 (1928), 133.
  *11. Core of Holman-dependent/incestuously-cross-referenced anti-Rosenow literature: MacNevin, M.G. and Vaughn, H.S., Mouth Infections and Their Relation to Systemic Disease, New York, Joseph Purcell Research Memorial, 1930, 78-91; Blayney, J.R., Dental Cosmos LXXIV, 635-653 (July 1932); Appleton, J.L.T., Jr., Bacterial Infection, Lea & Febiger, Philadelphia 1933, 565-577/ Reiman, H.A., and Havens, W.P., J.A.M.A., 114, 1 (1940); Woods, Alan C., Am. J. Opth. 25 (Dec. 1942), 1423-1444; Grossman, Louis I., Root Canal Therapy, 1946, 154-172.
  *12. e.g. Newman, H.N., J. of Dental Research 71(11), Nov., 1992, p. 1854, and Periodontal Abstracts Volume 41 Number 3, 1993, 73-77; Navazesh M and R Mulligan, Special Care in Dentistry, 1995, Jan-Feb, 15(1): 11-9.
  *13. Bryan AH, Bryan CA and Bryan CG, Bacteriology, 6th edition, Barnes and Noble, New York 1968, p. 22-24; Cvitkovitch DG and Hamilton IR, Oral Microbiol. Immunol. 9:200-217, 1993; Kaufmann SH, Annual Review of Immunology 1993, 11:129-63; Chalkey L et al., Fems Microbiology Letters, 1991 Dec. 15, 69(1):35-42.
  *14. De Long, R. J. theor. Biol. (1977) 64, 761-764; Madoff, Sarabelle, ed., The Bacterial L-Forms, Marcel Dekker, Inc., N.Y. and Basel, 1986; Weiser JN, et al., J. Infect. Dis., 1993 Sep, 168(3);672-80; Weiser JN, et al., Infection and Immunity, 1994 Jun, 62(6):2582-9; Rosengarten R and Wise KS, Science, 1990 Jan 19, 247(4940):315-8; Bove JM, Clin. Infect. Dis., 1993 Aug, 17 Suppl 1:S10-31; Pavolva IB, et al., Zhurnal Mikrobiologii,

Epidemiologii i Immunobiologii, 1990 Dec. (12): 12-15]; L. H. Mattman, Cell Wall Deficient Forms -   Stealth Pathogens, CRC Press, Boca Raton Fla. 1993.

*15. e.g. in stomach ulcers, as discussed by Monmaney, Terence, New Yorker, Sept. 20, 1993, 64-72, "Marshall's Hunch"

*16. L.T. Austin and T.J. Cook, J.A.D.A. 16, May 1929, 894-6; P.S. Rhoads and G.F. Dick, J.A.D.A. 19, November 1932, 1884-93; and W.F. Swanson and L.E. Van Kirk, J. Dent. Research 15, September 1936, p. 315; Rosenow, E.C., Cincinnati J. Med. 25: 329-339, Oct. 1944.

*17. Rosenow, E.C., J. Dental Res. 1:205-267, 1919.

*18. Rosenow, E.C., Kentucky M. J., Oct. 1927, 592-597.

*19. Rosenow, E.C., Studies on specific prevention and treatment of diverse diseases shown due to specific types of nonhemolytic streptococci, Am. Practitioner and Digest of Treatment (Philadelphia), 9(5), May 1958, p. 755-761.

*20. Rosenow, E.C., Arch. Path. 26: 70-76, July 1938; Rosenow, E.C., J. Nerv. and Ment. Dis. 122: 238-247, Sept. 1955.

*21. Rosenow, E.C., JAMA LXIII (Sept. 12, 1914), 903-908.

*22. Marshall, E., Science, Vol. 269, 25 August 1995, 1050-55, p. 1950, quoting NIH Director Harold Varmus, May 1995..

*23. Wilson, D., Body and Antibody, 1972, p. 257.

*24. Conrad B, et al., Nature 371 (22 Sept. 1994), p. 351.

*25. Rosenow, E.C., J. Nerv. and Ment. dis. 120: 196-206, Sept.-Oct. 1954, 204

*26. Rosenow, E.C., Proc. Staff Meetings of Mayo Clinic 8:500-502 (Aug. 16) 1933. (With Charles Sheard and C. B. Pratt.); Protoplasma 23:24-33 (March) 1935. (With C. B. Pratt and Charles Sheard); Postgrad. Med. 8: 290-292, Oct. 1950.

*27. Rosenow, E.C., JAMA 44:871-873, (March 18) 1905, 871-3; Jour. Infect. Dis. 17:403-408, 1915; Jour. Infect. Dis. 16:240-268, 1915; Jour. Infect. Dis. 19:333-384, 1916; Jour. Dental Res. 1:205-267, 1919, p. 243; Proc. Staff Meetings of Mayo Clinic 8:500-502 (Aug. 16) 1933 (with Charles Sheard and C. B. Pratt); Proc. Staff Meet., Mayo Clin. 12: 252-256, April 21, 1937 (with Heilman, F.R.); Am. J. Clin. Path. 15: 135-151, April 1945; Postgrad. Med. 2: 346-357, Nov. 1947; Postgrad. Med. 124-136, Feb. 1948; Postgrad. Med. 3: 367- 376, May 1948; Ann. Allergy 6: 485-496, Sept.-Oct. 1948; South Dakota J. Med. and Pharm. 5: 243-248; 262; 272, Sept. 1952; South Dakota J. Med. and Pharm. 5: 304-310; 328, Nov. 1952, p. 309; Ohio M.J., 53(7), July 1957, p. 783-5.

*28. INDEX MEDICUS, QUARTERLY CUMULATIVE INDEX MEDICUS, CUMULATED INDEX MEDICUS; 1902-1958; see AUTOMED A to Z -- The Automedical Index, available through instituteofscience.com, IoS BOOKS.

1.1 EDWARD CARL ROSENOW - BIOGRAPHICAL INFORMATION

Born: July 14, 1875; Alma, Wisconsin; D.: March 7, 1966

M.D.:1902; Rush Medical College

1903-1904: Intern at Presbyterian Hospital, Chicago

1904-1915: Research bacteriology and practice of internal medicine, Chicago [staff member, McCormick Memorial Institute for Infectious Diseases; worked with Drs. Ludvig Hektoen and Frank Billings.

1915-1944: Head of Division of Experimental Bacteriology and professor of experimental bacteriology, Mayo Foundation.

Married to Lydia B. Senty, Aug. 1, 1906

WHO'S WHO: "Research in transmutation of pneumococci and streptococci, localization of bacteria, lobar pneumonia, poliomyelitis, influenza, focal infection, epilepsy, schizophrenia; in-vitro production of antibodies to streptococci; first to point out focal infection of teeth."

Dr. Rosenow died on March 7, 1966, of the effects of a fractured hip suffered some time earlier (Am. J. Clin. Path. 46 (1966).

1.2 SOME ROSENOW TESTIMONIALS

   Many writers, over a period of many years, saw fit to highly praise Rosenow's accomplishments. The sampling exhibited below, from 1915 through 1958, may begin to convey just how special Rosenow and his legacy may turn out to be:

   "Rosenow ... demonstrated in his laboratory an experiment on a single rabbit which was infected with material from a patient who had died under violent encephalitic hiccoughs. Already 48 hours after the injection, the animal died in front of the visitors eyes after having hiccoughed violently for several hours."
      Jarlov E., Brinch O, Danish Section, *Assoc.Internationale Pour les Recherches sur la Paradentose, Copenhagen: Lassen and Stiedl*, 1938; abstr.- JAMA 111 (1938), 290

   "Illingworth, working in my clinic, was able to show that, using Rosenow's special medium, streptococci could be grown from the wall of the gall bladder in quite a large percentage of cases in which the bile was sterile. He further showed that the organisms of the 'coli' group are relatively infrequent except in active supprative cases.
   "... Dr. A. L. Wilkie ... has shown that cholecystitis is almost invariably an intramural streptococcal infection, and that Rosenow's contention of a selective affinity of this organism for the gall bladder is strikingly true. ... He has brought to light

the illuminating and remarkable fact that bile inhibits the
growth of this streptococcus. ... This fact accounts for the
widespread failure to confirm Rosenow's findings. ...
     Wilkie DPD, *Brit. Med. J.* 1, 1928, 481

"Frick [A. Frick, *JAMA* 82:595 (Feb. 23, 1924] stated that
according to his clinical experience there seems to be no doubt
that Rosenow's theory of the elective affinity of a specific
streptococcus, of a certain grade of virulence, for the gastric
or duodenal mucosa is correct and that a specific streptococcus
is the common cause of peptic ulcer."
     "Eusterman [Eusterman GB, *Minn. Med.*, 6:698 (1923)] summarized
the clinical evidence for the infectious origin of peptic ulcer
in the light of recent experimental work and expressed the
opinion that in certain types of ulcer it is the only tenable
theory at this stage of medical progress." ...
     "The streptococcus which we have isolated consistently in these
cases is identical with that first described by Rosenow as having
etiologic importance in the production of peptic ulcer in man,
and it provides a means for active immunization with specific
autogenous vaccine."
     Nickel AC & AR Hufford, *Arch. Int. Med.* 41 (1928), 215.

"Rosenow has shown us the various gradations of variety and
morphology that different oxygen-pressures bring about, and has
caught and held for our inspection the missing links of the chain
of relationships between both acute and chronic bacillary and
coccogenous affections."
     C. H. Pierce, *Journal-Lancet*, Minneap., Aug. 1915, 414-9.

"It has long been known that the tendency of organisms to
localize depends to a certain extent on virulence, and that the
virulence of an organism is changed by environment. Rosenow's
elaboration has been so extensive, however, as to almost
revolutionize former views concerning infection."
     William W. Duke, *Oral Sepsis in its Relationship to Systemic
     Disease*, C.V. Mosby, St. Louis, 1918, 74.

"[Rosenow's] work has been so scientific, and his facts so firmly
established that I believe we must either repudiate his facts, or
in a general way accept his conclusion ... in regard to the
elective affinity of bacteria for different organs and
structures."
     George W. McCaskey in A.R. Barnes and A.S. Giordano, *Journal
     of the Indiana State Med. Assoc.*, Ja 15, 1922, 5.

"Rosenow made a fundamental contribution to bacteriology in
demonstrating that the bacteria concerned in chronic foci of
infection are very sensitive to oxygen tension, ... that the
cultivation of the organisms and the reproduction of lesions in
animals is largely dependent upon the use of proper laboratory
technique. [and] that the organisms in chronic foci vary greatly
in their affinity for different tissues of the body."

Russell L. Haden, *Dental Infection and Systemic Disease*, Lea and Febiger, Philadelphia, Pa., U.S.A. 1928, 159.

"the tenets of both [bacteriology and immunology] offer definite confirmation regarding [specific tissue affinity and elective tissue localization], and perchance it is safe to assume that the 'Rosenow heresy' may yet become the medical guide of the future."
Walter L. Bierring, 87th President of the A.M.A. (1934), in the *Journal of the A.M.A.* 111 (Oct. 29, 1938), 1626.

"[Rosenow] was adept at securing organisms from focal lesions, culturing them, and in reproducing the clinical syndromes of the patients in animals. repeatedly by intracerebral injections [Rosenow] set off syndromes in rabbits the exact counterparts of the clinical manifestations observed in the patients - especially tics of one kind or another. When the patient and the rabbit were placed side by side the resemblance of syndromes [was] often unbelievable and at times almost ludicrous and suggestive of plagiarism. ... he prepared autogenous vaccines that worked miracles in innumerable patients."
Leonard G. Rowntree, *Amid Masters of Twentieth Century Medicine*, Charles C. Thomas, Springfield Ill. 1958

1.3 BACTERIAL-GENETIC INTERFACE - THE TRUE CUTTING EDGE

We are inundated these days with reference to so-called "hereditary" or "genetic diseases", which when properly cited are referred to as diseases to which there is or appears to be a genetic predisposition. Otherwise, everyone with a suspected defective gene would get the disease, and that does not occur. The factors contributing to actual onset of disease are many, including the quality of the air we breathe and food we eat. But there is also commonly thought to be some environmental cause yet to be identified. Often some form or combination of microorganisms is suspected, or even so-called "auto-immune" processes alone or in concert with some organism or "toxin". Modern perspectives generally recognize that the genetic factor is essentially a predisposition and does not itself cause disease, but that some undisclosed environmental factor triggers the actual onset of disease. Similarly, Rosenow discussed both onset and identity of disease conditions as attributable to a combination of (a) infection by micro-organisms and (b) constitutional or inherited predisposition. Thus, Rosenow's successful therapeutic regimens would at a minimum be expected to be complementary to gene therapy, and particularly attractive in light of the acknowledged general failure of gene therapy thus far to produce beneficial results Marx [Science 247, 1540] points out that "genetic susceptibility is apparently not the only determinant of whether an individual actually gets sick [from] ... diseases of more complex inheritance." Among these are listed heart disease, cancer, high blood pressure, obesity, diabetes, multiple sclerosis, Alzheimers, schizophrenia and manic depression. "Environmental influences, such as diet, smoking,

chemical exposures, viral infections, and <u>the all too common</u>
<u>'unknown'</u> [this writer's emphasis] must also play a role." Marx
lists number of persons in the U.S. affected with some of these
conditions:

```
--cancer                    6.0 million
--coronary heart disease    5.0   "
--diabetes                  0.5   "
--high blood pressure      60.0   "
--manic depression          1.0   "
--schizophrenia             1.8   "
```

   Coincidentally, Rosenow had worked with these very same disease
conditions, as well as arthritis, multiple sclerosis, ulcerative
colitis, epilepsy, thyroiditis, etc.; and had consistently
isolated specific organisms with which he was able to replicate
symptoms in laboratory animals; and then isolated the organisms
from the laboratory animals and was able to pass the disease
conditions on to other laboratory animals. Insodoing, Rosenow
appears to have fullfilled the Henle-Koch postulates for
establishing the cause of these diseases.
   Perhaps some future generations of geneticists will succeed in
creating conditions for the evolution of perfect human specimens,
people without genetic "flaws", totally impervious to any
possible attack by bacterial, viral or other pathogenic forms.
Whether such is either remotely possible or desirable could and
will fill several volumes if this has not already occurred.
   More likely, it is at the bacterial-genetic interface that the
future of medicine and improved - perhaps even ultimate - control
over disease conditions will come. Thus, while continuation of
studies aimed at improved understanding and control of the
genetic component are to be encouraged, it would be as or even
more foolish to ignore the bacterial side pending completion of
genetic studies as would be the reverse, particularly when so
much useful work has already been accomplished on the bacterial
side.
   Genetic predisposition to disease, e.g. M.S., may be viewed as
a greater vulnerability (or simply the existence of vulnerability) to attack by particular (strains of) microorganisms. This
particular weak link or opening might someday be closed by -
organism can be kept out or otherwise precluded from establishing
its intended colony, then so much the better - for you.
   Therein lies the importance, the immediacy, of reviving the
works or Rosenow and associates. Or we can ignore them and try
to reinvent the wheel. And where is this colony, this nest of
invaders? Usually in, under and/or around diseased or non-vital
teeth.

Chapter 2.   ORAL FOCUS AS CAUSE OF DISEASE

A general negative effect of oral infections on the overall health of an individual seemingly cannot be denied; beyond this, the idea that diseased teeth may cause other diseases has been recognized throughout the history of medicine - the concept of "oral focal infection".

Rosenow's work has gone even further, in demonstrating how organisms in oral foci acquire therein the ability to target specific tissues and cause specific diseases. Rosenow has:

1) proved the truth of this concept beyond all doubt, through extensive bacteriological studies that were invariably validated by numerous other investigators;

2) showed that the relationship is causal, i.e., that organisms emanating from diseased teeth, and secondarily tonsils, are the essential microbial cause of many diseases elsewhere in the body;

3) proved that this cause is specific for various specific diseases, i.e., that organisms from an "oral focus" (e.g. diseased teeth or tonsils) of a person with appendicitis, for example, tend to "electively locate in appendices of laboratory animals and cause appendicitis in them;

4) showed that "symptomless foci", e.g. diseased teeth or tonsils which are not inflamed or painful, etc., may be even more dangerous than those with symptoms, in that the former are indicative that the organisms have ready access to the circulatory system and are thus less likely to get "backed up" and cause symptoms within the oral focus, but for this same reason are more likely to escape and cause damage elsewhere;

(5) proved that non-vital teeth, i.e., teeth on which root-canal therapy has been performed, are invariably infected, and, insofar as these are often symptomless, are of paramount concern as a major contributing factor in the causation of a wide range of systemic diseases (as "nests" from which disease-causing organisms continually seep out into the bloodstream).

Rosenow's work in this area is summarily illustrated below in Table 1.1, in the case of more than 11,000 laboratory animals. For associated discussions, see APPENDIX A - 40R3.

For further examination of others' related works, see list of fifteen confirming studies, APPENDIX A - 48R2.

Table 2.1: LOCALIZATION OF STREPTOCOCCI IN 11,479 ANIMALS*

LESIONS IN ANIMALS'	SOURCE: DENTAL/OTHER FOCI IN PERSONS WITH	ROSENOW		ELEVEN CO-WORK.		TWENTY OTHERS		TOTALS	
		#	%	#	%	#	%	#	%
Stomach	Stomach/duodenum ulcer	1539	65	1231	52	280	60	3050	57
	Other diseases	3341	8	1798	6	996	3	6135	06
	No systemic disease	1329	14	665	7	300	7	2294	11
Joints	Arthritis	1447	53	1225	58	415	59	3087	56
	Other diseases	3433	13	1804	7	861	39	6098	15
	No systemic disease	1329	18	665	11	300	31	2294	18

Eyes	Iritis, other eye dis.	272	42	328	43	186	53	786	45
	Other diseases	4608	1	2701	1	1090	1	8399	01
	No systemic disease	1329	8	665	0	300	2	2294	05
Myocardium	Myocarditis	36	61	39	38	94	59	169	54
	Other diseases	4844	3	2990	7	1182	11	9016	06
	No systemic disease	1329	6	665	3	300	17	2294	07
Muscles	Myositis	891	72	50	58	86	56	1027	70
	Other diseases	3989	6	2979	9	1190	12	8158	08
	No systemic disease	1329	3	665	7	300	13	2294	05
Kidneys	Pyelonephritis	168	73	96	83	96	58	360	72
	Other diseases	4712	6	2933	3	1180	16	8825	07
	No systemic disease	1329	9	665	7	300	19	2294	10
Colon	Ulcerative colitis	527	58	60	60	119	42	706	56
	Other diseases	4353	2	2969	0	1157	1	8479	01
	No systemic disease	1329	5	665	0	300	0	2294	03
	TOTALS	6209		3694		1576		11479	

*   Rosenow, E. C., Dental Centenary Proceedings, Maryland State
    Dental Association and A.D.A., March 1940, p. 261-82.

Illustrative explanation of Table 2.1:
    In the case of stomach ulcers, 57% of animals, injected with
the organism from foci of stomach ulcer patients, were found to
have lesions of the stomach; vs. 6% of animals injected with
organisms from patients with other diseases.

2.1 IMPORTANCE OF SYMPTOMLESS FOCI INCLUDING PULPLESS TEETH

    In response to those who may assert "my teeth are fine"; "my
tonsils were taken out long ago", or "I had a "root-canal" years
ago, and it's no problem", in the presence of systemic disease
that has been linked to oral foci, Rosenow and others have
repeatedly urged practitioners to search for a focus that may not
be so obvious but is none the less insidious. See particularly
discussions in APPENDIX A:
    --29R1, 506: "SYMPTOMLESS FOCI IMPORTANCE";
    --29R1, 511: "REMOVAL OF FOCI NECESSARY EVEN WITH SPECIFIC
    VACCINE";
    --44R8, 329: :HIDDEN FOCI IN X-RAY NEGATIVE VITAL TEETH;
    "PULPLESS TEETH MUST GO: 8 SUPPORTING REFERENCES

Table 2.2:   Foci of infection in:
[29R1-506]   tonsils, teeth, pulpless
                            teeth
Diseases:
encephalitis   70%   56%   87%
arthritis   51   69   61

torticollis	60	75	76
MS	78	67	89
chronic polio	65	71	92
gastroduod.ulcer	74	74	52
lesions of eye	53	53	50
lesions of skin	74	56	77
prostatitis	63	54	69

2.2 PULPLESS TEETH: INFECTION SITE AND DISSEMINATION SOURCE

In 1940, speaking at the Dental Centenary Celebration, Rosenow discussed at length the issue of non-vital teeth, with reference to three supporting studies:

(a) P.S. Rhoads and G.F. Dick, J.A.D.A. 19, November 1932, 1884-93, reported that the number of colonies from apexes of pulpless teeth was 700 to 1000 times greater than the number obtained from identically treated vital teeth; and

(b) W.F. Swanson and L.E. Van Kirk, J. Dent. Research 15, September 1936, p. 315, found that 96% of 1220 root-filled pulpless teeth and 98% of 582 non-root-filled pulpless teeth yielded a growth, chiefly green-producing streptococci.

(c) L.T. Austin and T.J. Cook, J.A.D.A. 16, May 1929, 894-6, found that 89% of 100 pulpless teeth vs. 4% of 100 vital teeth yielded characteristic implicated streptococci.

> [40R3: Rosenow, EC, Proceedings Dental Centenary
> Celebration, Maryland State Dental Association, 1940,
> 261-282, p.266]

Rhoads and Dick 1932 concluded that all pulpless teeth are probable foci. For further details of their report on studies involving more than 3000 persons, please see APPENDIX B: Rhoads and Dick 1932, "PULPLESS TEETH - SUMMARIES OF 3000 PERSONS" and "ALL PULPLESS TEETH ARE PROBABLE FOCI".

Swanson and Van Kirk, 1936, obtained positive cultures in 96.4% of 1220 root-filled teeth and 97.8% of 582 not-root-filled teeth for an overall 96.8% of 1802 pulpless teeth. They concluded that "the sterile pulpless tooth under any circumstances may be an extreme rarity." For further details of their study of 1800 pulpless teeth, please see APPENDIX B, Swanson and Van Kirk 1936, "PULPLESS TEETH - 1800 OBSERVED"

Further details on Austin and Cook:
Austin and Cook 1929 sought "to secure a control for the large number of pulpless teeth cultured at The Mayo Clinic, and to determine the correctness of the opinion that a large percentage of normal vital teeth yield cultures of streptococci". They used normal vital teeth being removed because a full denture was being advised, with no more than two teeth from any one case, using extremely careful, described in detail, sterile methods. The vital teeth were compared with identically-treated pulpless teeth, both roentgenically negative and positive.

Table 2.3:   Cultures from 100 vital and 100 pulpless teeth

| | | Cultures G-B Broth | | Cultures in Glucose-Brain Agar | | | | |
| | | | | Zero | Numbers of Colonies | | | |
Teeth	Number	%yes	%no	Growth	0-20	20-50	50-100	100+
Vital	100	4	96	96	3	--	1	--
Pulpless	100	89	11	11	2	9	3	75
X-ray negative	50	84	16	16	4	8	2	70
X-ray positive	50	94	6	6	--	10	4	80

Austin & Cook

As seen in the above Table 2.3, most of the pulpless teeth, both x-ray negative and positive, were shown to be generally infected, and grossly so, when compared to the vital teeth. Fully 96% of the vital teeth yielded no bacterial growth sought by both of two culture methods. In three percent minimal growth was obtained and in only one was moderate growth obtained.

   "... A possible explanation for the 4 percent of positive cultures may be that some of these cultures were obtained from patients who were not only harboring a large number of infected teeth, some of which were immediately adjacent to the vital tooth cultured, but were also suffering from infective diseases.

   "In the pulpless group, which was used as a control, it was interesting to note that there was not a great difference" between x-ray negative and x-ray positive groups."

   Of the pulpless teeth, not only did 89% yield a positive growth of streptocci, but also "of this series, 75 per cent yielded more than 100 colonies in agar, which indicated that considerable infection was present in most of the cases."

CONTEMPORARY ACKNOWLEDGEMENT THAT PULPLESS TEETH ARE INFECTED
   It has been reputably acknowledged in modern times by Samuel Seltzer, head of the Endodontics Section of the venerable journal Oral Path., Oral Surg. ..., that nonvital teeth are infected:
   Seltzer 1987 [in Cohen, S. and R. C. Burns, Pathways of the Pulp, C.V. Mosby, St. Louis, 1987, a prominent endodontics (root-canal-therapy) text, p 1] concedes that in the early 1970s "more sophisticated techniques, such as those using strictly anaerobic conditions, revealed the presence of micro-organisms that hitherto had been unreported in root canals. ... The emphasis on obtaining negative cultures began to be dissipated." (That is, the fact that treated root canals are commonly infected is known but generally ignored by root-canal treatment advocates.)

2.3 FAVORABLE RESULT AFTER BOTH FOCUS REMOVAL AND VACCINE

   Rosenow emphasized the importance of removing foci in conjunction with vaccines.

   In 1929 he provided summary data for 358 cases of various diseases, comparing results where vaccines were or not used, and foci were or were not removed:

Table 2.4: All foci removed   All foci not removed
Vaccine   (% improved)   (% improved)
-Used: 61   25
-Not used: 54   21

For further discussion, please see APPENDIX A - 29R1, p. 510.

2.4   HOLMAN'S FRAUDULENT MANIPULATION OF ROSENOW'S RESULTS

Consideration of the correlation between diseased teeth and various systemic diseases reached a high level of prominence and sophistication in the first part of the Twentieth Century. But despite the conclusively refining studies of Edward C. Rosenow, Weston Price, Russel Haden, former A.M.A. Presidents Frank Billings and Charles Mayo, and others, the concept of focal infection has been playing "Rip van Winkle" for the past half-century.

This deplorable situation must in part be attributed to a carefully-constructed 1928 fabrication by W. Holman, which has come to occupy a critical position in the history of medicine. Holman's handiwork comprises the key and indispensable foundation for layers of subsequent denial of the importance of, and general disregard for, the revolutionary works of Rosenow and associates, as well as for the venerable concept of focal infection in general. Holman's deception thus continues to comprise the fraudulent foundation on which rests an inverted pyramid of ignorance and unnecessary speculation as to the cause of a range of human diseases.

DOCTORING THE NUMBERS*

Consideration of similarities between such diseases as multiple sclerosis, arthritis, diabetes, and thyroiditis [1] might as a matter of course refer to the monumental body of work of E.C. Rosenow [2], were it not for continuing effects of a gross distortion of his (early) research results [3] by W. L. Holman in 1928 [4]. Rosenow, who served with the Mayo Clinic from 1915-1944 and published nearly 300 articles spanning the period 1902-1958, conducted extensive series of animal experiments and other tests which evidenced the phenomenon of elective localization of bacteria (emanating from oral foci) as a factor in these and diverse other diseases [2, 3, 5].

A 1928 article by Holman challenged the significance of Rosenow's results with a so-called "rearrangement of Rosenow's data", and subsequently has served as a common and key reference in literature underlying the modern relationship between medicine and dentistry. [6] On examination, Holman's "rearrangement" is seen as a cleverly-designed deception. For example, Rosenow reported that 60% of 103 animals injected with bacteria as isolated from stomach ulcer patients had developed lesions with hemorrhages in the stomach/duodenum, compared with an average 17% of 405 animals injected with strains from other diseases (see Table 2.5 below). Holman calculated from this that lesions in the stomach had developed in 62 animals injected with bacteria from stomach ulcer patients and in 68 other animals, exhibited these as percentages (48% and 52%) of the sum 130 animals with lesions, and simply omitted all reference to the actual total number injected (508). Such was the basis for Holman's carefully-worded statement "that it is roughly a 50 per cent chance whether any particular localization occurs with a 'specific' or 'non-specific' strain" and for his improperly consequent claim that "the specificity of bacteria involved has not been proved".

Holman's continuing legacy is exemplified in Paul B. Beeson's 1976 [7] exclusive reference to a 1940 article by H. A. Reiman and W.P. Havens as concerns "decisive" rejection of Rosenow and "the focal infection fad"; Reiman and Havens [6], in turn, exclusively credited Holman with having refuted elective localization. Similarly, numerous works up to modern times, [8] seemingly including virtually the whole of key supporting literature for modern endodontics [9], are fundamentally reliant on Holman or works which themselves depend on Holman [6]. For the most part, as a result of cumulative years of negative regard largely (directly or indirectly) traceable back to Holman, Rosenow's work has been generally maligned and consequently ignored.

In 1940, Rosenow published composite results of more extensive series of experiments by himself and thirty-one others, involving more than 11,000 animals and emphatically confirming Rosenow's earlier work (Table 2.1, above) [4]. Yet neither this nor continued assertions of the value of the focal infection concept [10] have sustained major interest in Rosenow or the field in general.

The extent to which Rosenow's work has been wrongfully discredited argues for its reconsideration, particularly as concerns the essential type of non-hemolytic streptococcus used in his experiments (consistently isolated only in media affording a gradient of oxygen pressure, such as dextrose-brain broth), the purported etiologic importance of infected tonsils and teeth (including symptomless pulpless teeth, now independently acknowledged as commonly infected) [11], and the advocacy of autogenous vaccine-therapy.

*As proposed to <u>Nature</u>, London, 20 Oct. 93; returned 2 Nov. Details and implications are discussed in a separate report, *MEDICINE'S GRANDEST FRAUD PHD)*.

Table 2.5: INJECTION INTO LAB ANIMALS OF BACTERIA "AS ISOLATED"; ROSENOW'S 1915 RESULTS (J.A.M.A. LXV 1688) VS. HOLMAN'S 1928 "REARRANGEMENT" (Arch. Path & Lab. Med. 5, 133).

LESIONS IN ANIMALS' \/ \/	SOURCE \/ \/ PATIENTS WITH:	Rosenow's Data		Holman	
		ANIMALS INJECTED	% WITH LESIONS	(NUMBER) (W/LESIONS)	
Joints	Rheumatic fever	71	66%	(= 47)	36%
	Other diseases	437	19%	(= 84)	64%
				131	
Endocardium	Endocarditis	44	84%	(= 37)	30%
	Rheumatic fever	71	46%	(= 33)	27%
	Other diseases	393	13%	(= 52)	42%
				122	
Myocardium	Rheumatic fever	71	44%	(= 32)	38%
	Myositis	40	35%	(= 14)	17%
	Other diseases	397	9%	(= 36)	44%
				82	
Muscles	Rheumatic fever	71	27%	(= 19)	24%
	Myositis	40	75%	(= 30)	38%
	Other diseases	397	7%	(= 29)	37%
				78	
Stomach/Duodenum (w/hemorrhages)	Stomach ulcer	103	60%	(= 62)	48%
	Other diseases	405	17%	(= 68)	52%
				130	
Stomach/Duodenum (with ulcer)	Stomach ulcer	103	60%	(= 62)	67%
	Other diseases	405	7%	(= 30)	33%
				92	
Gallbladder	Cholecystitis	41	80%	(= 33)	43%
	Other diseases	467	9%	(= 43)	57%
				76	
Appendix	Appendicitis	68	68%	(= 46)	71%
	Other diseases	440	4%	(= 19)	29%
				65	
Kidneys	Rheumatic fever	71	39%	(= 28)	52%
	Other diseases	437	6%	(= 26)	48%
				54	
Skin	Erythema nodosum	20	90%	Not listed	
	Herpes zoster	61	70%	by Holman	
	Other diseases	427	4%		
Parotid	Mumps	19	73%	Not listed	
	Other diseases	489	0%	by Holman	
Pancreas	Mumps	19	42%	Not listed	
	Other diseases	489	4%	by Holman	

BIBLIOGRAPHY

    1. Utz, U., etal, Nature 364, 243 (1993); Waksman, B.H., Nature 337, 599 (1989).
    2. Rosenow, E.C., Streptococci in etiology of diverse

diseases, including diseases of nervous system, J. Nerv. and Ment. Dis. 117: 415-428, May 1953; 122, 238-247, 321-331 (1955).

3.   Rosenow, E. C., J.A.M.A. LXV 1688 (1915).

4.   Holman, W.L., Archives Path & Lab. Med. 5 (1928), 133

5.   Rosenow, E. C., Dental Centenary Proceedings, Maryland State Dental Association and A.D.A., March 1940, p. 261-82.

6.   MacNevin, M.G. and Vaughn, H.S., Mouth Infections and Their Relation to Systemic Disease, New York, 1930, 78-91; Blayney, J.R., Dental Cosmos LXXIV, 635-653 (July 1932); Appleton, J.L.T., Jr., Bacterial Infection, Lea & Febiger, Philadelphia 1933, 565-577; Reiman, H.A., and Havens, W.P., J.A.M.A., 114, 1 (1940); Woods, Alan C., Am. J. Opth. 25 (Dec. 1942), 1423-1444; Grossman, Louis I., Root Canal Therapy, 1946; Easlick, K. A., J.A.D.A. 42 (1951).

7.   Beeson, Paul B., in Bowers, J. & E. Purcell, eds., Advances in American Medicine: Essays at the Bicentennial, 1, (N. Y., J. Macy Found. 1976), 151-2.

8.   Bellizi, R. and W. P. Cruse, Journal of Endodontics Vol. 6 (May 1980), 576-580; Burket, Lester W., Oral Medicine 6th Ed., J.B. Lippincott Co., Phila., 1971, 550-556; Chase, A., Magic Shots, 1980, 424-431. Coolidge, E. D., J.A.D.A. 61 (Dec. 1960) 676-688; Crowley, M.C., Am. J. Orthodontics (Oral Surg. Sect.) 32, 126-130, Feb. 1946; Grossman, Louis I., Root Canal Therapy, 1940; Grossman, Louis I., JADA 93 (July 1976), 78-87; Jawetz, E., Oral Surg., Oral Med., Oral Path. 8 (1955), 1069-1073; Sharp, George C., JADA and Dental Cosmos, 24 (August 1937), 1231-124; Topazian 1962, D.S., Indian J. of Med. Sci. 16 (1962), 1072-1083; Wolfson, B.L., Cal. State Dental Assoc. 25 (1949), 106.

9.   Ingle, John I., Endodontics, Third Edition, Lea and Febiger, Philadelphia, 1985, 1; Grossman, Louis I., Seymour Oliet and Carlos E. Del Rio, Endodontic Practice, Eleventh Edition, Lea & Febiger, Philadelphia, 1988, p. 234-240; Wiene, Franklin S., Endodontic Therapy, C.V. Mosby Company, St. Louis 1989, 1-2.

10. Editorial: "Focal Infection", J.A.M.A. 150, 490-491 (1952); Thoden van Velzen, S.K., L. Abraham-Inpijn and W.R. Moorer, J. Clin. Periodont. 11 (1984) 209-220; Morse, D. R., in Cohen, S. and R. C. Burns, Pathways of the Pulp, C.V. Mosby, St. Louis, 1987, p. 378; Newman, H.N., J. of Dental Research 71(11), Nov., 1992, p. 1854, and Periodontal Abstracts Volume 41 Number 3, 1993, 73-77; Navazesh M and R Mulligan, Special Care in Dentistry, 1995, Jan-Feb, 15(1): 11-9.

11. Seltzer, S., in Cohen, S. and R. C. Burns, Pathways of the Pulp, C.V. Mosby, St. Louis, 1987, p. 1.

2.5 FOCAL INFECTION UPDATES: MEDLINE ON FOCAL INFECTION

From 1966 through 1993, MEDLINE carried some 1400 citations on the subject of "focal infection" in conjunction with the keyword "dental", many involving a continuing or recurring interest in the (causative) correlation between dental foci and various disease conditions.

Table 2.6: FOCAL UPDATE - MEDLINE ON FOCAL INFECTION
---subject "FOCAL INFECTION"; keyword "DENTAL"----

years:	1966-74	1975-9	1980-5	1985-9	1990-4
no.items	544	303	222	205	140

Diseases discussed in contemporary articles & thought to be
caused by oral foci include:
--alopecia areata (Zivkovic 1990)
--arthritis, meningitis, endocarditis, uveitis (Lens '88) --brain
abscess (Andrews 1990)
--cavernous sinus thrombosis (el Fakir etal 1993; Goscinski 1991)
--conjunctival tumor (Ruban 1991)
--coronary atherosclerosis (Mattila etal, 1993)
--disseminated intravascular coag. (Carter etal 1992)
--endocarditis (Lieberman 1992; Godeau 1992; Preda & Pasetti
1990)
--erythema nodosum (Kirch & Duhrsen 1992)
--fever (Pernice etal, 1990; Samra etal, 1986)
--ischaemic heart disease (Paunio, etal., 1993)
--mediastinal abscess and pneumonia (Petrone '92)
--metastatic processes (Störtbecker 1967)
--myocardial infarction (Mattila 1993; Asikainen & Alaluusua
1993)
--necrotizing fasciitis (Stoykewych etal 1992; Rapoport etal
1991)
--optic neuritis (Chaabouni etal 1991; Philippe etal 1992;
Ilewicz etal 1990; Bocca etal 1989)
--pulmonary embolism (Martinez, etal., 1994)
--pyrexia (Laine etal, 1992; Editorial *The Lancet* May 31, 1980)
--rheumathoid arthritis (Newman 1993)
--scleroderma (Wood & Lee '88, Janssens etal 87)
--septicemia (Kansenshogaku, 1994; Ocampo etal '91)
--sinusitis (Neupokoev and Neupokoeva, 1991)
--subfertility in males (Bieniek & Reidel, 1993)
--swollen finger (Wallace 1991)
--trigeminal neuralgia (Barrett and Buckley 1986).
 (see MELVYL MEDLINE for citations)

   Note that many of these conditions had been shown by Rosenow to
be related to an oral focal infection, including even
subfertility. For full listing of disease conditions and
citations, see INDEX).

2.5.1 FOCAL INFECTION - 1980
   A *Lancet* 1980 editorial (see APPENDIX B) on the focal infection
concept concluded "The ætiological role of chronic dental
infection in systemic disease has probably been underestimated in
the past"; and in 1984 a particularly forceful call was made for
formal reappraisal of the focal infection concept (see APPENDIX
B, Thoden van Velzen, 1984).
   In each of years 1992, 1993, and 1994, articles with the title
"Focal Infection Revisited" were listed in MEDLINE, two by Newman

and one by Hughes; we shall revisit these below, plus a 1995 article on the same subject by two U.S.C. professors and a Dec. 1996 article by Newman.

Particular attention is invited to the 1994 article by Hughes and associated commentary. Hughes has detailed many of the "standard" objections which continue to be raised in opposition to the concept of oral focal infection; a detailed rebuttal to these points, with specific reference to Rosenow's works, has been integrated.

2.5.2 FOCAL INFECTION - 1992

Newman 1992 [*J. of Dental Research* 71(11), Nov., 1992], p., 1854, "Guest Editorial: Focal Infection Revisited - the Dentist as Physician", notes that "Ever since the original concept of focal infection led to an excess of extractions over 70 years ago, the theory has been in relative disrepute. And yet to ignore focal infection is to refuse to recognize an abundant literature, all of medical significance." Beyond evidence that many conditions may be the result of "bacteremia of oral origin", "There is also some evidence that microbial fractions, rather than whole cells, may play a part, perhaps in some form of immune complex, in systemic forms of inflammation not overtly infectious in nature - for example, some forms of arthritis."

Newman noted that "One problem is that inflammatory periodontal diseases and caries are so common, that sequelæ are much less frequent, and their possible systemic significance is easily overlooked."

Newman 1992 concludes "The mouth may be more boring ... than other body orifices, but its medical significance has been underestimated for too long. It is time to re-examine the role of focal oral infection in systemic disease."

Reference: Miller WE (1890).

2.5.3 FOCAL INFECTION - 1993

Newman 1993 proclaimed "... it is now as opportune as ever it was to consider oral flora control ... in terms of prevention of systemic infection of oral origin. It is also conceivable that diseases (including types of arthritis) not heretofore considered infective may have some link with oral bacteria ... . The most common pathways are direct ... [but] organisms can also spread along the fascial planes of the head and neck, through the bloodstream and lymphatic system, and along nerves, as well as along mucous surfaces ... ."

Newman discusses and provides citations concerning a number of systemic infections of probable or possible focal oral origin, including brain abscesses, meningitis, acute hemiplegia, acute orbital infection (eyes), uveitis, endophthalmitis, lung abscesses, arthritis, necrotizing mediastinitis, necrotizing fasciitis, anaerobic septicemia and thrombophlebitis of the internal jugular vein, leukemia, pyrexia, endocarditis, and neurological problems including selective anesthesia of peripheral branches of the trigeminal nerve.

"... it behooves us to reflect on the fact that the organisms

of most interest to the dental researcher and clinician ... may
have effects on organs and systems near to or far from the mouth.
 We may expect increasing attention from our medical colleagues
concerned with such infections, and with diseases such as
rheumatoid arthritis, in which there may be a more complex
microbial involvement ... . The similarities between chronic
inflammatory periodontal diseases and chronic systemic
inflammatory disorders have been noted, and the rheumatologists
and the periodontologists have already begun to share ideas
(Newman and Williams, 1992)." [Newman, H.N., *Periodontal
Abstracts* Volume 41 Number 3 1993, 73-77]
 We are reminded of a similar awakening that occurred 8-decades
ago, when Billings 1912 and 1913 presented papers on focal
infection as a causative factor in chronic arthritis. [See
APPENDIX B for detailed historical discussions].

2.5.4 FOCAL INFECTION - 1994

 Hughes 1994 conceded that "scientifically sound research ...
[was] performed by a small number of highly motivated
bacteriologists", this being the work from 1904 by Dr. Frank
Billings and associates, particularly E.C. Rosenow, and Charles
Mayo. Hughes relates a remarkable story told by Ejnar Jarlov, a
previously skeptical Danish rheumatologist, of how Rosenow had
replicated symptoms of an expired patient's violent hiccough in a
rabbit.
  Hughes' presentation overall seems a bit prejudiced by still-
prevailing negative attitudes against Rosenow, e.g., he states
"attempts to repeat the isolation [and elective localization]
work of Rosenow often failed to confirm his findings".
Remarkably, a bit further into his article he goes on to concede
that the requisite "stringent, specific culture conditions ...
were rarely observed by later investigators."
  Whereas, when these conditions were met, Rosenow's work was
invariably substantiated, including his demonstrations of the
elective localization of streptococci.

2.5.5 FOCAL INFECTION - 1995

 Navazesh M and R Mulligan, *Special Care in Dentistry*, 1995 Jan-
Feb, 15(1):11-9. "Systemic dissemination as a result of oral
infection in individuals 50 years of age and older."; discuss
"the role of oral infection as the etiology of systemic
disorders" and provide a review of the literature published
during the period 1980-1994, "focusing on well-documented cases
... [of] oral infection as the cause of disease at sites remote
from the oral cavity".
 Navazesh and Mulligan report that "The number of edentulous
individuals aged 75 years or older has drastically declined from
67.3 in 1958 to 47.3 in 1985. The increasing trend for retention
of teeth into older age puts older adults at continued risk for
systemic complications of oral origin."
 The authors lament the relative lack of attention in recent
years to the "role of oral infection as the etiology of systemic
complications".

The authors devote specific sections to discussions of brain abscesses, meningitis, mediastinal abscesses, bacterial endocarditis, aspiration pneumonia, vertebral osteomyelitis, prosthetic joint infection, gastritis and ulcers, hepatobiliary diseases, chronic urticaria, fever of unknown origin, tetanus, and gangrene of the tongue. It was noted that the onset of the disorders commonly occurred from a few days to a few months after dental manipulations.

2.5.6   FOCAL INFECTION - 1996

H.N. Newman, *J. Dent. Res.* 75 (12) 1996, "Focal Infection", notes a "resurgence of interest ... in recognizing the relationship between oral foci of infection and a wide range of diseases." Newman reviews historical and current work in the field, referring to Rosenow's "theory of elective localization". Recent reports of correlation between oral foci and various types of diseases are cited, concluding that "We certainly need to realize that there are links between oral and systemic health and oral and systemic disease." Extensive references are given.

Chapter 3.
INNATE INSTABILITY OF BACTERIAL TYPES: DISSOCIATION & MUTATION

Although the popular contemporary view holds that the realm of bacteria is distinctly separate from that of viruses, and within each realm numerous separately distinct entities exist, the reality of the situation is not so clear cut. The facts of mutation and dissociation of bacterial species are well established and instrumental to Rosenow's work.

Rosenow's initial work with dissociation of bacterial species built on the prior works of Flexner, Amos and others on the etiology of poliomyelitis, as well as others on variability and dissociation in general, e.g. P. Hadley 1927, Kendall (Science).
 For example, Kendall stated "It is postulated that a majority, if not all, known bacteria can and do exist in a filterable and in a non-filterable state."
In his studies of transmutation, Rosenow drew upon the works of T. Smith (Assn. Am. Physicians, Trans. ix, 1894, 85-89) and his discussions of the role of microbial variability in epidemics and infectious diseases. Rosenow has related that his experimentation with transmutation of bacterial species (e.g. see APPENDIX A - 14R4) had led him to the definitive recognition of the phenomenon of "elective localization".
In the process of altering virulence of strains, increasing it through animal passage and decreasing it through cultivation on artificial media, Rosenow noted some peculiar patterns of localized lesions in postmortem examinations of laboratory animals. He subsequently experimented with strains associated with specific human diseases, and found that these tended to localize in corresponding tissues of laboratory animals.
This work highlighted the importance of proper isolation and culture technique in preserving virulence and specificity of disease-causing organisms.

Some historical items on the subjects of dissociation and mutation are highlighted below. For further reading on the subjects of microbial variation and transformation, the reader is kindly referred to APPENDIX C.

3.1 DISSOCIATION - Hadley's review

The line between what is considered a bacteria and a virus is essentially determined by the capabilities of man-made filters, while true size is actually a continuum from larger organisms which get caught in a filter to smaller ones that pass through. Microscopic and submicroscopic organisms commonly grow smaller or larger depending on environmental conditions.   In other words, it would appear that most or even all bacteria may dissociate into smaller, filtrable (viral), forms under favorable conditions, and vice-versa in the case of viral forms, i.e., revert to larger forms.
The book-within-a-journal (312 pages!) published by Hadley in

1927 provides a comprehensive discussion of the immense body of prior work on the occurrence of dissociation of bacterial forms, including much work even prior to the start of the Twentieth Century. Hadley discussed in detail "an ever-increasing mass of evidence pointing to the instability of bacterial species [which] ... may have a more significant bearing on problems of virulence, infection and immunity than many have supposed." (See APPENDIX C1 - Hadley 1927, for further discussion.)

3.2 CHICK EMBRYO MEDIUM
ROSENOW'S VIRUS-MAKING RECIPES

CHICK EMBRYO MEDIUM - OLD CULTURES YIELD FILTRABLE AGENTS
   Autoclaved chick embryo infusion was found (a) to "not turn acid from growth of streptococci", (b) "to be highly favorable for rapid growth and maintenance for a very long time of viability of streptococci."; and (c) "As cultures in this medium became old, extremely small and filtrable forms of the streptococci appeared, and in some instances, filtrable transmissible agents resembling in their effects in animals those of the respective viruses were demonstrated. Moreover, on prolonged storage of cultures in this medium at room temperature or in the incubator, changes in agglutinative titer and in virulence were found to occur seasonally in accord with the streptococci isolated in studies of current epidemics of poliomyelitis, encephalitis, and respiratory infection."

   See APPENDIX A - 50R1 and 35R5 for instructions for preparing chick-embryo medium.

3.3 TOXINS

   It has recently been shown that endotoxins in "sepsis syndrome" may not be directly responsible for the presumed "toxic" effects observed in their presence, but rather may serve as a "marker" for dissociation of bacteria into smaller, cell-wall deficient forms. In view of the apparent general ability of microorganisms to exist in dissociative forms, one might speculate that toxins in general might be subject to such reappraisal. (See APPENDIX C1 - 1993, Hurley JC)

3.4 CONTEMPORARY UPDATES: DISSOCIATION/REVERSION; MUTATION

   A number of contemporary discussions of dissociation of bacterial species are featured in APPENDIX C1; and of current work on mutations in APPENDIX C2. These encompass considerations of dissociation as a form of reproduction, relation to virulence, dissociation as a reversible phenomenon, the role of environment in size and phase variation, and the relation between streptococci and pneumococcci, all work compatible with that of Rosenow in these areas.
   On the subject of dissociation, a notable measure of attention

in recent years has been given to cell-wall deficient forms of bacteria -- so-called "L-forms".

Not surprisingly, when this work is traced back to its origins, we find the work of P. Hadley and coworkers prominently cited, along with that of F.R. Heilman of Mayo. In turn Hadley's classic work refers back to work by Rosenow a decade earlier, and Heilman and Rosenow co-authored five articles in the 1930s. Therefore, current work with L-forms is to some extent both a continuation and validation of the prior works of Rosenow in this area.

A scan of citations in MEDLINE with keyword "L-form" discloses that L-forms are being implicated in the current literature in a number of conditions, e.g., secretory otitis media, idiopathic hematuria, tuberculosis, lymphadenitis, staphylococcic sepsis, burn wound infection, in bone marrow, and in diseases in fish and pigeons.

For the period 1990-1994, MEDLINE lists 71 items on the "subject" of "l-forms"; 2001 items with "l-forms" as a "keyword" and 202 items with "l-forms of bacteria" as "keyword". These include reference to the possible role of oral foci as a reservoir for systemic disease; e.g., Avdonina LI, etal., 1992 noted that "The regularities of the pathologic process development in periodontal tissues of subjects without tuberculosis were found to fully conform to the current concept of a latent tuberculous infection. The periodontal foci of infection may be regarded as reservoirs of persistent mycobacteria, whose main form, L variant, was detected in 71.68 % of cases." See APPENDIX C1 for further discussions of dissociation, reversion, L-forms, etc.

And recent work by Chalkey etal 1991 (see APPENDIX C2 for futher discussion) on transformations between viridans streptococci to pneumococci looks like a fairly clear confirmation of Rosenow's work 1n 1914 (see APPENDIX A - 14R4).

Chapter 4.   ROSENOW'S REQUISITE METHODOLOGY
  Oxygen Gradients, Serial Dilutions, Glycerol-Salt Menstruum

The methods utilized by Edward C. Rosenow evolved over a span of more than a half-century and nearly 300 published articles. Even in his last published articles in the late 1950s we do not find Rosenow resting on his laurels; rather, he continued probing still-unresolved questions. Each recounting thus did not and could not possibly incorporate every relevant detail discussed over the entire prior period; however, (1) the overriding importance of a medium which affords various <u>gradients of oxygen pressure</u> (see 4.1), consistently emphasized by him as essential for more than four decades; (2) the highly desirable refinement of using <u>serial dilution cultures</u> (see 4.3) in conjunction with that special medium; and (3) the importance of storage at 10 degrees C. in a menstruum of <u>glycerol and saturated saline</u> (see 4.4); comprise three consistent and indispensable components of his work. Rosenow's methodology is not particularly simple; however it does represent the most simple manner in which he was finally able to assuredly isolate a causative organism in a number of diseases, many of which are still considered "idiopathic" perhaps simply due to a failure to utilize proper methods. The serial dilution method, as complicated as it may appear to be, is the single most preferable way to virtually guarantee that the correct organism will be obtained, when used in conjunction with the dextrose-brain-broth culture medium. And the use of a glycerol-saline menstruum and 10 degrees C. storage proved to be incomparably effective in preserving specificity over long periods of time.

As Rosenow has shown, many still-mysterious disease conditions are neither "idiopathic" nor of immaculate conception (the so-called "auto-immune" fad); they are caused by an organism which can be called forth with Rosenow's methods - from lesions, often from blood, and from oral foci (primarily non-vital teeth or diseased teeth or tonsils).

As for short-cuts that might yield comparable results, we are reminded that Rosenow was nothing if not thorough; were short-cuts to be had, he would have so informed us. Perhaps some day short-cuts will be found which are as effective as Rosenow's methodology; perhaps not. To date, it seems evident that shortcuts which do not comply with Rosenow's detailed <u>instructions</u> (see 4.5), which some latter-day investigators have insisted on taking, are self-defeating, and readily explain why such negligent investigators have failed to isolate the proper organism. The fact is that Rosenow's methodology does work and has invariably resulted in success by investigators who have used it. Further, Rosenow's constant empirical finding over a half-century regarding the importance of gradients-of-oxygen-pressure also makes perfect common sense; after all, actual conditions within the living being are neither strictly aerobic nor strictly anaerobic.

Beyond the isolation, production and preservation of properly-specific strains, Rosenow's vaccines are the result of decades of study and have reportedly "worked miracles" [L.Rowntree, 1958].

For those persons who steadfastly refuse to give up their poisonous, endodontopathological nests, the Rosenow vaccines are probably the best hope of keeping the offending bacteria at bay.

Thus in the case of a number of disease conditions was Rosenow reportedly able to provide a hopeful measure of therapy. Nonetheless, his work clearly establishes that it is better to extract and clean out the nests. (See discussion above in 2.2.)

4.1 OXYGEN GRADIENTS - IMPORTANCE IN CULTURE METHOD (to obtain causative organism from blood and tissues in many diseases)

As Rosenow repeatedly asserted over a period of more than four decades, attempting to culture, under aerobic conditions the same pathogens he had grown using reduced oxygen gradients, is flawed from inception. Even if a suspected pathogen had been correctly identified in the first instance, propagation under strictly aerobic conditions would require adaptation by the organism to the extent that a meaningful relation to its former human-pathogenic form could easily have been, indeed apparently is, destroyed.

This phenomenon had been described during the 19th century by Louis Pasteur, in response to difficulties in culturing the "septic vibrio" of septicemia. Pasteur had referred to "the destruction of the septic vibrio by the atmospheric oxygen dissolved in the [culture] fluids", which was avoided through use of anaerobic techniques. As per Pasteur, "... It might be said that the air burned the vibrios." [Pasteur, Louis, (and Jourbert, and Chamberland) "The Germ Theory and its applications to medicine and surgery", Comptes Rendus de L'Academie des Sciences, lxxxvi., (1878), 1037-43]

IN OTHER WORDS: In order to grow the harmful organisms in test tubes, Rosenow (and Pasteur) have noted the importance of replicating conditions that exist in the human body -- particularly including reduced oxygen gradients.

As early as 1914, Rosenow noted that "in many chronic conditions the cultures [from bodily fluids] are usually sterile and demonstration of bacteria in the tissues usually fails." At this time Rosenow first described "methods for making cultures particularly from excised tissues and from the blood and other fluids in which due regard is paid to the question of oxygen pressure, particularly in the primary culture ..."

Rosenow described the use of tall tubes of culture medium "in which there is afforded not only aerobic and anaerobic conditions but a gradation of oxygen pressure between those two points, a gradation of H and OH ions, and a wide range of nutrition [wherein] positive cultures have been obtained frequently while cultures made in the usual way remained sterile."

"Thus certain non-hemolyzing streptococci [or diphtheroid organisms] have been isolated from the blood repeatedly when the usual method failed or showed much fewer colonies" in leukemia, rheumatic fever, occasionally arthritis deformans, puerperal sepsis, infectious endocarditis, Hodgkin's disease, erythema nodosum, rheumatism, bronchopneumonia; and from tissues in rheumatism, arthritis deformans, duodenal and gastric ulcers, cholecystitis, goiter, etc."

At this early stage, Rosenow stated that "the common isolation of bacteria from tissues which have been considered sterile is of definite importance, lends support to the contentions of Adami and others that certain ill-understood conditions are due to a low-grade infection and not merely intoxication, and calls for an extensive study of the whole question by this or similar methods." [14R12]

Over the following forty-plus years Rosenow would strive to simplify his methods and increase the likelihood of obtaining the proper causative organism. But the lesson of the importance of a medium affording a gradient of oxygen pressure did not substantively change from his initial 1914 statements on the subject. (It is noted that the key to Barry Marshall's contemporary work with stomach ulcer is the use of reduced oxygen gradients (see 4.2, below).

4.2 OXYGEN GRADIENTS UPDATE (STOMACH ULCER BACTERIA)

Monmaney, Terence, New Yorker, Sept. 20, 1993, 64-72, "Marshall's Hunch", notes that notwithstanding earlier indications that an organism might be involved in stomach ulcers (with no reference Rosenow, "in the fifties, a supposedly definitive study of human gastrointestinal flora concluded that the stomach was microbe-free, and thus it came to be viewed as a 'sterile' organ. ...

"Meanwhile, during the 1970s ... microbiologists developed new techniques for identifying and culturing fastidious bacteria like Heliobacter, which requires a trace of oxygen but drowns in air."

In fact, Rosenow had emphasized the importance of such oxygen gradients from 1914 through 1958, and had conducted definitive studies implicating the role of bacteria in stomach ulcers from 1915.

4.3 SERIAL DILUTION

It may appear a bit strange - needing a more dilute solution of an organism in order to grow it, but that's what the serial dilution method is all about. For some reason growth of the sought-after causative organisms is stunted by other organisms at lower dilutions, but is enabled preferentially at higher dilutions. Rosenow's explanation of why he adopted the serial dilution culture method, i.e., "the use of serial dilutions of the inoculum in dextrose-brain agar and dextrose-brain broth": "When this is carried out in multiples of ten, it may be frequently observed that although little or no growth occurs in the first or second tube, at still higher dilutions growth is

shown. Absence of growth in the low dilutions may be due, it is
thought, to inhibiting substances in the inoculum which are
rendered inactive by serial dilution."   38R5
    Rosenow later offered that this occurred because at higher
dilutions, "the specifically virulent streptococci outgrow the
avirulent streptococci, staphylococci and E. coli." [55R1]

    Some meticulous workers may be able to obtain the proper
organism without the use of the serial dilution method; indeed,
Rosenow and others consistently did so during the three decades
prior to his initiation of the serial dilution method. However,
once he discovered the great value of its use, he invariably
employed it through the succeeding two decades. Yes, it seems a
little complicated at first, but choosing to not employ it
carries a far greater risk of wasting one's time and efforts.
Let us benefit from Rosenow's 50 years of experience in growing
this organism.

    The serial dilution method apparently guarantees success.
Whereas in the past some complex crosschecks, sometimes involving
injections in lab animals and checking for lesions therein, were
employed by Rosenow in order to assure that he and the right
organism, the serial dilution method seems to ha e removed the
guesswork. The bacteria which grew predominantly in dilute
cultures, e.g. at 10^{-6}, 10^{-10} or beyond, were the ones being
sought.

4.4   GLYCEROL/SALINE MENSTRUUM

    The preservation of streptococci in glycerol-NaCl menstruum
(dense suspension of glycerol, two parts, and saturated sodium
chloride solution, one part) and preferential use of such
streptococci in vaccines was to become standard operating
procedure for Rosenow [29R1].
    Rosenow reported that streptococci stored in such menstruum
preserved specificity over periods of as long as 8 years [34R3];
"corresponding strains, grown aerobically, had lost elective
localizing power in the course of several daily transfers."
Moreover the toxicity of the bacteria was found reduced upon
storage in glycerine-salt menstruum, without loss of specificity.

4.5   ROSENOW'S RECIPES: VACCINE & ANTIBODY

DEXTROSE-BRAIN BROTH; GLUCOSE BRAIN BROTH/AGAR

    The painstakingly-derived culture medium, used consistently by
Rosenow and associates over the period of several decades, was
described in several articles (e.g., see INDEX: dextrose ...).
    Attention is invited to two particularly-detailed recipes for
this culture broth medium -- one given by Haden in 1928, for
glucose-brain broth (see APPENDIX B - Haden 1928); and one from
Rosenow in 1938, for dextrose brain broth (see APPENDIX A -
38R5). Cultures in this type of broth were generally used in

production of vaccines and in animal experiments; the cultures in agar were useful in obtaining counts of discrete numbers of colonies.

ISOLATION OF STREPTOCOCCI (DIVERSE DISEASES) [58R1]

   We find a particularly thorough explanation of isolation and production of streptococci in Rosenow's last article, published in 1958. The serial dilution method seems to have been perfected - three tubes suffice to pull out the offending organism, usually from the second tube.
   Once a pure culture of the finicky organism was isolated, as per above, it could be readily grown in larger lots. This allowed for production of a quantity of autogenous vaccine for later administration, or for production of large lots of vaccine for distribution in the case of infectious diseases.
   Rosenow repeatedly asserted that the organisms in very different diseases were virtually indistinguishable in terms of "size, chain formation and staining reactions".
   For further details, please see excerpts in APPENDIX A, 58R1: "ISOLATION AND PRODUCTION OF STREPTOCOCCI"; "PRODUCTION OF STREPTOCOCCI (DIVERSE DISEASES)"; "SIMILAR ORGANISMS, DIFFERENT DISEASES"; or full reprint in APPENDIX D4.

"THERMAL" ANTIBODY PREPARATION

   The production and use of thermal antibody was a late development in Rosenow's career, and may represent the grand prize of his treasure chest of discovery. In particular, Drs. Rosenow and Rappaport reported on the successful use of thermal antibody alone, sans vaccine, in therapy and prophylaxis of polio (see Chapter 6. POLIO; and Rosenow's last article in 1958 discussed beneficial results from the use of thermal antibody in diverse diseases (See APPENDIX A - 58R1, THERMAL ANTIBODY PREPARATION; see also full article, reprinted as APPENDIX D4).

*****.

VACCINE PREPARATION & ADMIN.

   Rosenow discussed vaccine preparation and administration in a number of articles. Particular attention is directed to discussions from three articles, excerpted in APPENDIX A1: 55R2, "VACCINE PREPARATION SUMMARY" (Schizophrenia) 34R3, "VACCINE PREPARATION DETAILS" (COLDS, INFLUENZA) 57R1, "ADMINISTRATION OF VACCINE AND ANTIBODY" (M.S.); full article reprinted as APPENDIX D3.

Chapter 5. ANTIBODY CATALYSIS THEORY

5.1 OVERVIEW; WHY A LITTLE ANTIBODY GOES A LONG WAY

Rosenow's work on the subject of antibody production is based on and supportive of a catalysis theory, whereby within the bacterial or streptococcal cell is a substance severely antigenic to the outer surface, Dr. Rosenow's attempt to create auto-antibodies gives primary credit to two sources: (1) Tyler 1942 and (2) Pauling 1942. These two primary sources are briefly summarized here, and discussed in greater detail below.

Tyler 1942 explains why so little initial antibody may serve to counteract a large infection. If the substance inside an infecting organism is itself simply antibody and is liberated through the penetrating and priming, catalytic, action of a small amount of identical substance [homologous antibody], a large effect on the infecting organism may be explained. The larger amount of substance thus released would have a like, catalytic effect on the infecting organism. Tyler thus argues that antibody can be manufactured from the antigen itself. However, when the total organism including its exterior is consumed intact or agglutinated, the inside substance may not be liberated, whereas cooking antigen converts 'neutral' globulin in antigen into (positively-charged) antibody construct (through addition of oxygen). Oxygen attacks (oxidizes) the streptococci. They can't grow in it.

Pauling 1942 cooks the antigen with normal serum globulin and thereby creates a specific antiglobulin. Pauling's involvement in this area was the direct result of solicitation by the great Karl Landsteiner.

It is noted that Hooker, whose 1931 work with Boyd was associated with development of the catalysis theory, subsequently was involved with formative work on the concept of protein folding with Follensby in 1947, which concept is of great interest in modern times.

MOLECULE AGGLUTINATES >600 BACTERIA; CATALYSIS THEORY IMPLICATED

Hooker and Boyd, 1931, p. 115, reported "From quantitative data relative to the weight of injected antigen and to the potency of resulting antibody it is conservatively estimated that one molecule of active antigenic substance gives rise to an amount of agglutinin capable of flocking 600 bacteria. This result is difficult to reconcile with the hypothesis that antibody is a conjugate of antigen and body globulin. The surface relationship (implicated in the mechanics of agglutination) between one globulin molecule and 600 bacteria is 1:25,000,000 [visualized as a dime on an acre and a half]. Even with the assumption of multiple nonspecific determinants in a single molecule of antigen the above discrepancy is extreme. A theory of antibody formation involving catalysis would seem more promising."

5.2   FOUNDATIONS: FOSHAY & SABIN

The nature of antibody produced by Rosenow was repeatedly
validated through use of Foshay's classic antiserum/antibody
test. Additionally, no discussion of the development of current
understanding of antibody is complete without reference to the
works of Florence Sabin.

FOSHAY'S CLASSIC ANTISERUM/ANTIBODY TEST   Foshay 1936

"In tularemia the bacterial-specific intradermal antiserum
reaction is due to an antigen-antibody reaction involving only
the species-specific polysaccharide. ... Since the production of
positive reactions in patients is dependent upon the existence in
their skins of that part of the antigenic complex which
determines the species-specificity of the invading parasite, the
reaction serves as a confirmatory diagnostic test of great
precision and accuracy." [Foshay, Lee, J. Infectious Dis. 59
(1936) 330-339, "The Nature of the Bacterial-Specific Intradermal
Antiserum Reaction"]

PHYSICAL CHEMISTRY, OSMOSIS, CONDUCTANCE   Sabin 1939

Florence Sabin, 1939, p. 67, "... within the past decade,
evidence that antibodies are themselves protein has been steadily
accumulating. ... The development of [quantitative micro-methods
by Heidelberger and his collaborators ... led to accurate
investigations on the physical-chemical properties of antibodies
by the ultracentrifugal and electrophoretic methods. Since the
molecular weight and electrical mobilities found were
characteristic of proteins, the identification of antibodies as
modified serum globulins may be considered accomplished."
Therefore, "the cellular mechanisms which give rise to antibodies
must be concerned in their normal functions with the synthesis of
globulin. For some years evidence has been presented implicating
the cells of the reticulo-endothelial system in the formation of
antibodies. The present report seeks to make our understanding
of this function more definite.
p. 67, "Aschoff formulated the concept of the reticulo-
endothelian system. Though this name has been used in different
ways, the idea is based on the fact that certain specific
endothelia and certain mononuclear cells of the tissues have high
phagocytic power and react toward the same materials. With these
studies as a basis there has grown up an extensive literature
implicating the reticulo-endothelial system in the formation of
antibodies. It includes observations involving the spleen, the
lymph nodes, and macrophages or clasmatocytes. ...
"Many recent studies on the origin of the serum proteins have
also been pointing, in our judgment, toward the reticulo-
endothelial system. Most of these studies have implicated the
liver, but have also suggested that the liver is not the sole

source of these proteins. The involvement of the liver is due, it would seem, to the presence of the Kupffer cells, a part of the reticulo-endothelial system.

SERUM PROTEINS COME FROM CELL CYTOPLASM Sabin 1939

   p. 69, "In the present studies some evidence will be presented in support of the concept that throughout life the serum proteins, certainly as far as globulin is concerned, come from the sacrifice of a part of the cytoplasm of cells. This process has no relation to the function of secretion, in which case a material formed by the cytoplasm but clearly distinct from it, appears within the cell and is cast out of it with no loss of cytoplasm whatever."
   p. 77, "... the production of antibodies within lymph nodes was proved by McMaster and Kidd in 1937."
   p. 78, "The present data thus provide an example of a functional reaction of both neutrophiles and monocytes within the bloodstream, whereas it is true that they function for the most part within the tissues, using the bloodstream for transport.

DOSAGE AND FREQUENCY - THEORETICAL CONSIDERATIONS - Sabin 1939

   "These experiments throw some light on the importance of dosage and spacing of the injections of antigens as developed in the experience of immunologists. The cells require time for two processes, namely, the preparation of the antigen for introcudtion into the cytoplasm and the synthesis of the new globulins. ... Massive doses ... served to load the cells with much larger aggregates of the dye protein, which presumably cound not be taken up by the cell as easily as the smaller particles. Thus these data suggest a [p. 79] justification for the practice of small, divided doses, in that several daily injections of moderate amounts of antigen serve to bring into action a sufficiently large number of phagocytic cells to assure an effective production of antibodies. Studied from 6-24 hours after such a series of injections, the cells were found to be filled with antigen in relatively unchanged state and there were no antibodies in the serum. An interval of from 4-7 days allows for the produciton of antibodies and reveals the cells with only a small amount of residual visible antigen."

CONCLUSIONS: RETICULOENDOTHELIAL SYSTEM & ANTIBODY Sabin 1939

   p. 79, conclusions:
"1. The use of an antigen which can be seen within the cell demonstrates that one may stimulate the phagocytic cells either of the liver and spleen or of the tissues and lymph nodes to produce antibodies.
   "2. The appearence of antibodies in the serum correlates with the time when the dye protein is no longer visible within the cells and with the phenomenon of a partial shedding of their surface films.

"3. It is thus inferred that the cells of the reticulo-
endothelial system normally produce globulin and that antibody
globulin represents the synthesis of a new kind of protein under
the influence of an antigen.

"4. An antigen is a substance which can specifically modify the
synthesis of the cytoplasm of the cells of the reticulo-
endothelial system."

5.3   TYLER ON ANTIFERTILIZIN AND AUTOANTIBODIES

Tyler 1942, p. 128, indicated that fertilizin "comprises a part
or more probably the whole of the gelatinous coat that is present
on the surface of the [sea urchin] egg. This coat swells and
slowly goes into solution as the eggs stand in sea water ..."

"... the supernatant seawater (called eggwater) ... has the
property of agglutinating the spermatozoa of the same species."

p. 130 "...the agglutination of sperm by fertilizin is a
spontaneously reversible reaction.... egg water also has the
property of increasing the activity of spermatozoa."

p. 131, "It is clear that there must be present on the surface
of the sperm a substance with which fertilizin reacts in causing
the agglutination. This substance has been extracted from sperm
[and] termed antifertilizin [with the] ability to destroy the
sperm agglutinating property of fertilizin. ....

p. 132,"... an antifertilizin has also been obtained from
below the surface of the egg. ...

p. 133, "The finding of antifertilizin below the surface of the
egg means that below the surface of the cell there is present a
substance that is essentially an antibody to the surface
substance. ... This situation, if it be found to hold for cells
in general, has some interesting implications in regard to
general immunology [i.e.,] an explanation of auto-agglutination
and the possibility of obtaining auto-antibodies ...

Such a mechanism might explain why "suspensions of blood cells
and bacteria may agglutinate in response to changes in
temperature, acidity, salinity, etc. ... [whereby] If the surface
substance is partially removed by any agent, the patches of
subsurface substance is left exposed [and may combine' with the
surface substance of several others [etc.] causing agglutination.

THEORY ON GENERATION OF ANTIBODY FROM ANTIGEN   Tyler 1942

"If pathogenic bacteria likewise have complementary surface and
sub-surface substances, then the antibody to the organism should
be obtainable simply by appropriate extraction of the sub-surface
substance without the necessity of producing an anti-serum in
some laboratory animal."

p. 135, "The mechanism that we assume for agglutination is the
lattice theory of antigen-antibody reaction of Heidelberger
[1939] and Marrack [1938], which is strongly supported now by the
chemical investigations of Pauling etal [1941]. According to
this view antigen and antibody molecules are multivalent with
respect to the mutually complementary groups by which they

combine. ...

p. 136, "... the concept of univalent antibodies ... postulated by Heidelberger [1935] and more recently by Pauling [1940] ... [may] account for many apparent failures of immunization in certain species of animals and with certain antigens .... It is already being taken into account in investigations into the basis of allergy [Sherman 1941].

p. 137 "Fertilizin has been found to serve as an aid to fertilization .. . To serve as an aid to fertilization the fertilizin must be present on the surface of the egg. In solution fertilizin acts as a barrier to fertilization. In regard to antifertilizin, experiments in which varying amounts are removed show that the sperm are impaired in their fertilizing power... . Here, too, fertilization is inhibited when anti-fertilizin is present in solution or when the eggs are first treated with such solutions. To be effective in fertilization it appears that the reaction between fertilizin and antifertilizin must take place while both are still essentially part of egg and the spermatoön respectively. ...

"In conclusion it may be said that certain specific substances are extractable from eggs and from sperm of various animals. These substances are evidently complementary proteins and they interact in a manner analogous to that of the complementary substances involved in the usual serological reactions, namely antigens and antibodies. They appear to be concerned with the initial stages of the fertilization process, and their specificity of action can account in part at least for the degree of species and tissue specificity exhibited in fertilization."

5.4 LANDSTEINER-PAULING & ANTIBODY

ANTIBODY PRODUCTION   Pauling 1940-5
CHEMISTRY OF DISEASE   Pauling 1940-5

More than a half-century ago, polio-virus-co-discoverer Karl Landsteiner asked the world's preeminent chemist, Dr. Linus Pauling, to investigate the chemical basis of disease. After years of consequent study of the problem, Pauling contributed a "highly appreciated" chapter to Landsteiner's book [THE SPECIFICITY OF SEROLOGICAL REACTIONS (Harvard U. Press, Cambridge 1945)] entitled "Molecular Structure and Intermolecular Forces".
 Thus did Pauling build towards better-known later work on the alpha helix and on the molecular structure and significance of Vitamin C. But it is the work that was directly associated with Pauling's early association with Landsteiner that is of interest here. In the period 1940-1945, Pauling and associates built on earlier works relating to the catalysis theory of antibody formation, which work consequently was integrated into the medical synthesis of Edward C. Rosenow.

ANTIBODY PRODUCED IN RETICULO-ENDOTHELIAL SYSTEM Pauling 1940
ANTIBODY IS RECONFIGURED, NORMAL GLOBULIN   Pauling 1940
ANTIBODY IS BIVALENT Pauling 1940

ANTIGEN IS MULTIVALENT   Pauling 1940

p. 2643, "When an antigen is injected into an animal some of its molecules are captured and held in the region of antibody production (There is some evidence that this is the cells of the reticuloendothelial system; see Florence Sabin, J. Exptl. Med. 70 67 (1939), and references quoted by her.)"

p. 2644, "I assume .... that all antibody molecules contain the same polypeptide chains as normal globulin, and differ from normal globulin only in the configuration of the chain; that is, in the way that the chain is coiled in the molecule. ... The number of configurations accessible to the polypeptide chain is so great as to provide an explanation of the ability of an animal to form antibodies with considerable specificity for an apparently unlimited number of different antigens, without the necessity of invoking also a variation in the amino-acid composition of amino-acid order."

Note 9: "It has been pointed out by A. Rothen and K Landsteiner, Science 90, 65 (1939) that the possibility of different ways of folding the same polypeptide chain to obtain different antibodies is worth considering."

p. 2646, Theory is based on assumptions of bivalence of antibodies and multivalence of antigens.

p. 2647, "An ideal structure of the antibody-antigen precipitate for N=12 may be described as having antigen molecules at the positions corresponding to closest packing, with the 12 antibody molecules which surround each antigen molecule lying along the lines connecting it with the 12 nearest antigen neighbors."

"Similar ideal structures can be suggested for other values of the antigen valence. ....

"It is not to be inferred that the actual precipitates have the regularity of structure of these ideal arrangements."

2656, "An interesting possible method of producing antibodies from serum or globulin solution outside of the animal is suggested by the theory. The globulin would be treated with a denaturing agent or condition sufficiently strong to cause the chain ends to uncoil; after which this agent would be removed slowly while antigen or hapten is present in the solution in considerable concentration. The chain ends would then coil up to assume the configurations stable under these conditions, which would be configurations complementary to those of the antigen or hapten. ...

"It seems not unlikely that certain processes auxiliary to antibody formation occur. The reported increase in globulin (aside from the antibody fraction) after immunization suggests the operation of a mechanism whereby the presence of antigen molecules accelerates the synthesis of the globulin polypeptide chains.

"The mechanism for catching the antibody molecule and holding it in the region of globulin synthesis may be closely related to that of antibody production - possibly a partially liberated globulin chain which forms a bond or two bonds with an antigen molecule directly above it is prevented from freeing its central part from the cell wall, and so serves as an anchor.

"The renewed production of antibody in the serum after bleeding is to be attributed to the presence of trapped antigen molecules in the cells. [This surely sounds like a description of autohemotherapy.] The greater duration of active than of passive immunization may be attributed to this or to the presence of complexes of antigen and surrounding antibodies, the outer ends of which could combine with additional antigen."
[The renewed production of antibody in serum could be explained alternately as resulting from antigen in the blood being introduced to the tissues in which antibody is formed, with resulting infusion of antibody into the system. Such production would likely not take place within the bloodstream for reason of lack of an "anchor".]

ANTIBODY MOLECULES BIVALENT Pauling 1942b

p. 3014, Pauling 1942b summary cites analyses of precipitates between various dyes as evidence taken to indicate bivalence of most of the antibody molecules.

MANUFACTURED ANTIBODY Pauling 1942

Pauling 1942, p. 215, Method of preparation of modified protein: "A solution containing 0.01% of dye and 1.0 % of protein at approximately pH 7.8 was placed in a water bath at 57°C, which is about 10° below the denaturation temperature of the protein. After 3 or 4 days, depending on the temperature, concentration of reagents, and pH, precipitate began to appear... . The amount of precipitate increases for several days." After 11-14 days, the mixture is dialized against 1.0 % NaCl solution to remove most of the free dye. It is then placed in a fresh bag and dialized against 0.5N arsanilate solutions for about 4 days, and the remaining solution dialized against 1.0% NaCl solution "until free of hapten." (about 3 or 4 days.)
p. 216, "... under the best conditions only about 15% of the manufactured antibody was precipitated. ... It will also be noted that only about 15% of the dye antigen was precipitated under optimum conditions, which agrees closely with results obtained with the same dye and natural antibodies."
Pauling 1942, p. 215, "the modified protein, which will subsequently be referred to as manufactured antibody, behaved like natural antibody in forming specific precipitates and in the fixation of complement. It was specific in that it reacted with specific homologous antigens..."
p. 220, "By heating solutions of 'y'globulins and antigen to 57°C for several days antisera homologous to the antigens have been prepared."

MANUFACTURE OF ANTIBODIES IN VITRO Pauling & Campbell 1942

"The Manufacture of Antibodies in Vitro", with H2O2 and Heat, Pauling and Campbell, 1942, p. 211, report having "succeeded in endowing normal serum globulin with the properties of a specific antibody..."

this is based on the theory [Pauling 1940] whereby "globulin would be treated with a denaturing agent or condition sufficiently strong to cause the chain ends to uncoil; after which this agent or hapten is present in the solution in considerable concentration. The chain ends would then coil up to assume ... configurations complementary to those of the antigen or hapten."

p. 212, Of the five methods of denaturation used in the preliminary investigations, treatment with sodium hydroxide solutions gave the most promising results.

p. 213, "heat denaturation at various temperatures up to 80°C with slow cooling produced approximately the same effect as alkali denaturation."

p. 218, cites experiments with pneumococcus polysaccharide, wherein a [manufactured antibody] solution agglutinated Type III pneumococci but did not agglutinate either Type I or Type II pneumococci."

MECHANICS OF IMMUNITY Pauling 1943

Pauling 1943, p. 203, refers to Arrhenius's 1904 lectures on immunology at U.C. Berkeley, citing Arrhenius's observation that Ehrlich and others, "because of incomplete knowledge of the phenomenon of chemical equilibrium, had been led to invent artificial hypotheses in order to explain their observations in the field of immunology."

Pauling cites advances in physical chemistry and structural chemistry that now "allow for a more penetrating interpretation....

"Two important advances in the attack on the problem of the nature of immunological reactions were the discovery that the specific [antigen-antibody] precipitate contains both antigen and antibody and the discovery that antibodies, which give antisera their characteristic properties, are proteins."

p. 205, Pauling cites the van der Waals attraction which varies inversely with the 7th power of interatomic distance.

p. 208, complementariness theory - similar to Ehrlich's "lock and key"; "particles can be agglutinated by an amount of antibody very much smaller than the amount required to cover their surface..."

p. 210, azoerythrocytes can be agglutinated by less than .02% as much antibody as would cover their surface with a layer 3.5A thick. ...

p. 211 "The fact that slides can be coated with alternate unimolecular layers of antigen and antibody in specific combination indicates effective bivalence of antibody molecules as well as antigen molecules.

"It has long been known that in antigen-antibody precipitates molecules of antibody are present in larger numbers than those of antigen, the antibody-antigen molecular ratio being considerably greater than unity for nearly all systems."

   p. 212, Pauling cites presence in rabbit and horse antisera of univalent antibodies able to combine with antigen but unable to form precipitates.

   p. 213, discusses probable conversion from multivalent to univalent antibody through destruction of one of combining regions due to a denaturing agent.

   p. 217, Summary: Specificity of interaction/combination of antigen and antibody arises from structural complementariness which allows weak forces to bind, i.e. van der Waals, Coulomb and electric dipole/multipole attractions, hydrogen bonds, etc. Evidence indicates that the precipitation reaction is specific, precipitating antigen and antibody must be multivalent or at least bivalent.

MECHANICS OF IMMUNITY Landsteiner 1945

   p. 148, "Antibodies combine with a much larger quantity of antigen than that necessary for their production. According to a calculation made by Hooker and Boyd [<u>JI</u> 21, 113, 1931] the discrepency may be so great that a single antigen molecule gives rise to a quantity of antibodies sufficient to agglutinate several hundred bacilli, and in determinations by Pappenheimer the weight of the resulting antibody was 10,000 times that of the antigen injected."

   p. 150, cites Pauling's proposition that "antibodies differ from normal serum globulins only in the way in which the two end-points of the globulin polypeptide chain are coiled..."

   p. 256, "the first attempt, by Arrhenius, at a theoretical treatment of precipitin and agglutinin reactions was rationally based on the mass law but included a number of quite improbable propositions."

   p. 259, "It was brought out by Hooker and Boyd [1934, 1939] that the ratio, by weight, of antigen to antibody in precipitates in the equivalence zone diminished with increasing molecular weight of the antigen."

MECHANICS OF IMMUNITY Pauling in Landsteiner 1945
   p. 275, "It is ... probable that the high specificity which often characterizes physiological activity is in most cases specificity of intermolecular interaction rather than primarily of chemical reaction..."

   p. 277, refers to ions with opposite charges and strong inverse-square Coulomb attraction: "In water or other medium of high dielectric constant the Coulomb forces between ions are very greatly reduced in magnitude, so that they no longer lead to the formation of strong chemical bonds." [perhaps because the attraction for water of solvation is greater]

   p. 285, "It is hydrogen-bond formation between water molecules which gives to water its unusual physical properties - abnormally high melting point, boiling point, heat of fusion, heat of vaporization, dielectric constant, etc."

p. 289, "The theoretical discussion of the interaction of molecules in solution is complicated by competition with solvent molecules. A solute molecule may have as strong electronic van der Waals attraction for the solvent molecules as for other solute molecules. The effective van der Waals attraction of two solute molecules in aqueous solution may be very small, since the close approach of the two molecules involves the replacement of the water molecules adjacent to teach molecule."

p. 291, "A molecule would show strong attraction for that molecule which possessed complete complementariness in surface configuration and distribution of active electrically charged and hydrogen-bond forming groups, somewhat weaker attraction for those molecules with approximate but not complete complementariness to it, and only very weak attraction for all other molecules."

[such complementariness may be relevant to considerations of the origin of Flint's hydration methodology, e.g., groupings of 23- see Secret Code of the Universe (www.hydration.com)]

PROTEIN MOLECULES UNFOLDING - Follensby & Hooker 1947

p. 215 "If the proteins are made up of peptid chains held together by different types of cross-linkages and by hydrogen bonds as postulated by Pauling and by Chibnall, it is conceivable that the molecules can unfold partially or even completely due to the breaking of these linkages."

p. 206, "When glycerol, sugars, OH ions or urea are added to heated immune sera, some investigators have found that they exert a protective effect upon antibody." [JR Marrack, 1938]

PAULING THEORY MOST STIMULATING

Cushing and Campbell 1957 refer to Pauling's 1940 work as "the most stimulating theory within recent years." [Pauling, L., J. Am. Chem. Soc., 62:2643 (1940)] Pauling's work, in turn, refers to the 1938 work of F. Sabin regarding the production of antibodies in the reticuloendothelial system.

BIBLIOGRAPHY - CATALYSIS THEORY

  --Arrhenius, Svante A., Immunology, MacMillan Co. 1907
  --Cushing, JE and DH Campbell, Principles of Immunology, McGraw-Hill, New York, 1957.
  --Follensby EM and Hooker SB, JI 55 (1947), 205-218, "The Effect of Heat upon Anti-Hemocyanin"
  --Hooker, Sanford B, and William C. Boyd, J.I. 21 (1931), 113-115, "A Quantitave Aspect of the Hypothetical Incorporation of Injected Antigen in Resulting Antibody"
  --Landsteiner, Karl, The Specificity of Serological Reactions, Revised Ed., Harvard U. Press 1945
  --Pauling, Linus, "Molecular Structure and Intermolecular Forces", in Karl Landsteiner, The Specificity of Serological Reactions, Revised Ed., Harvard U. Press, 1945, 275-293.
  --Pauling & Campbell, 1942, p. 211, "The Manufacture of Antibodies in Vitro", w/H2O2, heat

--Pauling, Linus, <u>Am. Chem. Soc., J.</u> 62 (1940) 2643-2657, "A Theory of the Structure and Process of Formation of Antibodies"

--Pauling, Linus and Dan H. Campbell, <u>Journal of Experimental Medicine</u> 76 (1942), 211-220, "The Manufacture of Antibodies in Vitro".

--Pauling, Linus, David Pressman and Carol Ikeda, <u>J. Am. Chem. Soc.</u> 64 (Dec. 1942), 3010-3014, "The Serological Properties of Simple Substances. III"

--Pauling, Linus, Dan H. Campbell and David Pressman, <u>Physiol. Reviews</u> 23 (1943), 203-219, "The Nature of the Forces Between Antigen and Antibody and of the Precipitation Reaction"

--Rothen A. and K Landsteiner, <u>Science</u> 90, 65 (1939) per Pauling 1940, 2643.

--Sabin, Florence, J. EXPER. MED. 70, 67-82, "Cellular Reactions to a Dye-Protein with a Concept of the Mechanism of Antibody Formation", 1939

--Tyler, Albert, <u>West. J. Surgery</u> 50 (1942), 126-138, "Specific Interacting Substances of Eggs and Sperm".

Chapter 6.   POLIO AND "POST-POLIO SYNDROME"

To some extent, Rosenow's work may have fallen into disfavor because his work on polio did not culminate in a generally used prophylactic (preventive) polio vaccine. Five points are noted:

(1) Rosenow from 1916 had emphasized polio therapy, and was quite successful in his efforts (6.1);
(2) he had developed a successful prophylactic polio vaccine before Salk or Sabin, but did not gain widespread acknowledgement (6.2);
(3) his apparent understanding of the pathology of polio should be particularly welcome in view of modern medicine's lack of same (6.2);
(4) he implicated "peculiar" tonsillar abscesses in severe and fatal cases of poliomyelitis, and described the general significance of tonsils and other foci in aggravating attacks of acute infectious diseases (6.3); and
(5) he predicted the resurgence of polio in polio victims, and prescribed therapeutic measures to be taken (6.4).

6.1   ROSENOW'S SUCCESSFUL POLIO THERAPY

(a) as of 1940
  As summarized in JAMA 114, 2253, from 40R1, Rosenow compares the results obtained for 221 acute poliomyelitis patients treated with his antistreptococcus serum, versus 116 similar patients not receiving this treatment, from 1928 to 1940.

Table 6.1:   RESULTS OF ROSENOW'S POLIO THERAPY AS OF 1940

	Rosenow Therapy	Not Receiving Rosenow Therapy
	# (%)	# (%)
Total Number	221	116
Died	10 (5)	23 (20)
Remainder	211 (95)	93 (80)
No Paralysis	161 (73)	34 (29)
Slight "	29 (13)	10 (9)
Moderate "	14 (6)	17 (15)
Severe "	7 (3)	32 (28)

It is noted that less than ten percent of the treated group suffered moderate or severe paralysis, compared with 43% of the group not receiving Rosenow's treatment.

(b) 1948 - Rappaport, B. [Journal-Lancet, 68 (October 1948), 395-7, "Acute Poliomyelitis Treated with Thermal Antibody":
  Rappaport 1948 discussed 20 cases of epidemic poliomyelitis treated during the 1946 polio season. The author relates that during the current season some untreated preparalytic patients had developed paralysis after a few days, untreated patients with paralysis did develop more paralysis, and others with paralysis and treated with convalescent poliomyelitis serum continued to

develop more paralysis and several died.

In contrast, none of the 20 patients treated with Rosenow's "thermal antibody" died, only one with paralysis had temporarily worsened, but within 5 days of injection could breathe and swallow normally and was regaining use of muscles in both legs. None of the other six patients with paralysis worsened, and all improved, after inoculation of thermal antibody. None of the 13 preparalytic patients developed muscular weakness or paralysis. Within 5 days all five patients with difficulty in swallowing, were able to. Sixteen of the total 20 were noted as discharged with "no muscular weakness"; the four others were noted as gradually improving.

Rappaport concluded: "This thermal antibody for acute poliomyelitis contains no horse serum, and delayed reactions did not occur. With the pH adjusted to between 6.0 and 6.5 this artificial antibody caused small local reactions and in some cases no reactions. This antibody would seem to have curative effects in poliomyelitis and in returning the patient to normal activity in a relatively short space of time." ...

"The thermal poliomyelitis antibody was given intramuscularly into the lateral aspect of the thigh in all twenty cases. The amount varied from 15cc to 40cc. Eight patients received 15cc each, two received 20cc each, one received 25cc, eight received 30cc, and one received 40cc. The dose varied with the severity of the illness and somewhat with the size of the patient." [p. 395]

(c) 1954 - Rappaport, Benjamin, QUARTERLY BUL., NORTHWESTERN U. MED. SCHOOL 28:57 (1954), "FURTHER OBSERVATIONS ON ACUTE POLIOMYELITIS TREATED WITH THERMAL ANTIBODY"

In 1954 Rappaport discussed an additional 26 cases of acute poliomyelitis, for a total of 46 consecutive cases treated with Rosenow's thermal poliomyelitis thermal antibody. The first 20 occurred in 1948 and are discussed above.

Of the 26 later cases, paralysis or weakness was present in 12 and reflexes were lost or absent in six of the remaining 12; 5 could not swallow or could do so only with difficulty.

Charts given for the 26 patients note discharge with "no muscular weakness" in 23 of the 26 and the remaining three with some residual weakness in one leg only, one slight, "but can walk alone" (the above-mentioned 6-year-old), one with "some weakness ... Can walk alone with leg brace", and one with "right leg weak, but can walk with a cane."   Time between date of injection of antibody and discharge ranged from 7 to 37 days, averaging 17 days.

6.2 THE FIRST SUCCESSFUL PROPHYLACTIC POLIO VACCINE

The safe inoculation of 30 contacts, as per Rappaport 1954, at a minimum speaks to the question of the safety of administration of antibody to well contacts. As all of these reported cases occurred from 7-17-47 to 10-24-51, these (limited) tests occurred

prior to the trials of Salk vaccine, and thus may therefore be
considered the first successful instance of prophylactic
vaccination against polio.

(In 1952 Salk used monkey kidney cells, and inoculated 161
persons. In 1953 experiments were extended to 5000 persons, in
1954 trials and in 1955 vaccination began.)

Far more important than such questions of priority, Rosenow's
work provides answers to questions concerning polio that are
currently generally considered unknown. Notably, Bernard N.
Fields has recently pointed out that the discovery of a
prophylactic vaccine for polio caused the abrupt discontinuation
of further research into the pathology of polio, leaving it still
a mystery. [Nature 369 (12 May 1994), 95-96]

6.3 ROSENOW ON TONSILS AS TEST TUBE; ABSCESSES AND POLIOMYELITIS

Rosenow particularly emphasized the danger, not of actively
inflamed tonsils, but rather of "small atrophic tonsils with deep
pockets which cannot heal for mechanical reasons", characterizing
these as virtual "test tubes" for the manufacture of harmful
pathogens.

For further discussions of tonsils as test tubes and in
particular their role in polio and acute diseases, please see
APPENDIX A1:

16R4 ORGANISM FROM TONSILS CONSISTENTLY PRODUCES POLIO IN ANIMALS
16R7 TONSILS AS TEST TUBES
17R7 TONSILLAR ABSCESSES AND POLIO
18R2 TONSILLAR ABSCESSES AND POLIO
27R9 FOCI IN TONSILS AND SEVERITY OF ACUTE INFECTIOUS DISEASES

6.4 ROSENOW PREDICTION OF RESURGENCE OF POLIO, AND THERAPY

[Rosenow, E.C., Further immunological and clinical studies on
importance of neurotropic streptococcus in etiology of epidemic
poliomyelitis and its relation to natural virus, J. Nerv. and
Ment. dis. 120: 196-206, Sept.-Oct. 1954, 204]

"... it is suggested that the administration of the poliomyelitis
streptococcal thermal antibody used with favorable results in the
treatment of acute epidemic poliomyelitis be extended to persons
having severe paralytic poliomyelitis long after onset and who
according to the cutaneous tests have antigen in excessive titer
and, according to cutaneous and agglutinative tests, have
antibody in deficient titer."

As Rosenow had predicted, P. Elmer-Dewitt [Time, March 28,
1994, 54-55] recently discussed "post-polio syndrome", or "acute
paralytic poliomyelitis sequelae", noting that "Doctors aren't
certain what causes it or how best to treat it .... Before the
end of the decade, by one estimate, postpolio syndrome will

strike 40% to 50% of the polio survivors ... .   What can be done
to help the postpolio sufferers? Not much, unfortunately. There
are only experimental treatments. A steroid called prednisone,
usually used to treat immune-system diseases like MS, seems to
help in postpolio as well, reducing fatigue and increasing
endurance. ..."

Chapter 7. AIDS AS A TYPICAL "FOCAL DISEASE"
      - A Proven Autogenous Vaccine-Therapy
      - HIV-AIDS Controversy Resolved

"It can be said, regarding Medicine, that one who knows only
current information about Medicine does not even know that."
      SIR WILLIAM OSLER, in J. F. A. McManus, The Fundamental
      Ideas of Medicine, Charles C. Thomas, Springfield, Ill.,
      1963, p.6

   How can it be, in the presumably brilliant intellectual climate
of 1998, that two groups of well-respected medical and scientific
experts have essentially opposite views on the role of HIV in
AIDS? On the one hand, influential researchers including Anthony
Fauci of the National Institutes of Health and Robert Gallo of
claimed HIV- discovery fame assert that HIV causes AIDS; on the
other hand, a number of equally creditable researchers, including
Peter Duesberg of U.C. Berkeley and Nobel laureate Carey Mullis
of U.C. San Diego, assert that HIV does not cause AIDS. Neither
position is based on frivolous conjecture; both groups
essentially KNOW that they are right. And essentially, they may
both be essentially correct. How can this be? Rosenow's work
holds the key to understanding this riddle.

   Similarities between AIDS and MS (7.1) have long been
recognized, prompting the hope that future advances in AIDS
research might benefit investigations into MS and other
presumably related diseases. Ironically, the most important
advance in understanding AIDS in recent years provides a
seemingly decisive link to a long-ignored monumental body of work
on MS and other diseases, which work may well hold the keys to
unravelling the many mysteries surrounding the syndrome known as
AIDS.
   In the early years of the age of AIDS, initial infection by the
organism that causes AIDS was thought to be followed by a long
period of dormancy, prior to the actual outbreak of full-blown
AIDS. However, this view has been replaced in recent years by the
realization that the AIDS organism is actively replicating during
the long period between infection and visible onset of disease,
and both tonsils and teeth (7.2) have been identified as
reservoirs for this replication process. Aside from specific
designation as a "reservoir", or source for more generalized
infection, numerous reports address oral or dental manifestations
(7.3) as an early indication of HIV infection.
   Such discussions vividly bring to mind the monumental works of
Edward C. Rosenow (Chapter 1; APPENDIX A). During an active
professional career spanning more than a half-century and
including nearly three decades with the Mayo Foundation
(1915-1944), Rosenow detailed the role of bacteria (and/or their
derivatives) emanating from "oral foci" in the causation of MS
and a wide range of other diseases, including disease of "blood-
building tissues" (7.4), and emphasized the primary importance of
the removal of these foci (2.3).

It may also be noted that the recent work of Wolinsky etal. has apparently refuted the popular so-called antigenic-diversity-theory. Their study, published in the authoritative journal SCIENCE, found that progression of AIDS is associated not with a continually mutating virus population, but rather with a stable one, thereby debunking one of the major assumptions that has guided AIDS research in recent times. This new finding is fully consistent with the hypothesis that AIDS is a typical so-called oral-focal disease (7.5).

Rosenow's work also involved therapeutic vaccines which reportedly worked wonders in numerous patients with various conditions. [L.Rowntree, 1958] If the disease condition known as AIDS is correctly grouped with conditions with which Rosenow worked, we may expect similar results. This in turn may serve to revive public awareness of the depth and broad scope of Rosenow's contributions (Chapter 1) to understanding and combatting human disease.

In the case of AIDS, the proper use of Rosenow's culture methods (Chapter 4) would be expected to yield the pathogenic phase of the causative organism of AIDS (as demonstrated by Rosenow in so many other conditions), which organism would be capable of replicating the disease conditions in laboratory animals (the lack of a so-called "animal model" for AIDS has been cited as a key factor inhibiting AIDS research [B. Fields [Nature 369, 12 May 1994, 95-96; C. Holden, Science 269, 29 Sept. 1995, 1819].); and could also serve as the foundation for highly specific therapeutic vaccines.

Regarding a program of therapy for AIDS, beyond the indicated removal of offending oral foci of infection, particular attention may be given to Rosenow's regimen of autogenous "vaccine" (antigen) and antibody against MS (see reprint, APPENDIX D3).

At first glance, the hypothesis of AIDS as a typical "oral-focal" disease may seem far removed from the continuing controversy over the relationship between AIDS and HIV; in reality, the latter is readily explained by the former.

Over the past several years, the conventional view that HIV is related to the cause of AIDS has been challenged by a small but reputable group of scientists, notably Peter Duesberg of Berkeley who maintains that HIV is too weak to cause AIDS. In accord with the works of Rosenow, the entity commonly found to be associated with AIDS, HIV, could be a dissociative form or invasive phase of a pathogenic streptococcal form, or both. Such dissociations and possible reversions to parent forms (see Chapter 3.4), under favorable conditions, have been discussed by several workers up to the present.

Specifically, in the case of the HIV-AIDS controversy, Rosenow's methodology for effecting dissociation of streptococcal forms (see 3.2) into filtrable (viral) forms would be expected to yield a filtrable phase of the AIDS organism. Should this be found to be HIV and the process demonstrated as reversible, this would show (a) how HIV might comprise an essential invasive phase of the organism that conveys AIDS (as per the conventional "pro-HIV" view), but, at the same time, (b) explain why this same HIV (phase) itself may be incapable of directly causing AIDS (as asserted by Duesberg). The situation (concerning the possibly-common occurrence of the existence of multiple phases (see 3.1, 3.2) for a given bacterial species) may be viewed as somewhat analogous to the differentiation of roles for the different stages in the metamorphosis of the likes of the malaria parasite, slime molds, and butterflies; in the case of bacterial species, such phase transitions are apparently readily-reversible.

Pending the establishment of mechanisms for proper production of therapeutic (S. rosenow) vaccines in accord with Rosenow's methodology, an immediately available interim measure that might be utilized is "autohemotherapy" (Chapter 8) in its original and predominant form - the prompt intramuscular or subcutaneous reinjection of autologous (one's own) whole blood. Regardless of the identity or source of the organism that causes AIDS, it is known that some form of the causative organism is in the blood; thus, as first suggested by Cuyugan in 1988 (see 8.3), autohemotherapy would be expected to have therapeutic value, presumably acting to some extent as an autogenous vaccine. It is noted that a more complex, experimental form of autohemotherapy (see 8.4) has been proposed for AIDS, seemingly paving the way for trials of the simpler original method (see 8.3, 8.5).

7.1 SIMILARITIES: AIDS AND M.S.

A number of reports discussing similarities between M.S. and AIDS have been published over recent years. For example:

   --Gray, F., etal., Neurology 1991 Jan. 41(1):105-8, "Fulminating multiple sclerosis like leukoencephalopathy revealing human immunodeficiency virus infection".
   --Laurenzi, M.A., etal, "cerebrospinal fluid interleukin G activity in HIV infection and inflammatory and noninflammatory diseases of the nervous system." Clinical Immunology and Immunopathology, 1990 Nov., 57(2):233-41.
   --Berger, J.R., etal, Neurology 1989 March., 30(3):324-8, "Multiple sclerosis-like illness occurring with human immunodeficiency virus infection."
   --Waksman, BH, Nature 337 (16 Feb. 1989), 599, "Multiple Sclerosis: Relationship to a retrovirus?
   --Reddy EP,etal, Science 243 (27 JA 1989), 529-533

Waksman 1989 discussed studies suggesting "a relationship between a retrovirus related to HTLV and multiple sclerosis. ..." and the possibility that research aimed at arresting retroviral replication "being developed for the distantly-related AIDS virus might also be beneficial in the case of MS.
Waksman, commenting on Reddy etal's recent report suggesting a relationship between a retrovirus related to HTLV-1 and MS, "it is possible that these findings will stimulate attempts to

develop preventive viral vaccines or therapeutic investigation
with drugs which arrest retroviral replication, such as those
being developed for the distantly-related AIDS virus."

Reddy 1989, p. 532, "An association between the occurrence of
HTLV-1 related sequences in MS patients and the development of
the disease is implicated by our studies." The authors suggest
specifically that treatments similar to that with "antiviral
drugs such as azidothymidine ... might be effective in some cases
of chronic progressive myelopathies of humans."

Koprowski etal 1985 [incl. RC Gallo], discussed data suggesting
a relation between MS and the human T-cell lymphotropic viruses;
specifically, "Some MS patients respond immunologically to, and
have cerebrospinal T cells containing, a retrovirus that is
related to, but distinct from, the 3 types of human T-cell
lymphotropic viruses." [p. 154] ...
"We have discussed our data as though they indicated the
presence and involvement of a novel HTLV-related virus in MS. If
that is the case, our attempts to isolate the virus should
eventually be successful. For now, the data are suggestive, but
not conclusive." [p. 159]

In addition, both MS and AIDS have long gestation periods,
which in the case of MS and numerous other disease conditions has
been demonstrated by Rosenow to be attributable to a low-grade
infection of non-virulent streptococci emanating from oral foci
(generally teeth and tonsils). [48R3: Rosenow, E.C.,
Bacteriologic studies of multiple sclerosis, Ann. Allergy 6:
271-292, May-June 1948] Another similarity between the two
disease entities is the apparent difficulty encountered in
locating a causative organism.
In the case of AIDS, the existence of the disease in a given
individual is considered indicated by the presence in the blood
of antibodies to HIV, not the HIV virus itself; in MS and several
other disease conditions, the presence of antibodies coupled with
the problem of identifying a causative organism has fed the
notion that these may be "autoimmune" diseases, caused by the
body's immune system turning against itself. AIDS has also in
the past been grouped with the so-called "auto-immune" diseases,
although a viral etiology is now generally considered likely.
Nonetheless, it would appear that at least some of the current
confusion over AIDS might be attributed to the apparently
bankrupt concept of "autoimmune disease", and that in turn to the
defrauding of Rosenow.
In concert with Rosenow's work, it is possible that the
pathogenic phase of the causative organism for AIDS, which all
seem to agree is in the blood, may simply be undetectable by
ordinary culture procedures, i.e., perhaps it is identifiable
only through the use of careful culture techniques which foster
the growth of fastidious organisms in a reduced oxygen gradient.

7.2 TEETH AND TONSILS AS RESERVOIR FOR AIDS ORGANISM

HIV FOUND IN SEROPOSITIVE PATIENT'S NON-INFLAMED DENTAL PULPS
  Glick M, etal., Oral Surg., Oral Med., Oral Pathol. 71 (June
1991), 733-736, "Human immunodeficiency virus infection of
fibroblasts of dental pulp in seropositive patients", examined
dental pulps from 11 HIV-seropositive patients, from teeth
extracted for reasons other than pulpal disease, and confirmed
the presence of HIV in the pulps of all but one of the patients.
  The one negative result was obtained in the case of a patient
who "was clinically in an asymptomatic stage of HIV disease but
was seropositive for the virus. ... All controls, which consisted
of pulp tissue from HIV-seronegative patients, lacked evidence
for the virus..." The authors note "The lack of destruction and
function of the fibroblasts, as demonstrated by intact H-E-
stained specimens and clinically asymptomatic dental pulps,
suggests that the fibroblasts act as a reservoir for HIV in the
body."

  In a followup item, ibid. 73 (Feb. 1992), 135, Endodontic
section editor Samuel Seltzer noted that this had been "the first
study to document the presence of HIV in the fibroblasts of
noninflamed dental pulps of HIV-seropositive patients ... . The
diagnostic significance of this finding remains to be explored
and developed."

REPLICATION PROCEEDS IN PREVIOUSLY-ASSUMED LATENT PERIOD
  Maddox, J., Nature 362 (25 March 1993), 287, in an editorial,
discusses "Where the AIDS virus hides away". He notes two
independent studies indicating "that the long and variable
latency period between HIV infection and overt AIDS is explained
by replication of virus in the lymph nodes. ...
  "With hindsight, it is not surprising that the lymph nodes (but
also the spleen, adenoid glands and tonsils should be sites at
which the presence of HIV is most readily demonstrated....
  This suggests that the apparent latent period "is not clinical
latency at all, but rather a period in which the replication of
the virus proceeds apace in the lymph nodes and some other
tissues of the immune system."

TONSILS ARE FOCUS FROM WHICH HIV DISSEMINATES
  Pantaleo G, etal. 1993, including A.S. Fauci, "HIV infection is
active and progressive in lymphoid tissue during the clinically
latent stage of disease", Nature 362 (25 March 1993), 355-359,
note that "HIV disease is active in the lymphoid tissue
throughout the period of clinical latency, even at times when
minimal viral activity is demonstrated in blood." [355]. Authors
refer to this as "the first demonstration of a striking dichotomy
between peripheral blood and lymphoid tissue from the same
individuals in viral burden and replication. The authors suggest
that their work "may have important implications in the design of
therapeutic strategies." Of note, high levels of HIV expression
were observed in lymphoid tissue other than lymph nodes, such as
adenoids and tonsils, indicating a systemic dissemination of HIV

among lymphoid tissue and not a localization to lymph nodes."
    In other words, this seems to say that the lymphoid tissue is
not the target of localizing virus, therefore it may well serve
as a focal source.

    MORE LIKELY-VIRUS-PRODUCTIVE CELLS IN LYMPH NODES THAN IN BLOOD
    Temin and Bolognesi 1993 relate how Pantaleo etal 1993 "show
that in asymptomatic HIV-infected patients there are many
infected cells in the lymph nodes, more than in the blood, and
that these lymph-node cells are more likely to be virus-
productive than cells in the blood." Temin and Bolognesi 1993
conclude that "A clear message from the new work [Pantaleo etal,
etc.] is that HIV infection is a very complicated process and
that it will require the march of science, frustratingly slow as
it sometimes seems, to gain sufficient knowledge to control it."

    Heath, SL, etal., Nature 377, 26 October, 1995, note that
"Large amounts of human immunodeficiency virus (HIV) localize on
follicular dendritic cells (FDC in the follicles of secondary
lymphoid tissues following viral infection. During clinical
latency, active viral infection occurs primarily at these
sites"., citing among others, Pantaleo, G, etal., Nature 362,
355-358 (1993), who had implicated the tonsils as a reservoir for
HIV. Heath etal "report here that HIV on FDC is highly
infectious." This is determined with "an in vitro model of the
germinal centre", utilizing FDC from the tonsils of non-HIV-
infected individuals.

    HIV IN TONSILS, LYMPH NODES
    Fox, CH, etal, J. Infect. Dis. 164, 1051-1057 (1991), "Lymphoid
Germinal Centers Are Reservoirs of Human Immunodeficiency Virus
Type 1 RNA", asserts that "in the early stages of HIV infection,
germinal centers serve as important reservoirs of free virus in
the interstitial spaces, and this reservoir disappears as the
germinal centers involute with advancing disease." The authors
note HIV virus type 1 RNA was found in high concentrations in the
extracellular space in all of five tonsils examined: including
one from an adult CDC class III patient and four pediatric
patients with class IIa disease.
    p. 1055: "This study provides evidence at the molecular level
supporting a number of previous studies that have demonstrated a
reservoir of HIV-1 particles associated with the follicular
dendritic network of lymph node germinal centers. ... it appears
that the follicular dendritic cell network in lymphoid germinal
centers serves as a filter that retains virus, enclosed in immune
complexes, on the surface of the follicular dendritic processes.
 The virus-antibody complex would thus be available to any
susceptible cell that might migrate through the germinal center.

... The cases reported here, with the exception of autopsy cases,
all had lymphadenopathy or tonsillitis sufficient to warrant
surgical biopsy to rule out neoplasia or infection or to remove
obstructive hyperplastic tissue.

"The depopulation of germinal centers in late progressive disease and the disappearance of strong virus signals occur simultaneously with the disorganization of the follicular dendritic cell network. This effect may be due to infection and death of the follicular dendritic cells, since virus budding from dendritic cells in germinal centers is well described. ... It may be that the observed late-stage increase in circulating viremia reflects either decreased trapping or the release of large amounts of virus-antibody complexes from lymph nodes due to the death or disappearance of the follicular dendritic cells."

"... our finding of large amounts of HIV RNA in the germinal centers in the distribution of follicular dendritic cells suggests that this RNA may serve as a persistent source of infection for CD4+ cells."

ORAL MUCOSA NEGATIVELY AFFECTED DURING HIV INFECTION
Pimpinelli N, etal., J of Investigative Derm., 1991 Sep, 97 (3):537-42., "CD36(OKM5)+ dendritic cells in the oral mucosa of HIV- and HIV+ subjects.", suggested that "the antigen-presenting function of [CD36+ dendritic] cells in the oral mucosa [of HIV- subjects] is negatively affected during HIV infection."

SUSCEPTIBILITY OF TONSILLAR CELLS TO HIV INFECTION
Degrassi, A, etal, AIDS Research and Human Retroviruses 10, 1994, 675-682, 675: "Transfer of HIV-1 to Human Tonsillar Stromal Cells Following Cocultivation with Infected Lymphocytes": The authors assessed the susceptibility of normal human tonsillar stromal cells (HTSCs) to infection by HIV-1, and concluded "The infection of HTSCs may contribute to HIV-1-mediated pathogenesis indirectly as a viral reservoir or directly by structural and functional modification of the lymphoid microenvironment."
p. 680:
"The mechanism by which HIV-1 infects HTSCs is of considerable interest because it does not appear to involve the CD4 molecule commonly used by HIV-1 to infect human cells. ...
"The role of HIV-1-infected HTSCs in the pathological changes accompanying infection clearly depends on the normal in vivo function of these cells. To date, little is known about such function ...
"... an early consequence of HTSC infection could be virus release and its rapid spread throughout the host. ... In the final stages of disease, virus-induced death of HTSCs would lead to complete loss of LN (lymph node) architecture."

7.3 AIDS AND DENTAL ILLNESS

Numerous reports in the contemporary medical literature address the oral/dental manifestations of HIV infection, most notably severe periodontitis, suggesting such might be "the first sign [or indication] of HIV infection" [Navazesh & Lucatorto 1993; Holmstrup P & Westergaard, 1994; Chapple IL, Rout & Basu, 1992; Jones AC, Migliorati & Baughman, 1992], "an important clinical marker" [Levine & Glick 1991], "an early presentation" [Tenenbaum etal 1991]. Such reports imply, or explicitly conclude, that "HIV seropositivity ... may be a risk factor for gingival inflammation" [Barr C, Lopez & Rua-Dobles 1992].

Glick etal 1991 suggest that fibroblasts of the pulp may serve as a possible reservoir for HIV, reminiscent of Rosenow's monumental studies of the focal-infective role of such oral infections. One "well-documented" neurologic manifestation of HIV, peripheral neuropathy of the facial nerve, is seen as cause for early dental intervention; it is noted that Austin Flint, who would go on to become the 36th President of the AMA, had as early as 1868 discussed the correlation between this condition and diseased teeth.

Piazza etal [J. Med. Virology, 1994 Jan, 42(1):38-41] report a "significantly higher... concentration of hemoglobin" in saliva "in subjects with AIDS-related complex (ARC)/AIDS compared to asymptomatic/PGL subjects, and in subjects with stomatitis compared to subjects without stomatitis", and in other anti-HIV-positive groups compared to healthy controls. Piazza, etal focus on "possible implication in sexual transmission". Indeed, one of the unresolved questions in AIDS research, as per Fields 1994, is "How does HIV cross mucosal surfaces such as those lining the mouth, vagina and anus?" Piazza seems to have provided at least a partial answer.

The data also is consistent with the hypothesis of a possible role of oral infection as a focus for the insidious chronic and mysterious infections that characterize AIDS. Certainly the higher concentration of blood in saliva is an indication that the all-important barrier protecting the interior of the organism from the outside world has been breached, and apparently somewhere in the mouth.

7.4 ROSENOW AND 1940 DISEASE OF "BLOOD-BUILDING" TISSUES

40R3: Rosenow, E.C., Focal infection and elective localization in relation to systemic disease; review and results of further studies, Proceedings, Dental Centenary Celebration, Maryland State Dental Association, 1940, pp. 261-282, 1940, p. 271:

"The lesions most frequently seen in patients referable to focal infection are those of the locomotor system, joints, muscles, tendon sheaths and ligaments. The kidney, skin, heart, stomach, duodenum and eyes are often affected. Less commonly, other organs such as those of the nervous system and BLOOD-BUILDING TISSUES may be involved. Rarely, very unusual localizations of streptococci from dental and other foci of infection such as onychia occurred as shown by Haden and Jordan, thyroid disease (especially thyroiditis) as shown by Cantero and lesions of the gasserian ganglion produced electively in experiments of my own in cases of trigeminal neuralgia. The removal of foci in instances of trigeminal neuralgia (and in my experience their presence is constant in this condition) obviously should be done as a preventive measure ... ."

7.5 DEBUNKING OF ANTIGENIC-DIVERSITY THEORY SUPPORTS HYPOTHESIS THAT AIDS IS TYPICAL "FOCAL DISEASE"

S. M. Wolinsky etal. [SCIENCE 272 (1996), 537-541] reported finding "that a rapid rate of CD4 T cell loss was associated with relative evolutionary stasis of the HIV-1 quasispecies virus population". The authors go on to note that "stable viral population equilibrium can be found when the starting virus is relatively fit and replicating in a defined, relatively constant environment".

In a preceding commentary, F.M. Miedema and M.R. Klein, SCIENCE 272 (26 April 1996), 505-6, note that this work by Wolinsky etal. refutes the theory that increasing antigenic diversity underlies the development of AIDS, which "antigenic diversity theory ... has attracted significant attention and has even guided the discourse in the field." (In other words, Wolinsky etal. have refuted the popular view: that the ability of the AIDS virus to continually mutate allows it to keep a step ahead of the body's defenses and thereby cause AIDS.) Miedema and Klein offer "These intriguing new results leave us with several unanswered questions."

As disturbing as this might first appear, particularly to those who have come to accept the antigenic diversity theory, we may note that the works of Rosenow comprise a framework consistent with Wolinsky etal.'s observations. The oral focal environment, noted as comprising "reservoirs" (see 7.2) for replication of HIV (or related phases of it), constitutes just such a "defined, relatively constant environment" in which a stable viral quasispecies" could continue to replicate; i.e., it would not need or even be expected to mutate or otherwise vary in order to survive. Nor, in accord with Rosenow, would it need to be particularly virulent. As with MS, the long gestation period of AIDS would appear to reflect the chronic nature of the infective organism, its low overall virulence combined with high specificity.

Chapter 8.   TOWARD AN AUTOMEDICAL SYNTHESIS

AUTOHEMOTHERAPY: AN EXPEDIENT, IMMEDIATELY AVAILABLE THERAPY
-- Pending availability of Rosenow's vaccines
-- For hematogenous conditions not from oral foci

Autohemotherapy, the immediate extravascular (intramuscular or subcutaneous) reinjection of one's own blood, has been reportedly successfully employed in a wide range of disease conditions since its generally-regarded introduction by Ravaut in 1913. Several hundred articles on the subject have been published in mainstream medical journals, as discussed and indexed in the *AUTOHEMOTHERAPY RERERENCE MANUAL*. The subcutaneous or intramuscular reinjection of autologous blood or components is also often discussed in contemporary literature without specific reference to the term "autohemotherapy".

Autohemotherapy appears to comprise a desirable interim therapy option for the wide range of diseases linked by Rosenow to oral foci, pending the general availability of specific vaccines, insofar as (a) Rosenow has shown that the causative organism or its derivative(s) in a wide range of diseases is hematogenous, i.e., blood-borne (see 8.1, below) and (b) many of these same diseases have been addressed in the autohemotherapy literature (as shown in Table 8.2).

Regardless of the source of infective organism, autohemotherapy would appear to comprise an expedient and compelling therapy option in the case of any disease entity in which the causative organism is disseminated through or resides in the blood. Of particular interest in this regard are malaria and AIDS (see 8.2).

The term "autohemotherapy" also has been and continues to be used with reference to the more risky procedures involving intravascular reinjection of autologous blood (see 8.3). It is noted that currently accelerating trends in bone-marrow transplantation - - towards the use of (a) autologous [one's own] bone-marrow in the place of heterologous [someone else's] and (b) the use of blood or blood components in place of marrow - - are rapidly transforming a significant portion of the field of bone-marrow transplantation into a form of intravascular autohemotherapy.

8.1 ROSENOW EXCERPTS INDICATING PRESENCE OF ANTIGEN IN BLOOD
(See APPENDIX A2 for indicated citations):

PNEUMONIA-SECONDARY TO BLOOD INFECTION; NOT LOCAL   05R1
Rosenow demonstrated "That the pneumococcus [of lobar pneumonia] is not only present, but present in large numbers in the blood ..... In no instance could I demonstrate pneumococci in leukocytes. ... Invasion of the blood in this present series ... supports ... the view that pneumonia may be the secondary localization of a primary blood invasion and not a local disease."

STOMACH ULCER CAUSED BY STREPTOCOCCI IN BLOOD - 16R8-335
ULCER, INFECTIOUS ORIGIN OF - HISTORICAL PRECEDENTS- 16R8-334
   "The infectious origin of ulcer, while not generally accepted,
has had adherents for many years." Rosenow recounts various
studies from 1857 involving the experimental production of
stomach ulcer following intravenous injections of various
organisms, and demonstrations from 1874 of bacteria in edges and
floors of ulcers, which bacteria generally had been considered
secondary invaders. Rosenow asserts "It is a well known fact
that ulcer in the stomach in man occurs not infrequently during
severe or fatal infections of various kinds, particularly
streptococcal infections. ... Bolton [Ulcer of the Stomach, 1913,
p. 59] states that probably the commonest cause of necrosis of
the mucous membrane and resulting acute ulcer of the stomach is
bacterial infection, that the infection occurs through the blood
stream, and that the necrosis is due to the direct effect upon
the tissues of the bacterial poison, alone or together with the
gastric juice."

   "The supposed relation between infected tonsils or gums and
gastric ulcer may be due not to the swallowing of bacteria, as is
usually supposed, but to the entrance into the blood of
streptococci of the proper kind of virulence to produce a local
infection in the wall of the stomach. Many other observations
may be cited, such as associated infections of the gall bladder
and appendix, which suggest that gastric ulcer may be due to
streptococci."

ORAL INFECTIONS - DAMAGE THRU BLOOD/LYMPH, NOT SWALLOWING
   "It should be emphasized ... that the chief harm from these
conditions [infections of the gums and enveloping membranes about
the roots of teeth] comes from the absorption of the bacteria and
their products into the lymph stream or blood, especially if
drainage is inadequate, not from swallowing the infectious
material... " [19R6-243]

ANTIGEN IN BLOOD IN ACTIVE STREPTOCOCCAL INFECTIONS - PRECIPITIN
REACTION [37R1]
   "Patients with active streptococcal infections often appear to
have free bacterial antigen in the blood which gives a precipitin
reaction with the specific or related antiserum."[37R1]

STREPTOCOCCUS IN NASOPHARYNX, PULPLESS TEETH, SOMETIMES BLOOD IN
SCHIZOPHRENIA AND EPILEPSY- 52R2, p. 262, conclusions:
   "the consistent isolation of alpha streptococci in studies of
idiopathic epilepsy and schizophrenia, the reproduction in
important respects of the disease pictures in animals, the proof
of their serologic specificity by the special methods employed,
and the data obtained in these studies indicate: (1) that persons
suffering from epilepsy and from schizophrenia harbor in
nasopharynx, in pulpless teeth, and sometimes in their blood,
specific types of alpha streptococci of low general but high and
specific 'neurotropic' virulence; (2) that the streptococci

produce neurotoxins which have predilection for certain structures in the brain and thus may play a role in pathogenesis and (3) that attempts to combat such inapparent infections specifically by passive and active immunization with the respective antigens and antibodies are indicated in addition to present-day methods of prevention and cure." [52R2]

ANTIBODY ADMINISTRATION, EFFECT ON ANTIGEN IN BLOOD - 52R3-309
   Polio, multiple sclerosis, epilepsy, schizophrenia:
   "It has been found in previous studies that subcutaneous or intramuscular injection of respective thermal streptococcal antibody in therapeutic amounts is followed by a prompt improvement in symptoms and a diminution in specific streptococcal antigen and an abrupt increase in antibody titer in skin or blood of persons having influenza or other respiratory infections, poliomyelitis, multiple sclerosis, and epilepsy and schizophrenia. ...
   "The antibody solution injected subcutaneously was prepared by autoclaving at 17 lbs pressure, a suspension of NaCl solution containing 0.4% phenol. Two or three ml of the solution of antibody and of NaCl solution in controls depending on the age of patients were injected subcutaneously immediately after the primary intradermal tests had been made ...   [52R3 p. 309]

CUTANEOUS TEST RESULTS - MS [57R1]
   Rosenow conducted extensive series of skin tests, wherein reactions to injections of antibody (which indicated the presence of antigen in the blood) and antigen (which indicated presence of antibody) were measured and compared:
   Erythematous cutaneous reactions (sq. cm.) in persons having MS to the intradermal injection of thermal antibody-indicating antigen and of antigen-indicating antibody prepared respectively from streptococci isolated from the nasopharynxes of persons who had MS, neuroses, and arthritis:

Table 8.1: CUTANEOUS ERYTHEMATOUS REACTIONS IN MS PATIENTS [from 57R1 Table 1] (corrected to conform with narrative):

Persons who had multiple sclerosis	Cases	Reactions in sq.cm. to I.D. injection of				
		Antibody-indicating antigen	Antigen-indicating antibody			
Type of strain:		Multiple-sclerosis			Neurosis	Arthritis
Stain or case #:		8125	8125	7700	8126	8134
Not receiving either vaccine or	23	5.75	7.31	9.63	3.14	1.43
thermal antibody	20	6.25	8.07		5.04	2.15
Receiving both	13	7.86	3.15		3.85	1.86

   "Cutaneous erythematous reactions indicating antibody (5.75 and 6.25 sq. cm.) were significantly less in persons not receiving

such therapeutic injections than in persons receiving such
treatment (7.86 sq.cm.). ...

"It will be seen that the immediate erythematous reactions to
the intradermal injection of streptococcic antibody (taken to
indicate specific circulating streptococcic antigen in patients
not receiving antibody or vaccine therapeutically) were far
greater (7.31, 8.07, and 9.63 sq. cm.), respectively, than in
persons receiving therapeutic injections of antibody and vaccine
(3.15 sq. cm.). ...

"Erythematous reactions following intradermal injection of
control antibody solutions were uniformly minimal, but in each of
the three groups having multiple sclerosis reactions were greater
to injections of 'neurotropic' (8126) streptococcic thermal
antibody than to corresponding injections of "arthrotropic"
(8134) antibody prepared respectively from streptococci isolated
in studies of diseases of the nervous system and arthritis."

Table 8.2: Diseases addressed within literature of:
autohemotherapy (H); autovaccine (V); Rosenow (R)

Abscesses	HV	Psoriasis	HV
Acne	HV	Puerperal Infection	VR
Alcoholism	H R	Pulmonary Diseases	VR
Allergies	HVR	Pyelonephritis	VR
Anemia	H R	Pyogenic Infection	HV
Angina	H R	Respiratory Infect.	VR
Appendicitis	H R	Rheumatism	HVR
Arthritis	H R	Rhinitis	HV
Asthma	HVR	Scarlet Fever	VR
Bacterial Infection	HV	Septicemia	HV
Boils	HV	Stomach Ulcer	H R
Bronchitis	HVR	Streptococcal Infection	VR
Cancer	HVR	Typhoid	HV
Chorea	H R	Urethritis	HV
Colitis, Ulcerative	HVR	Verruca	HV
Common cold	VR	Virus Diseases	HVR
Diabetes	H R	Whooping Cough	HV
Encephalitis	H R		
Endocarditis	VR		
Epilepsy	H R		
Erythema	H R		
Eye Diseases	H R		
Furuncles	HV		
Glaucoma	H R		
Gonorrhea	HV		
Hayfever	HVR		
Headache	H R		
Herpes simplex	H R		
Herpes Zoster	H R		
Hypertension	H R		
Inflammatory Infection	HV		
Influenza	HVR		
Iridocyclitis	H R		
Leprosy	HV		
Leukemia	H R		
Lung Disease	H R		
Meningitis	VR		
Mental Illness	H R		
Migraine	H R		
Mouth Infection	H R		
Multiple Sclerosis	H R		
Nasal Infection etc	HV		
Nephritis	VR		
Nervous System Dis.	H R		
Ozena	HV		
Pancreatic Disease	H R		
Pemphigus	HVR		
Pneumonia	HVR		
Poliomyelitis	H R		
Prostatitis	VR		

8.2 AUTOHEMOTHERAPY: MALARIA, AIDS

In 1941 Filipino Dr. Eutiquiano Cuyugan treated approx. 40 malaria patients as follows: Blood (10 cc) was drawn from the arm, put in a culture dish for 2-3 mins. (swirled a bit to keep coagulation even), & injected into the same patient's buttock muscle. After 8-10 hours the site of injection became red. After 1 day chills would cease but fever remained. Over 2-3 days, fever would diminish and then disappear. By the 4th day patients could generally resume normal activity. A dose of about 3cc was not effective for a 10-year-old but a subsequent dose of about 5cc was. Cuyugan's son Roberto performed the procedure on others and self and believes it safe, suggesting possible use against AIDS.*

Cuyugan's method may be viewed [from the theoretical perspective] as a synthesis of elements of Sir Almroth Wright's studies** involving: (a) "auto-inoculation"{350-1} of blood (b) into the tissues where "bacteriotropic substances are manufactured"{353}; comprising (c) "vaccine-therapy" with preferred "vaccines prepared from the original patient"{375}.

*Interviews with R. Cuyugan, San Francisco, USA, Jan.,1988.
**WRIGHT, A.E., Studies on Immunization (1909).

Published as "Cuyugan's Malaria Treatment - Aid vs AIDS?" S.H.SHAKMAN [*Proc., Pacific Division AAAS* 7(1988), Part 1, 42]

8.3 AUTOHEMOTHERAPY FOR AIDS - COMPLEX METHOD PROPOSED IN 1992

Bocci V., Medical Hypotheses, 1992 Sep, 39(1):30-4., "Ozonization of blood for the therapy of viral diseases and immunodeficiencies. A Hypothesis."

Abstr: Bocci 1992 calls for investigation of his methodology by biologists and clinicians. "Once this is done, owing to the large range of medical applications and the simplicity of the procedure, autohemotherapy could become very valuable particularly in underdeveloped countries."[Medline] "If autohemotherapy can be understood on a scientific basis, it may become an acceptable practice in orthodox medicine".[Bocci]

Bocci lists a number of viral diseases that may benefit from so-called "major autohemotherapy" [intravenous reinjection, after exposure to ozone], including viral hepatitis; herpes simplex, zoster, labialis and genitalis; papillomavirus; respiratory diseases; CFS; common cold; AIDS, etc. He makes no mention of exhaustive body of literature discussing extravascular autohemotherapy, which practice he briefly refers to as "minor" autohemotherapy.

8.4 RAVAUT'S "AUTOHEMATOTHERAPY" - BIRTH OF AUTOHEMOTHERAPY

Notwithstanding the prior works of Elfstrom in 1898, Jez in 1901 and Bier in 1905, the main body of literature on the subject of the history of "autohemotherapy" generally refers to a 1913 article by Ravaut [13H2] as initiator of the field of autohemotherapy. Ironically, Ravaut's title referred not to autohemotherapy, but rather to "autohematotherapy".

Immediately following Spiethoff's initial discussion of the use of "eigenserum" or autoserum in 1913, Ravaut reported on the use of a simplified procedure comprised of immediate reinjection of whole blood. Spiethoff echoed with reference to both autoblood and autoserum therapy, and a distinct body of literature blossomed up through the 1920s and 1930s, generally acknowledging the "founding" role of Ravaut, which literature constitutes the heart of the *AUTOMED VOLUME II.*

AUTOHEMOTHERAPY: HERPES, TOXIC DERMATOSES OF PREGNANCY - 13H2

In his "classic" 1913 article, Ravaut refers to Mayer and Linser, 1910, who reported successful treatment of herpes gestations by injections of a serum from the blood of a pregnant woman, and to reports by them and several others of similar treatment of "toxic dermatoses" of pregnancy, including urticaria, pemphigus, dermatitis herpiformis, strophulus, prurigo, eczema and pruritus and various hemorrhagic diseases of the skin; Spiethoff, who was apparently the first in the series of investigators cited by Ravaut to use the serum obtained from the patient himself (autogenous), and who also in certain cases continued to advocate bloodletting; Hueck on Duhring's disease, psoriasis, eczema, urticaria and pruritus. [13H2; see also Jones and Alden, 37B3; Wein, 25E7]

Ravaut refers to his "more simple" method of reinjection as "autohématothérapie", and pointed out that there was less risk of infection than might be encountered as a result of manipulation of autogenous serum, or due to someone else's infected blood. Ravaut concluded that it was more useful to inject the total blood to insure the inclusion of all blood elements that might play a useful role.

Ravaut emphasized that it seemed preferable to inject the total blood prior to allowing it to coagulate so that the substances or microbial bodies will, when resorbed by the organism, provoke a useful reaction. Ravaut reported on the treatment of 3 acne, 3 psoriasis and seven other various skin disease cases.

AUTOHEMOTHERAPY COMPELS PRODUCTION OF ANTIBODY - 13H2

Ravaut suggested that the reabsorption of blood injected under the skin compels the organism to produce a greater quantity of antibodies.

Chapter 9. AUTOLYSIS OF AUTOIMMUNE CONCEPT

AUTOIMMUNE DISEASE OR
MUCH ADO ABOUT NOTHING

From autoimmune-disease-concept-pioneer Ivan Roitt to science writer Wilson to writer/professor team Mizel & Jarte, there is agreement on the failure of the "autoimmune disease" concept to have been substantiated. However, in that this very concept owes much of its early impetus to having been pressed into service to explain why cause(s) of a bunch of diseases had supposedly not been definitively identified, with the resultant building of a church around this nothingness ("autoimmune" disease), the realization that the explanation itself might be "nothing" may have been mathematically predetermined.

It is noted at the outset that many of the disease conditions that have been purportedly identified as "autoimmune diseases" or diseases in which an "autoimmune" mechanism is thought by some to be operative appear to be all conditions that in earlier times, and by some still currently, have been linked to foci of infection, predominantly oral. Indeed for example, pernicious anemia, one of the first conditions to be designated "autoimmune" was a half-century earlier linked by William Hunter to oral foci.

Substantiation of the validity of the etiological significance of oral foci would appear to invalidate the very need for an "autoimmune" hypothesis to explain why proponents of this hypothesis had not been able to isolate causative organisms for a number of disease conditions.

In fact, causative organisms had already been found, beyond all reasonable doubts; the Henle/Koch principles/postulates of causation had been clearly and incontrovertibly exceeded; and the theoretical concept of "autoimmune disease" was unnecessary, fictional and wasteful from its very inception. The essential and simple reason that perpetrators of this farce have failed to come up with the causative organism is that they have failed in their culture methods to replicate essential conditions found in the living body, i.e. particularly the existence of gradients of oxygen pressure; whereas the causative organism(s) may readily be isolated using the specific methodology repeatedly validated by Rosenow and followers over a period of several decades.

Nonetheless the fiction of an "autoimmune disease" explanation continues not merely to muster consideration, but to be taken as fact in a range of contemporary literature. For example, the 1993 Encyclopedia Britannica in "autoimmunity" and "disease" sections refer to "autoimmune disease ... triggered not by an outsider invader but by the body's own tissues" (Vol. 1 & 4); although elsewhere in the Encyclopedia Britannica L. Sokoloff incorporates a more carefully-worded statement: "A number of observations suggest that acquired connective tissue diseases are autoimmune diseases".

Likewise authoritative professional journals occasionally qualify but seem to accept as fact the concepts of "autoimmune mechanism" and "autoimmune disease". For example, in the British

journal Nature [364, 246 (1993)], Utz etal. initially qualify
that "the cause of MS is unknown [but] is thought to involve a T-
cell-mediated autoimmune mechanism; and unqualifiedly conclude
with reference to "other T-cell-mediated autoimmune diseases ...
".

   So onward with a brief survey of some seemingly significant
developments in the history of the autoimmune disease concept -
the "black box of immunology" [Mizel/Jarte 1985] that "seems to
blur at the edges and escape our grasp" [Wilson 1972] -
"distinctly confusing" and "very complicated" [Roitt 1977].
Fortunately all that that is truly essential is "nothing".

AUTOIMMUNITY REVIEW Waksman 1959

Waksman, Byron H. 1959 cites Rivers, TM, DH Sprunt and GP Berry
1933 as having "described the experimental production of
encephalomyelitis in monkeys injected repeatedly with nervous
tissue ..."
     ["Experimental Allergic Encephalomyelitis and the "Auto-
     Allergic" Diseases", International Archives of Allergy and
     Applied Immunology, Supplementum ad vol. 14 (1959);
     "Observations on attempts to produce acute dissseminated
     encephalomyelitis in monkeys."J. Exp. Med. 58:39-53 (1933);
     Rivers TM and Schwentker, FF, "Encephalomyelitis accompanied
     by myelin destruction experimentally produced in monkeys. J.
     Exp. Med. 61:689-702 (1933)]

   p. 3-4 "That the central nervous system contains several
antigens which are organ rather than species specific and can
give rise to auto-antibody formation has been amply demonstrated
in a long series of papers, beginning with the early studies of
Brandt Buth and Muller, Witebsky and Steinfeld, and Plaut and
Kossowitz in 1926-29. ... Early attempts to produce disease of
the nervous system by autoimmunization were largely
unsuccessful... . Auto-allergic encephalomyelitis was first
described in a convincing manner by Rivers and his colleagues in
monkeys given long courses of injections of rabbit brain. The
use of the Freund adjuvant ws introduced in 1946-7 by Morgan,
Kabat etal, Morrison, and Freund etal, and shown to produce
encephalomyelitis rapidly and reproducibly in a large proportion
of injected animals."

ACTIVE/PASSIVE IMMUNIZATION Witebsky 1967
CIRCUMVENTING "HORROR AUTOTOXICUS" Witebsky 1967

-"active immunization, in which vaccines consisting of infectious
material, either in attenuated or killed form, are used to induce
immunity."
-"passive immunization takes advantage of the presence of
circulating antibodies in the serum of actively immunized animal
or man to transfer immuinity directly to a non-immune
individual."

Witebsky refers to Ehrlich and Morgenroth 1900, their failure to observe auto-antibodies, and their assertion that "the failure to form harmful autoantibodies is based on the biological principle of self-preservation, called *horror autotoxicus*."

Witebsky noted that "the hypothesis of autoimmunization as a cause of human disease was suggested by clinical investigators, obviously challenging the validity of the horror autotoxicus or self-recognition concept", but that no such autoantibodies were actually encountered. However "when thyroglobulin [and other antigenic material] incorporated into complete Freund adjuvants (a mixture of mineral oil, a detergent and acid-fast bacilli) was injected, the picture changed and thyroglobulin antibodies appeared ... "

[And there you have it, only when mineral oil, detergent and bacilli are added to autologous material was an immune response elicited.]

MECHANISM UNCLEAR Witebsky 1967

To Witebsky's credit, he keeps qualifying the situation: "... Even then, the question remains as to the trigger mechanism which in the human disease would correspond to the important role the complete Freund adjuvants seem to have in the production of experimental thyroiditis. This important problem has not as yet been resolved, but preceding virus infections are at present under investigation."

Witebsky discusses other presumed autoimmune diseases, mentioning myasthenia gravis, pemphigus vulgaris, lupus erythematosus, Addison's disease and Sjögren's disease, noting that the presence of presumed autoantibodies "might very well be the result of the morbid process rather than its cause."

Witebsky concludes that "the exact mechanism [of autoimmunity] remains the topic of extensive investigations." Nonetheless he expresses the belief "that further investigations ... will reveal the mystery of the mechanism of autosensitization." [Not in Witebsky's nor your nor mankind's lifetime. There's no such thing. As Witebsky noted, the whole charade was invented by clinicians unable to accept that they were not able to pinpoint conventional causation for a wide range of diseases, and/or too lazy to utilize Rosenow's methods which had already established causation.]

AUTOIMMUNE PROOF MISSING Witebsky 1967

Witebsky, "reviewing the situation regarding the possible role of autosentitization in disease" cites as first possible explanation "the activation of potential autoantigens ... by preceding, presumably viral, infections of the target organ. ... we have to admit that the final proof of autosensitization as the etiological factor of disease in the human is still missing."

Witebsky, p. 1373, asserts that "the demonstration of organ-specific antigens remained an unsolved problem for many years.

"By definition, an organ-specific antigen, in contrast to the

species-specific antigen, occurs in one particular organ only.
Uhlenroth (1903) was the first to discover an organ-specific
antigen, in the lens of the eye, and many years later organ-
specific antigens were found in the brain. ... There is a second
type of organ-specific antigen which is not only characteristic
for the organ in which it occurs but is also limited to the
species. Such a second type of organ-specific antigen is found
with increasing frequency in many different tissues, secretions
and blood cells.

ROSENOW MENTOR CITED Witebsky 1967

   "An organ-specific protein of considerable interest was found
by Hektoen and Schulhof in the thyroid gland. Thyroglobulin ...
when injected into rabbits, elicited the formation of antibodies,
precipitating thyroglobulin but not the 'globulin' of any other
organ." It is noted, however, that:
   (1) Hektoen was an early mentor of Rosenow, with whom the
latter began his career in the late years of the 19th century,
and with whom he co-authored a paper on the treatment of
pneumonia with autolysed pneumococci [13R5].
   (2) Hektoen was, beyond an advocate of vaccine-therapy, a
supporter and to some extent inspiration for Rosenow's views as
pertains to the phasal nature of the poliomyelitis and other
organisms [Hektoen L, Mathers G and Jackson L, "Microscopic
demonstration of cocci in the central nervous system in epidemic
poliomyelitis", J. Infect. Dis., 22:87-94, 1918; Hektoen L.,
"Recent investigations on the bacteriology of acute
poliomyelitis", Boston M. and S. J., 176:687-695, 1917.
   (3) Thus Hektoen's findings relating to specificity may be
viewed within the context of the works of Rosenow, particularly
as pertains to the mechanics underlying localization of bacteria
or components as a causative factor in various diseases, issues
on which Hektoen and his McCormick Institute was extensively
involved with Rosenow, in contrast to its association by Witebsky
etal. with the hypothesized concept of autoimmunity.

AUTOIMMUNITY ESCAPES GRASP Wilson 1972

   David Wilson in 1972 cautions from the start that "The problems
of auto-immune disease, which began as a concept only in 1956
following work by Ivan Roitt and Deborah Doniach at the Middlesex
Hospital in London, are many and the answers available so far are
distinctly confusing. But the most common of the auto-immune
diseases is rheumatoid arthritis, and any work which helps
towards the relief of rheumatoid arthritis is bound to be
important. Thyroid diseases, certain forms of anemia, some forms
of kidney disease, and ulcerative colitis are all believed either
to be auto-immune diseases or at least to involve auto-immune
phenomena."
[Body and Antibody, Knopf, New York, 1972, p. 22]
   Wilson goes on to discuss the purportedly auto-immune-related
problems of allergy, which triggers an "exaggerated" response

from the body's immune system in which "an unwanted antibody is *probably* participating."

Wilson's introductory chapter continues with discussion of "intellectually interesting" questions posed by the "concept" of the "science of self"; touches on the transition from "older immunology" to the reign of and now disillusion with antibiotics, and then to the "new immunology"; refers to continuing challenges of influenza, the common cold and malaria; and concludes a quote from immunologist Sir Peter Medawar: "Ideas are the lifeblood of science. They can't be bought; they can sometimes be sold."

There you have it - right from the mouth of immunology. In this case the "idea" is a bill of goods - the concept of autoimmune disease. And contemporary medicine, in its desperate need to appear to know more than is commonly known and appear to at least be on the way-certain to figuring out presumably-still-unknown causes of various diseases, has herein bought - a bill of goods. Nice try.

To Wilson's credit, he clarifies "... note that I have been careful to avoid saying that the manufacture of auto-antibodies causes these ["autoimmune"] disease states. ... the present state of opinion about auto-immune diseases generally [is] a state of confusion and conflicting views. Auto-immunity ... seemed to offer prospects for progress against a number of conditions that had hitherto proved intractable largely because they lacked any obvious cause. ... but as we approach each separate 'auto-immune disease,' the concept seems to blur at the edges and escape our grasp."[257]

In discussing early historical work which had inspired Roitt and Doniach to postulate the existence of autoimmunity, Wilson seems to indicate that the earlier work did not hold up, but nonetheless the concept took off on its own. And there it stands still - a modern medical monument, to nothing.

DONIACH AND ROITT'S FICTION Wilson 1972

As related by Wilson, Deborah Doniach had noticed a great many plasma cells producing antibodies in the thyroid of people suffering from" Hashimoto's disease. [p. 261] She and Ivan Roitt had both read an abstract discussing the presumed production of "auto-antibodies", and this led to a test which purportedly established the first "clear case of auto-immune disease". They mixed autologous blood serum with thyroid tissue extracts of Hashimoto's disease patients, observed precipitation reactions, and interpreted this to "show that antibodies in the blood serum were binding together with constituents of the patients' own thyroid glands."

Wilson continues: "People began to look for signs of auto-immunity in almost every disease where the cause was unknown; and very rapidly they found it ... in systemic lupus erythematosus, nephrosis, multiple sclerosis, Addison's disease, ulcerative colitis,... chronic liver disease ... haemolytic anemia ... pernicious anemia ... [and] most exciting of all, ... rheumatoid arthritis and rheumatic fever.

"But ... remarkably little progress followed. ... It now appears likely in more and more cases that the auto-immune reaction may only be a consequence of some other disease process.[262-3] Take the case of ulcerative colitis, a by no means rare disease of the intestines. Auto-antibodies can clearly be shown here but it is considered probable that this is simply a cross-reaction to the presence of gut-bacteria antigens. Cross-reaction between antibody and antigen for which it is not specific is only to be expected ... Similarly, in many of the other cases of auto-immune disease there is now scientific controversy over whether the aetiology is auto-immunity or whether the auto-immune reaction is ... something that appears in the course of events but is non-causative." [p.265]

Wilson cites a "growing body of evidence that the actual tissue damage in cases of auto-immune disease - the damage to cartilage and bone surface in cases of rheumatoid arthritis, for instance - may be caused by antibody-antigen complexes rather than by the auto-antibodies themselves." In this case a "lump of antibody and antigen remains in the tissues", presumably causing the problems of arthritis. [And the antigen must have a source, which Rosenow showed to be bacterial; so once again we come back to Rosenow's having established the etiology of these diseases.]

Wilson wraps up his discussions of auto-immunity, with "The very latest developments ... seem... to suggest even more confusion"; concluding with an expression of "sympathies for the scientists who are trying to unravel the tremendous problems of auto-immunity."

Wilson's final chapter addresses "the future of immunology", including a single notation which suggests that aging may be due to the same mechanism as "autoimmune disease"; presumably Wilson's "sympathies" would go to limb-climbers in that area as well.

In summary, Wilson describes, rejects, and then conveniently chooses to ignore the concept of "autoimmune disease". Good advice.

FICTIONAL AUTO-IMMUNE EMPIRE Roitt 1977

Roitt dedicates his ninth and concluding chapter of ESSENTIAL IMMUNOLOGY, 3rd Ed., Blackwell, Oxford 1977 to "autoimmunity"and the "spectrum" of autoimmune diseases. At the outset, he concedes that "the role of autoimmunity in many disorders is still not defined", this coming some two decades after he and D. Doniach played a significant role in instigating the autoimmunity flurry. Here Roitt refers to the difficulty in distinguishing between secondary harmless "autoantibodies" following tissue damage, e.g. heart infarction, and presumed-pathogenic "autoantibodies" in the case of true "auto-immune" diseases. Among these latter Roitt lists a number of disease entities which coincidentally had been implicated by Welsh [46R1], Rosenow and others as related to oral focal infection, including pemphigus vulgaris and systemic lupus erythematosus, ulcerative colitis, rheumatoid arthritis, opthalmia and uveitis, myasthenia gravis,

multiple sclerosis, nephritis, thyroiditis and some forms of
infertility.

Roitt discusses these presumed "autoimmune" diseases as
covering a spectrum from "organ-specific" to "generalized", their
tendency to overlap in a given patient, and evidence for a
genetic component. But the possibility of a bacterial or
microbial contributant appears to have been given short-shrift,
at least as portrayed in his last chapter - i.e. only as a
rejected alternate (v.s. a genetic) explanation for familial
clustering; as a cross-reacting or other stimulant to creation of
autoantibodies; or as adjuvants.

Most significantly, Roitt states "A strong case can be made for
the fairly straightforward view that an autoimmune response to
the Fc portion of IgG gives rise to complexes which are
ultimately responsible for the pathological changes
characteristic of the rheumatoid joint." [Tilt again! Time to
flush this stuff.]

We may note that the works of Billings and Rosenow involved
exhaustive studies of arthritis and establishing the role of oral
focal (streptococcic) infection in its etiology. To the extent
that hypothesized "autoimmune" processes may also be involved,
these would clearly be secondary to an etiologically significant
bacterial infection in genetically predisposed individuals. The
implication is that this may be the generalizable case for all
presumed "autoimmune" diseases, i.e., that the very idea of
autoimmunity as a primary disease-causative factor may be flawed.

Regardless of the extent to which pathological mechanisms of
given diseases may be imaginatively intrepreted as involving a
self-destructing immune system (i.e. autoimmunity), these
mechanisms are in any case in fact the direct result of a
causative bacterial infection; that this is not more widely known
appears to reflect the failure to use proper methods (of Haden,
Rosenow, etc.) which disclose the existence of the causative
microorganisms.

Overall, it would appear that the hypothesized explanation of
autoimmunity for these diseases becomes somewhat superfluous in
the presence of a known bacterial cause. Superfluous and, as
Roitt himself had described so-called "autoimmune" reactions (p.
166), "Very complicated." [Indeed!!].

THORAZINE MAKES PEOPLE CRAZY Roitt 1977

Roitt's self-described "very complicated" explanation of
"autoimmune" reactions invokes the example of chlorpromazine-
induced haemolytic anemia, wherein the drugs are assumed to
couple with body components, and this cell-drug complex provokes
the generation of (auto-) antibodies. [166]

We may note that Rosenow had also discussed the effect of
chlorpromazine on the blood, showing that the presence of
chlorpromazine in the blood if anything lowers the level of
antibodies against the streptococcus etiologically linked to the
mental illness condition. In other words, if indeed a given
mental condition were caused by a bacterial infection,

chlorpromazine actually aggravates the underlying disease
condition.

   Just how the "drug-coupling" effect discussed by Roitt might
relate to Rosenow's work is not clear; in any case the former
shows how chlorpromazine can make you sick (anemic) and thereby
leave your blood and overall being in a deficient condition,
while the latter specifically demonstrates that chlorpromazine
does not make you well but rather worsens your condition with
respect to the infection that apparently causes mental problems.
   In any case this would appear to be "medication" to avoid.
   Rosenow's work in particular helps explain why people have been
known to "go off" when abruptly taken off these types of
"medication". Perhaps any outwardly beneficial action merely
involves a drug-lobotomizing (thorazinging/zombifying) reduction
of the patient's ability to function, period.
   Fortunately Rosenow has also provided a worthy detailed
exposition of the clear connection between the likes of Cotton's
1919 demonstration of the connection between oral foci and mental
illness, and the likes of Reddick 1955 and many earlier writers
who reported the successful use of autohemotherapy. This would
be explained by the existence of an appropriate "antigenic" form
of the infecting organism or toxin in the blood, which when
reinjected intramuscularly or subcutaneously acts as a vaccine;
however if the offending infectious (often oral) focus is not
removed, effects of autohemotherapy would be expected to be
temporary.

HORROR AUTOTOXICUS Mizel/Jarte 1985
BLACK BOX OF IMMUNOLOGY Mizel/Jarte 1985

   Mizel and Jarte identify as the "first theory of autoimmuity"
Paul Ehrlich's "horror autotoxicus", suggesting that an
experiment in the 1930s involved "an immune response [to virus-
free rabbit-nervous-system tissue] that also turned against the
central nervous system of the monkeys themselves...", causing a
disease "which came to be called experimental encephalomyelitis"
and which "was almost identical in its symptoms to a naturally
occurring disease - multiple sclerosis." The authors seem to
imply that this work did not hold up, but nonetheless the seed
was planted. [SB Mizel, P Jarte, In Self-Defense, Harcourt Brace
Jovanovich, San Diego 1985]
   The authors then survey "progress" being made in with MS using
experimental encephalomyelitis as an animal model; touch on
correlations of geography and with measles; discuss the "never
observed ... latent form" of herpes virus; ride the "viral" theme
to rheumatoid arthritis - a "highly complex disease" in which
"the autoimmune attack ... even turns against antibodies
themselves"; concede that "we do not understand fully what sets
these mechanisms off in the first place"; correlate arthritis
with EBV, and systemic lupus erythematosus with "beige" (inbred)
mice models and sex hormones; and cite the apparently single-
common factor in "autoimmune disorders" - genetic predisposition.

Their conclusion: "Autoimmunity remains one of the great unsolved mysteries - the "black box" of immunology, as some investigators have called it." [An empty black box.]

Mizel and Jarte do not identify their single 1930 reference purportedly involving autoimmunity, but we may assume these to be the same items discussed by Waksman 1959 above; that this and other subsequent related efforts did not involve an actual or anyway near pure "autoimmune" response seems clear. Rather we have a response against a combination of tissue and adjuvant, which consequently may have involved autologous tissue and hence was incorrectly interpreted as involving autoimmunity. In any case on related subjects we may note (1) Rosenow's definitive bacteriological work on multiple sclerosis (e.g., see 16R7, 53R1, 55R1, 57R1, 58R1, and particularly 48R3); (2) his involvement with equine encephalomyelitis (37R3, 37R5, 53R1); (3) his production of several experimental diseases on numerous occasions, including encephalitis and allied conditions from 1922, and (4) his use of oxygen gradients in culture methods which often brought forth unsuspected organisms.

And as for Mizel and Jarte's admission that "Scientists don't know exactly how" the "never-observed" latent form of "clever" herpes simplex viruses "literally ... hide out" in nerve cells and "after a period of latency, ... make their way back to the site of infection and once again induce lesions ..." -- guess what!? The suspected virus may comprise a filtrable phase of Rosenow's streptococcus, which resides in oral foci in "off-season" and rides the blood stream to dinner (secondary foci) "in season". Presence of the organism in blood explains the often-reported and consistent success of autohemotherapy in treating herpes simplex. And they don't hide out in nerve cells at all; they "hide out" in oral foci, and they or their toxin continually spill out through the blood stream and cause herpes simplex and other "viral" diseases.

Mizel and Jaret have offered: "One of the great debates in immunology and in cancer research has focused on the question of whether of whether or not the immune system can recognize and destroy cancer cells that arise spontaneously in the body." [160]

What if there's no such thing as "spontaneously"-generated cancer cells or spontaneously-occuring "autoimmune disease"? Would it then be possible to escape the conclusion this "great debate" was above all a great waste of time?

AUTOIMMUNE INERTIA Morse 1987

Morse 1987 in Cohen and Burns, 378, discussed the possible relation of the concept of oral focal infection to the concept of auto-immunity, in the case of such conditions as diseased joint tissues and rheumatic fever: "... oral microbes (e.g. alpha-hemolytic streptococci) may sensitize tissues at a secondary site, such as joint tissues. The sensitized tissue antigens may then evoke an autoimmune type response, and a secondary disease could result. This could occur even though the original inciting microbes were destroyed. A similar autoimmune mechanism has been

proposed for the development of rheumatic fever. ..."
   We may note that arthritis and rheumatic fever are disease
conditions for which Dr. Rosenow exhibited apparently conclusive
results as relates to the causative role of elective localization
of bacteria from oral foci, decades prior to the invention of the
"auto-immune" hypothesis. It would appear that the concept of
"autoimmune disease" may have become popular in part due to the
failure to definitively locate a causative organism in various
disease conditions, which failure may be simply attributed to the
failure to utilize Dr. Rosenow's very specific instructions for
culturing the causative organisms.
   In 1948, Dr. Rosenow, referring to the possible connection
between his work on MS and that of others on experimental
encephalomyelitis, had spoken of how in the absence of the
original inciting microbe, an "autogenous sensitizing
streptococcal-nervous-tissue complex" might form [48R3].   Thus
did Dr. Rosenow seem to uncannily anticipate Morse's discussion -
a contemporary fall-back position of advocates of the autoimmune
disease concept, this several years prior to the very advent of
the concept of autoimmune disease [by Roitt in 1956]. However,
within the context of Dr. Rosenow's half-century of work, the
concept of autoimmunity in the strict sense is immediately placed
in its proper perspective as clearly surperfluous; to the extent
that autogenous tissue may become integrated into a disease-
related complex, it is no longer strictly autogenous. We may
therefore regard this as Dr. Rosenow's attempt to explain how the
facts concerning his MS work might be reconciled with studies of
experimental encephalitis, which in the absence of a proper
context have spawned such wasteful concepts as "autoimmune
disease".
   It is commendable that Dr. Morse has discussed the idea that
oral focal infections may be the underlying cause of diseases
which are curently considered as possibly caused by
"autoimmunity", and somewhat interesting if not amusing that the
medical profession is nonetheless compelled to retain the
consequently irrelevant concept of "autoimmune mechanisms". It's
not easy to admit to chasing a foul ball for as long as most
current medical practitioners have been around; it's not easy to
say goodby.

AUTOIMMUNE MILESTONES Medawar 1991

   Peter Medawar, The Threat and the Glory, Oxford U. Press 1991,
p. 196, note 9:
"The study of "auto-immunity" and of autoimmune diseases has
been particularly associated in recent years with the names of J.
Freund and E. Witebsky. That Hashimoto'[s thyroiditis is
essentially the consequehce of a self-immunization was
demonstrated by I.M.Roitt and D. Doniach. For a general review
of these matters, see B.H. Waksman, Experimental allergic
encephalomyelitis and the Auto-Allergic Diseases (Basle, Karger,
1959).

MYASTHENIA GRAVIS MISGUIDE Keesey 1994

J.C. Keesey and R. Sonshine, in A PRACTICAL GUIDE TO MYASTHENIA GRAVIS, a handbook for patients and families, circa 1994 indicate that "the vast majority of MG cases are autoimmune", and list as autoimmune diseases MG, thyroid disease, lupus, rheumatoid arthritis and juvenile diabetes, without mention of the theoretical and controversial nature of the very concept of autoimmune disease.

Meanwhile the "autoimmune disease" concept continues to serve as theoretical foundation for the only two "long-term treatment options" generally known as available to MG patients (aside from 20% spontaneous remissions) - "potentially dangerous" drugs and surgical removal of the thymus gland. On the use of such drugs, we may note that Harris and Sinkovics have raised "serious doubts about the rationale" [J. E. Harris and J. G. Sinkovics, The immunology of malignant disease, C.V. Mosby, St. Louis, 1970, 193; likewise the rationale for surgical removal of the thymus would appear doomed with the demise of the concept of "autoimmune disease", except as any surgical procedure may inadvertently involve autohemotherapy.

Fortunately for all concerned there is another option, a specific therapy for MG and related diseases; as developed at Mayo Clinic within a body of work produced there during the period 1915-1944; by E.C. Rosenow; and apparently no one is paying attention. The reader is referred to some of Rosenow's articles which address myasthenia gravis - 36R3, 36R4, 39R1, 53R1, 55R1, 58R1. The first two of these citations discuss serology and the bacteriology of MG specifically; the others discuss Rosenow's evolving methodology for treating diverse diseases including MG. The very fact of Rosenow's having addressed serologic findings suggests a possible role for autohemotherapy.

Keesy and Sonshine also describe two "expensive" and temporary therapies involving intravenous manipulation of the blood - plasmapheresis and IVIG (intravenous human immune globulin). Plasmapheresis involves the removal of blood and return of red blood cells in artificial plasma; IVIG, which "may be thought of as the opposite of plasmapheresis ... swamps the body with pooled gamma globulin antibodies from many donors." At a minimum it may be stated that both are, by definition, forms of intravascular hemotherapy. Plasmapheresis, which in fact is directly derived from and comprises a modern form of bloodletting, is by virtue of its autologous nature a form of (intravascular) autohemotherapy.

This and other approaches involving therapeutic use of blood or blood products are discussed further in the AUTOHEMOTHERAPY REFERENCE MANUAL.]

SUPERANTIGENS OR SUPERCROCK? Conrad 1994
The persistence of the concept of autoimmunity in the face of its obsolescence is exemplified in the invocation of an hypothesis of a "superantigen". Nature 371 (22 Sept. 1994), v., introduces a featured article [Conrad B etal] thusly: "Insulin-

dependent juvenile diabetes is an autoimmune disease triggered by unknown factors in genetically predisposed individuals. ... Rather than a conventionally processed antigen, a superantigen in the cell membrane of pancreatic islet cells seems to be involved."

Nature adds to the hype by soliciting the views of MacDonald, MR and Acha-Orbea H, ibid p. 283, who join Nature in cheering for the superantigen.

Conrad B, etal, Ibid, p. 351, state "Insulin-dependent diabetes mellitus is a T-cell-mediated autoimmune disease whose onset is believed to be triggered by unknown environmental factors acting on a predisposing genetic background."

The authors suggest [p. 355] "the involvement of a superantigen rather than a conventional antigen in the aetiology of IDDM. Superantigens are unique products of ubiquitous bacteria and viruses. [*1-Marrack, P and Kappler J, Science 248, 705-11, 1990]

In the light of historical findings [*12 Notkins AL and Yoon, JW in Notkins and Oldstorm, Concepts in Viral Pathogenesis, p. 241-247, Springer New York, 1984,], viruses might be the modifying agent responsible for the superantigen presence on the diabetic islets. Superantigens can also be the product of endogenous or integrated retroviral genes ... .

"Thus we can hypothesize that if the first exposure to the superantigen is at a very early age, potentially autoreactive T-cell clones are inactivated. ... If instead the first exposure to this superantigen is years after birth, ... In a genetically predisposed individual, some of these T cells are able t initiate the process that eventually results in destruction of the B-cells of the pancreas. ... Continuing studies are aimed at determining whether the superantigen (and perhaps the responsible virus is actually present on the *B*-cells of the pancreas or was brought into the islets by infected lymphocytes. Exposure to superantigens as the triggering event in the pathogenesis of IDDM is a compelling novel hypothesis in which the diverse observations made in the fields of immunology, virology, genetics and epidemiology coalesce."

It all seems so ridiculous. Generations of investigators, and their students, ignore Rosenow's proven methods, claim there's no organism to be found, conclude therefore the cause is an autoimmune mechanism, then admit there must be something causing the autoimmune mechanism, but nonetheless retain the now superfluous mechanism.

OK, call the causative factor a superantigen. And if you want to see what it looks like, cook it up in tall tubes of Dr. Rosenow's dextrose-brain broth [see RECIPE]. Then refer to it properly, as "Streptococcus rosenow", clean out oral foci, and prepare autogenous vaccine. And watch the concept of autoimmunity, and many diseases, disappear.

KOCH PRINCIPLES V. AUTOIMMUNE HOCUS

If there's any room in Ehrlich's grave, he's probably doing flips over the suggestion that his "horror autotoxicus" is being

used in part as theoretical base for what it purported to say is
impossible. Moreover, the imposition of the concept of
autoimmune disease by definition renders untenable Koch's
postulates of causation (because there's presumably no causative
organism with which to reproduce disease in laboratory animals).
  Thus the theoretical invention of "autoimmunity" by
autodefinition exempts itself from the scrutinous purview of
known scientific principles that have come to be generally highly
regarded as among the fundamental building blocks of medical
progress.
  In sharp contrast to the hocus basis of the autoimmune fad,
Rosenow's standard procedures routinely equated to fulfillment of
Henle's principles/Koch's postulates; i.e. the implication and
culturing of a causative organism grown from oral foci, and
reproduction of symptoms in laboratory animals, etc.
  The discovery of a worthwhile principle, such as Kepler's laws
or Henle's principles, is not routinely followed by a rush to
modify or clarify, but rather a respectable period of assessment
and validation.
  In contrast, the autoimmune hypothesis has been characterized
by the need to re-adapt it to fit emerging facts which might
otherwise and logically leave it in the dust. As per Roitt, his
[1974] "second edition has been dictated by the breakneck
increase in immunological knowledge [since 1971]; and of his 1977
third edition he wrote: "The indecent speed at which we lurch
forward has necessitated radical revision."

AUTOIMMUNE DISEASE FAD - R.I.P.
  It is commendable that the medical profession appears to be
knowledgable, for it would be most disconcerting to patients if
they were constantly greeted with "I don't know" in response to
their complaints. However, when the pretention of knowledge may
keep false dead-end theories in the forefront and at the same
time inhibit consideration of true or prospectively hopeful
information, it's time to pull the plug. A good first step, for
example, would be to cancel all funding for research into so-
called "auto-immune" mechanisms; if the concept of "auto-immune"
disease is fictional, why put more tax money down this rat hole,
except as a social welfare program for unfortunately, apparently-
mistrained researchers? All is not lost; there are other
government welfare programs to pick up the slack.
  And while acknowledging the fictional status of "autoimmune
disease", we may also wish to note that the term "genetic
disease" continues to be improperly applied in the popular press
to many of these same disease conditions, conditions for which
there may be a genetic predisposition. Predisposition does not
guarantee aquisition of the disease; rather, such a genetic
"weakness" would appear to predispose its possessor to infection
by a bacterial or other organism with an affinity (taste) for the
type of tissue exhibiting such a weakness. We may note again
that the works of Rosenow and others have demonstrated the role
of bacteria emanating from oral foci as a key etiologocal factor
in many of these same disease conditions.

It is not surprising that simple terms are easier to grasp than detailed explanations. But since there's already so much to know, logic would dictate forgetting what is unneeded, including the simple and flawed concepts of "auto-immune disease" and "genetic disease".

Unfortunately, since so much has already been invested in these concepts, we can look forward to their being gradually reworked to fit the facts of an underlying bacterial etiology. Nonetheless it may be confidently predicted that somewhere in the next millenium, current purveyors of "autoimmune disease" will be likened to witch doctors of the past, and the true significance of the genetic-bacterial interface will be more generally and maturely integrated into medical research methodology.

Summation: If we have identified the known cause of a disease, we don't need an autoimmune concept to explain causation. Perhaps down the road a concept incorporating consideration of the secondary involvement of autogenous tissue, in combination with a foreign toxin or organism, might shed some light on the mechanics of the infected lesion. But first comes the infection, and all that is known regarding eliminating it and treating it. And that is why we must consult Dr. Rosenow.

APPENDIX A1: E.C. ROSENOW CHRONOLOGY - ANNOTATED EXCERPTS

PNEUMONIA SECONDARY TO BLOOD INFECTION/NOT LOCAL DISEASE 05R1
Dr. Rosenow demonstrates "That the pneumococcus [of lobar pneumonia] is not only present, but present in large numbers in the blood ..... In no instance could I demonstrate pneumococci in leucocytes. ... Invasion of the blood in this present series ... supports ... the view that pneumonia may be the secondary localization of a primary blood invasion and not a local disease."-871

ACID INTOXICATION/PNEUMONIA 05R1-872
Dr. Rosenow shows that pneumococcus grown in pneumonic serum produces a marked acid reaction, supporting the view that some of the symptoms of pneumonia are due to an acid intoxication. Dr. Rosenow notes that investigators have uniformly found a diminished alkalinity of the blood late in pneumonia after powers of resistance fail, and after death.
Dr. Rosenow indicates that in cooperation with Frank Billings, "In the treatment of 7 cases of pneumonia by the administration of large doses of alkalines, it was noted that the urine became strongly alkaline in reaction and remained so until the time of crisis. At this time, however, when the products of resolution were being rapidly absorbed, the urine [either became acid or neutral] in reaction for a period of time varying from 24 to 48 hours ... but with an increased dosage of alkali, in all cases the urine subsequently became alkaline."

ALLERGY VS. IMMUNITY 08R3-643
"Pirquet advises that the term 'immunity' be limited to indicate the condition of complete resistance in which no clinical reaction occurs, when poisons [such as diphtheria, tetanus, etc.) are introduced into the organism. He suggests the term 'Allergie' to indicate conditions of acquired immunity associated with anaphylaxis, such as that induced by vaccinia against variola, that of the luetic vs. syphilis, or of that produced by one attack of some of the acute specific infections."

TRANSMUTATIONS; STREPTOCOCCI TO/FROM PNEUMOCOCCI 14R4,28-9
Through the imposition of special conditions involving variations in oxygen tension and salt concentration, growth in symbiosis with other bacteria and injections into animals' cavities, Dr. Rosenow was able to commonly call forth mutational forms in streptococci. The below table summarizes Dr. Rosenow's 1913-1914 work on the subject of transmutations, listing original organism types and numbers and types into which these were transformed.

Table A1: TRANSMUTATIONS; STREPTOCOCCI TO/FROM PNEUMOCOCCI
[14R4-p. 28-29]

Original strain	Mutation (and number of strains so mutated)
\/ \/ \/ \/	\/ \/ \/ \/ \/ \/
S.hemolytic to	S.rheumatism (1)
	S.viridans (21)
	pneumococci (3)
	S.mucosis (1)
S viridans to	pneumococci (17)
	S.mucosus (2)
	S.hemolytic (10)
pneumococci to	S.hemolytic (11)
	S.rheumatism (3)
	S.viridans (7)
S.mucosis to	hemolytic S. (5)
	S.viridans (2)

14R4 - PROOF OF VALIDITY AND COMPLETENESS OF TRANSMUTATIONS

"In order to meet the objection [that claimed mutations may be the result of mixed cultures from the start] cultures of each main variety were obtained from single organisms by the Barber method. The same results were obtained with three of these 'pure line' cultures of hemolytic streptococci, 6 of *Str. viridans*, and 2 each of Str. mucosus and pneumococcus. Hence the changes observed are not due to mixtures nor to so-called "mass selection" but to actual changes wrought under the influence of changed environment.

"The transformation of some of the strains has been found to be complete by every test known. Thus the morphology, the presence of capsule, the fermentative powers, the solubility or insolubility in NaCl solution, the behavior toward the respective broth culture filtrates (Marmorek's test), the specific immunity response, as manifest by the production of opsonin and agglutination by antipneumococcus and antistreptococcus serum and the more or less specific pathogenic powers have been studied." ... [p. 29]
... "The changes observed have frequently the characteristics of true mutations because they appear suddenly, under conditions more or less obscure and because the newly acquired properties persist unless the organisms are again placed under special conditions. A pre-mutational stage seems to be necessary because the same strain will not yield mutants when placed under what seem to be identical conditions at different times. The underlying conditions which tend most to call forth changes are, first, favorable conditions for luxuriant growth and then unfavorable conditions - under stress or strain. This seems to call forth new or latent energies which were previously not manifest and which now have gained the ascendancy and tend to persist. ...

Figure A1: RELATION OF STREPTOCOCCUS GROUP MEMBERS   14R4

```
   streptococci<══>streptococcus
     from                viridans
   rheumatism
        ║                   ║
        ║                   ║
        ║                pneumococcus
        ║                   ║
    hemolytic               ║
  streptococcus             ║
        ║                   ║
        ║                   ║
        ║                   ║
        ║                   ║
        ║                   ║
        streptococcus
        mucosus
```

FOCI SITES FOR ACQUIRING AFFINITIES, BACTERIA WITH TASTE 14R4

   "The bearing these results have on bacteriology, epidemiology, and medicine might be discussed at length; only the following point will be mentioned: the fact that variations in oxygen tensions, and salt concentration, that growth in symbiosis with other bacteria and that injections into cavities in animals commonly call forth mutational forms in streptococci suggests strongly that similar changes might occur in various foci of infection where such conditions may prevail. It would seem, therefore, that focal infections are no longer to be looked upon merely as a place of entrance of bacteria but as a place where conditions are favorable for them to acquire the properties which give them a wide range of affinities for various structures.

   "From this study [the apparent position of the various members of the streptococcus group may be illustrated by the position of the fingers in a partially flexed hand, in which hemolytic streptococcus occupies the position of the little finger, the pneumococcus the place of the index finger (the opposite extreme), Str. viridans (representing the group of more or less saprophytic, non-hemolyzing streptococci) the middle finger, the streptococci from rheumatism the fourth finger, and Str. mucosus, having some of the properties of both pneumococci and streptococci, the position of the thumb. In this grouping there is in general an increase in parasitism and virulence as we approach the thumb (Str. mucosus). Being members of the same family, the sign of reversible chemical reaction (<══>) between each might be used to indicate their transmutability." [14R4-31]

FLEXNER ON BACTERIAL GROWTH IN ORGANS VS. ORGAN EXTRACTS 15R9-1690

   "Flexner [Simon, J. Exper. Med. 1896, i, 211] has shown that the functioning organ may be especially favorable to the growth of certain bacteria although the organ extracts may inhibit their growth; hence the growth of bacteria in various organs may be related to function and blood supply. Strep...

OXYGEN/BLOOD SUPPLY AND VIRULENCE

TRAUMA AND RESPIRATION
RIGHT VENTRICLE, WHY LESIONS IN 15R9-1690
"Streptococci of low virulence but highly sensitive to oxygen are
found to produce lesions in tissues whose blood supply and
therefore oxygen and food requirements are low (heart valves,
tendinous portion of muscles and the structures about joints).
Streptococci of greater virulence are found to produce lesions in
tissues whose blood supply and therefore oxygen and food
requirements are high (kidney, lung, etc.); hence localization
and production of injury seem to be closely related to the amount
of available oxygen in a given tissue. The fact that lesions
occurred far more frequently in the right ventricle (containing
venous blood) than in the left ventricle (containing oxygenated
blood) is in accord with this hypothesis. Might not the
predisposing action of trauma (locus minoris resistentiae), of
exposure to cold and of a drunken bout, to infection be best
explained on the basis of lack of oxygen? The changes observed,
as hemorrhage, cloudy swelling and necrosis, from a purely
chemical as well as from a colloid-chemical point of view, are
identical with the changes of tissue asphyxia. I have found that
pneumococci when grown and autolyzed under anaerobic conditions
produce a much larger quantity of toxic material than when grown
or autolyzed under aerobic conditions. Moreover, pneumococcus
extracts proved to be toxic to warm-blooded animals (guinea-
pigs), have the same inhibitory effect on the development of
fertilized eggs of arbacia as does lack of oxygen. Since
bacteria and their products are powerful reducing agents, one of
the chief effects of the bacteria and their products very likely
is interference with the normal cell respiration, and possibly
the greater the virulence the more powerful this interference."

AUTOGENOUS VACCINES PREFERABLE 15R11
  "The use of vaccines of any kind presupposes an accurate
bacteriological diagnosis. ... It is perfectly obvious ... that
it is more desirable to use the autogenous vaccine.'

DANGER OF INTRAVENOUS INJECTION OF ANTIGEN 16R1-1929
"The treatment of disease by the intravenous infection of nonspecific substances [e.g. and including relatively nontoxic
autolyzed pneumococcus extracts] which call forth severe chill
and accompanying severe reaction, while of apparent benefit in
some instances, as pointed out especially by Jobling and
Peterson, would for obvious reasons appear to be dangerous;
therefore we warn against their indiscriminate use, especially in
lobar pneumonia, until the nature and the degree of reaction are
better understood and can be accurately controlled." 16R1-1929

FLEXNER AND NOGUCHI 1913 WORK CITED [16R4, p. 1202]
  "In 1913 Flexner and Noguchi cultivated and demonstrated
microscopically a small filterable microorganism with which they
produced poliomyelitis in monkeys. They note that 'the cultural
conditions are those that apply more particularly to the

bacteria' but do not attempt definitely to classify the microorganism."

L-FORMS DESCRIBED BY ROSENOW 20 YEARS BEFORE "DISCOVERY" 16R4
   Poliomyelitis organisms consistently isolated "resemble pneumococci, but are usually smaller and free from demonstrable capsule" 16R4-1202
   "A peculiar polymorphous streptococcus has been isolated, often in large numbers, from the throat, from the material expressed from tonsils, and from abscesses in tonsils of a large series of cases of epidemic poliomyelitis. ... It is remarkably polymorphous, and appears to grow large or small according to the medium in which it is grown... .16R4-1202
   "Using the organism in its large form, poliomyelitis has been consistently produced in animals known to be unsusceptible to inoculation with [polio virus]."16R4-1202

AVIRULENT STRAINS MADE VIRULENT BY ANIMAL PASSAGE 16R7-662
VIRULENT STRAINS MADE LESS VIRULENT BY CULTIVATION 16R7-662
VIRULENT STRAINS CAUSE HEMORRHAGE, BRONCHOPNEUMONIA 16R7-662
   "During my studies on the transmutation of pneumococci and streptococci in which relatively avirulent strains were made virulent by successive animal passages, and highly virulent strains less virulent by cultivation, marked changes in localization following intravenous injection in animals were noted. At certain lower grades of virulence, endocarditis, arthritis, cholecystitis, ulcer of the stomach, myositis and iritis, respectively, occurred, while when the virulence was high, hemorrhages and edema of the lung and bronchopneumonia commonly occurred. The latter observation is in accord with the results of Wadsworth [A.B., Tr. Assn. Am. Phys. 1912, xvii, 72.]
   The results suggested the possibility that diseases of widely different symptomatology might be due to strains of bacteria of the same or closely related species, but having peculiar localizing or infecting powers."

DIFFERENT DISEASE, SAME BACTERIA 16R7-665
   "diseases of widely different symptomology might be due to strains of bacteria of the same or closely related species [with] peculiar localizing or infecting powers." 16R7-662

LIMITED BENEFIT, FOCUS REMOVAL 16R7-665
   "Too much benefit should not be expected from the removal of evident foci of infection, because a similar condition may be present in inaccessible foci and in others too small to be detected. Moreover, recovery may be made difficult by local tissue sensitivity or peculiar mechanical conditions, and living bacteria in a metastatic lesion may continue the process independently of the focal source."16R7-665

TONSILS AS TEST TUBES 16R7-666
   "The pus or other exudate containing the bacteria having

elective affinity is not from actively inflamed tonsils, but
usually from small atrophic tonsils with deep pockets which
cannot heal for mechanical reasons, and which are virtually test
tubes with a permeable wall."16R7-666

ULCER, INFECTIOUS ORIGIN OF - HISTORICAL PRECEDENTS- 16R8-334
   "The infectious origin of ulcer, while not generally accepted,
has had adherents for many years." Dr. Rosenow recounts various
studies from 1857 involving the experimental production of
stomach ulcer following intravenous injections of various
organisms, and demonstrations from 1874 of bacteria in edges and
floors of ulcers, which bacteria generally had been considered
secondary invaders. Dr. Rosenow asserts "It is a well known fact
that ulcer in the stomach in man occurs not infrequently during
severe or fatal infections of various kinds, particularly
streptococcal infections. ... Bolton [Ulcer of the Stomach, 1913,
p. 59] states that probably the commonest cause of necrosis of
the mucous membrane and resulting acute ulcer of the stomach is
bacterial infection, that the infection occurs through the blood
stream, and that the necrosis is due to the direct effect upon
the tissues of the bacterial poison, alone or together with the
gastric juice."

STOMACH ULCER CAUSED BY STREPTOCOCCI IN BLOOD 16R8-335
   "The supposed relation between infected tonsils or gums and
gastric ulcer may be due not to the swallowing of bacteria, as is
usually supposed, but to the entrance into the blood of
streptococci of the proper kind of virulence to produce a local
infection in the wall of the stomach. Many other observations
may be cited, such as associated infections of the gall bladder
and appendix, which suggest that gastric ulcer may be due to
streptococci."

SEASONALITY OF STOMACH ULCERS IN MALE HUMANS 16R8-356
"Since streptococci from certain foci of infection in patients
with ulcer tend to produce ulcer of the stomach in animals, might
not the frequency of ulcer in the male sex, in certain
localities, and during the winter months, be best explained on
the basis of a high incidence of throat and other infections?
Such infections would afford opportunity for streptococci to
acquire affinity for the stomach and to gain entrance into the
blood stream."

ALKALINITY & ULCER THERAPY: LOCAL OR SYSTEMIC ACTION? 16R8-357
   "Some ulcers in man may be made to heal when the acidity is
reduced by the administration of alkalies, as advocated
especially by Sippy, or by the alkaline contents of the duodenum,
following gastroenterostomy. Might not the good effect be due
partly to an alkalization of the tissues throughout the body,
rather than wholly to local action?"

ULCER, PROOF OF CAUSE OF   16R8-359

"The occurrence of acute ulcer of the stomach and exacerbations of the symptoms in chronic ulcer in connection with foci of infection; the improvement in symptoms following removal of foci of infection; and the development of new ulcers after excision of ulcer in patients in whom chronic suppurating foci have not been removed - all strongly suggest the etiologic relation between remote foci of infection and ulcer. None of these observations, however, prove the etiology of the ulcer. The demonstration of streptococci in foci of infection in patients with ulcer and in the ulcers themselves, and the fact that they localize in the stomach in animals, furnish what seems to me to be the final proof of the etiology."

TONSILLAR ABSCESSES/POLIO 17R7,994-5
"From July 21 to August 10, 1916, there were studied seven typical cases of epidemic poliomyelitis which occurred in Rochester. The cultures obtained from material expressed from the tonsils, injected intravenously in young animals ... was followed by flaccid paralysis in some of the animals in each case." In this and subsequent studies by Rosenow and others, "The extirpated tonsils of patients who were not convalescing as they should be and particularly those obtained in fatal cases were found to contain peculiar abscesses in which this streptococcus was present in enormous numbers. Cultures of the brain and cord in each of 12 fatal cases yielded the identical streptococcus ... . The same organism has been isolated from the brain and cord of every monkey paralyzed either with fresh human virus , with glycerinated human virus, glycerinated monkey virus or with filtrates of virus. ... Recently isolated cultures [of streptococcus] were found to protect monkeys against virus." [17R7, p. 994-5]

TONSILLAR ABSCESSES AND POLIO 18R2
"The results of the study of the tonsils and adenoids here reported indicate strongly that these structures afford important entrance ways for the microorganisms which we find consistently in the diseased tissues in poliomyelitis." [18R2, p. 308]

STREPTOCOCCI IN PNEUMONIA 19R5, 397
Rosenow and Sturdivant identified a "somewhat peculiar green-producing streptococcus or diplostreptococcus ....study of the sputum and other material [from patients during epidemic of influenza and accompanying pneumonia] shows that of all the bacteria isolated, the somewhat peculiar green producing streptococcus is the most important. This organism is present in large numbers at the very outset of symptoms of influenza and of the accompanying pneumonia; it is commonly present after death."
The authors reported that the mortality rate in a group inoculated three times with mixed vaccine which included this streptococcus was 1/5 that of uninoculated persons.

OXYGEN TENSION: IMPORTANCE OF VARIATIONS; CITATIONS 19R6-208-9

Streptococci and other bacteria in tissues and in chronic foci of infection, particularly those about teeth, are often extremely sensitive to oxygen. Many bacteria require partial oxygen tension and do not grow under strictly anaerobic or aerobic conditions."

BRAIN TISSUE IN DEXTROSE-BRAIN BROTH, SIGNIFICANCE OF 19R6-209
The particular benefits of the brain tissue within "dextrose-brain-broth" and "dextrose-brain-agar culture mediums, in tall tubes, are emphasized as early as 1919 [*19R6*]: "The brain substance renders the bottom of the tube anaerobic; the top necessarily is aerobic and it follows that every gradation of oxygen pressure occurs between these two points."
 Rosenow here cites his original 1914 work on methodology [14R12]; and the work on this subject by Gräf and Wittneben, Centralbl.f.Bakteriol. xkiv (1916), p. 97-110; & Wherry and Oliver, J.Infect.Dis. xx (1917), 28-34

METHOD: STUDY OF DENTAL INFECTIONS 19R6-210
"Two mediums, dextrose-brain broth and soft dextrose-brain agar, have been found especially useful. They are prepared from meat infusion or beef extract in the usual way, and titrated so that the final product is from 0.5 to 0.7 acid to phenolphthalein. In order not to interfere with the growth of sensitive bacteria and yet to indicate their number, the agar medium is made to contain only 0.5 per cent of agar, just sufficient to jell, instead of the usual 1.5 or 2 per cent. Both of these mediums are placed in test tubes so that the column of medium is at least 8 cm. tall. The mediums are then sterilized in an autoclave at 15 pounds pressure for fifteen minutes, or in an Arnold sterilizer on three successive days. Dextrose, from a concentrated sterilized solution, is added to both mediums after sterilization to make them 0.2 per cent dextrose; also decolorized acid fuchsin (Adraid's indicator). The addition of ascites fluid, blood, or serum, just before use, while advantageous in special instances, is found unnecessary for routine work. The brain substance renders the bottom of the tube anaerobic; the top necessarily is aerobic and it follows that every gradation of oxygen pressure occurs between these two points. The growth in these liquid mediums almost invariably begins at the bottom of the tube and then forces its way upward, in some instances to the top of the medium within twenty-four hours; in others, in forty eight or seventy-two hours, or not at all (text-fig.1). Tall tubes of broth made from meat infusion in the usual way, to which 5 per cent of blood is added and 0.5 per cent of dextrose from a concentrated solution just before use, have proved specially useful in studying the localizing power of bacteria from dental foci.
 "The liquid mediums are specially useful for studying the localizing powers of the primary culture, but they give little indication as to the number of bacteria present in the material inoculated, and one containing organism from the air or elsewhere

may outgrow the more parasitic organisms contained in the
material under consideration. The agar medium, in conjunction
with a study of smears of the material inoculated, furnishes
quite accurate information as to the number of bacteria contained
in the material inoculated and should be used as a control of the
liquid medium. [p.212] In the agar medium, contaminating
bacteria do not outgrow those contained in the material
inoculated. The bacteria live for a long time, and the
properties on which elective localization depends may be retained
in the deep colonies for a longer period than when grown
aerobically, so that transfers to the liquid mediums for animal
injectioins may be made at a considerable period after growth has
occurred.

"The material from a foul pulp or a dental canal may be
inoculated directly with a broach; effort should be made to carry
some of it to the deeper leyers of the mediums. A granuloma, or
other material from apical infections, may be emulsified in
sodium chloride solution in a mortar in a specially devised
sterile air chamber and then inoculated, or it mayb e dropped
into the broth directly. Transfers from these mediums to blood
agar or other mediums may be made for indentification and for
other studies.

"In the removal of teeth some danger of contamination with the
mouth flora exists even when extreme measures are adopted for
setrilizing the gum margins. This danger becomes slight in
proper hands and, if the agar medium yields many colonies, one
may be sure that the bvacteria were contained in the material
inoculated. If few bacteria exist in the tissue, as may be the
casei n chronic granuloma, control cultures in the agar medium of
the material contained in the pulp chamber of abscessed teeth,
for example, should always be made. This may be done
conveniently by sterilizing the surface of the tooth in a Bunsen
flame, or by dipping it in alcohol and burning the alcohol, care
being taken not to overheat the tooth and thus kill the bacteria
in the pulp. If cultures can not be made immediately, the tooth
should be wrapped in dry sterile gauze; it should not be placed
in sterile salt solution or other liquids as is so often done.
The pulp chamber may be entered from the seared apical end with
the aid of a flamed dental drill, or by splitting the tooth
wrapped in sterile gauze in the jaws of a rigid vise. Moreover,
the presence of bacterial is readily demonstrated by incubating
the granuloma or other tissue in the depths of the medium for
from eight to twelve hours, fixing the tissue in 10 percent
formalin, and cutting and staining sections. At the point where
living bacteria occur a colony containing many bacteria is formed
and, owing to the density of tissues, it is readily demonstrable
microscopically. This procedure has the advangage of showing the
location of the bacteria in their relation to the blood vessels.

"For details regarding inoculations of animals, reference
should be made to the original papers on elective localization.
Suffice it to state here that inoculations in animals should be
made intravenously, although specific [p.213] localization has

been obtained in some instances following intraperitoneal inoculation. The culture to be injected should be mixed so that the bacteria grown at the different levels are included. Control cultures of the material injected should always be made, since the freshly isolated organisms tend to die quickly and a negative result may be due to this cause. At least two animals, preferably medium-sized rabbits, should be inoculated with a given culture, one with a relatively amall dose (1 to 5 cc), the other with a large dose (5 to 10 cc). The dose in special instances may be made smaller or larger, depending on the type of bacteria at hand. If the bacteria are separated from the broth and suspended in salt solution, the dose should be increased. The animal should be anesthetized in from forty-eight to seventy-two hours after injection, and examined carrefully in a bright light for lesions. Animals seemingly well have rfrequently shown specific lesions. Repeatedly negative results have been reported by the inexperienced investigator when unmistakable lesions were found on closer examination, especially in the case of experiments in myositis and arthritis. Cultures and sections from the lesions should, of course, be made to determine the identity of the causative organisms, especially if the primary mixed cultures are injected. The nonpathogens disappear from the circulation and the tissues with remarkable rapidity, and the specific organisms quickly localizes and produces lesions. The animal often serves as an efficient plating, separating the pathogens from the nonpathogens. This fact was emphasized some years ago when it was shown that Streptococcus viridans from endocarditis was isolated in pure culture from lesions in the heart valves, and hemolytic streptococcus was isolated from the turbid joint fluid in animals after mixtures of the two strains had been injected intravenously."

ELECTIVE LOCALIZATION, MATERIAL DIRECTLY FROM TONSILS 19R6-215
   In response to "those who are inclined to minimize the importance of foci of infection as causes of systemic disease [who] have raised the objection that in animal experiments repeated large [IV] doses of cultures [cause localization which] under natural conditions ... does not occur, Dr. Rosenow made direct injections of bacteria that had grown in the tonsils. Thus it was found that bacteria in pus from tonsils and in emulsions of extirpated tonsils from persons with diseases of joints and muscles, stomach ulcers, kidneys, nerves, and skin, tend to localize in these same organs of injected laboratory animals.

DANGER: REMOVING MULTIPLE FOCI 19R6
   "The danger from the removal of too many foci at one time [in persons with chronic disorders who appear to be hypersensitive] was noted some years ago (1913) when a fatal exacerbation followed the removal and curettement of a number of abscessed teeth occurred in a patient suffering from chronic arthritis.
   "On Feb. 6, 1913, tonsillectomy was followed by a slight

increase in temperature for a day or two. On Feb. 16 a number of teeth were extracted, followed on the next day by fever from 102 to 105 degrees F for nearly 3 weeks, associated with pericarditis, pleurisy with effusion, bronchopneumonia, exacerbation of the joint sensitiveness, and successive crops of erythematous nodes of the skin chiefly over the forearms and legs, acute dilation with acute multiple ulceration of the stomach shortly before death Feb. 28."

ORAL INFECTIONS DAMAGE THROUGH BLOOD/LYMPH NOT SWALLOWING-19R6

"It should be emphasized ... that the chief harm from these conditions [infections of the gums and enveloping membranes about the roots of teeth] comes from the absorption of the bacteria and their products into the lymph stream or blood, especially if drainage is inadequate, not from swallowing the infectious material... " [19R6-243]

INFECTED TEETH, CORRECT FIRST; TONSILS MAY SELF-CORRECT 19R6

"Tonsillectomy as now so commonly practised before the condition of the teeth has been corrected is illogical. ... Some infections of the tonsils improve or even disappear following the extraction of infected teeth. The unnecessary sacrifice of vital teeth should be condemned." 19R6-246

HEMATOGENOUS ILLS: STOMACH GALL-BLADDER PANCREAS APPENDIX 21R2

Here Dr. Rosenow notes that diseases of joints, bones and endocardium are generally conceded to be hematogenous (blood-borne), whereas diseases of stomach, gall bladder, pancreas and appendix are thought by many to be due to infection through the mucous membrane or ducts which drain into it. "Many facts suggest that in these, too, the infection may be blood-born."

STOMACH ULCER - DIFFICULTY IN TRANSMITTING ORALLY - 21R2, 19

Efforts to produce ulcer of the stomach by feeding bacteria have been unsuccessful except in starving animals.

ORAL INFECTIONS AS PRECURSOR TO ACUTE DISEASE ATTACKS 21R2,21

Corroborative clinical evidence indicating causal relationship between the focus of infection and systemic disease is not leaking. the foci are present in demonstrable form in a high percentage of patients with the diseases under consideration. Acute attacks often follow exacerbations of infections in sinuses, tonsils, and teeth. Evans has noted a marked increase in the incidence of appendicitis during epidemics of sore throat.

RESPONSE TO CRITICISM OF LARGE INJECTIONS - SMALL DOSES INJECTED IN LAB ANIMALS   21R2, p. 21

"My original experimental studies in ulcer, cholecystitis, and appendicitis extended over a short period, and included a relatively small series of cases. ... The number of bacteria injected was relatively large and this has been objected to. I believed it worthwhile, therefore, to continue the studies in a larger and more varied series, including recurrent ulcer, and to the effect of the injection of smaller doses of bacteria. ... In all cases the symptoms were active at the time of the study and in all there were foci in which a [causal] relationship was suspected. Painstaking effort was made to obtain cultures from the depths of the focus and to eliminate as far as possible the more saphrophytic bacteria on the surface. Glucose-brain broth in tall columns was substituted for ascites-glucose broth. The dose for a routine injection consisted of from 0.1 cc to 0.25 cc for each 100 grams of body weight. Usually only one injection was given. In order to rule out all possible objections to dosage, the small amount of pus expressed from tonsils and emulsions of tonsils was injected directly.

   In this study, involving 183 strains of bacteria and 774 laboratory animals, bacteria from predominantly oral foci of persons with various diseases, including stomach ulcers, cholecystitis, appendicitis and myositis, were found to overwhelmingly electively locate in lab-animals' tissues which corresponded to the human systemic diseases.

   "... The conclusion that streptococci are the chief cause of ulcer of the stomach, cholecystitis, and appendicitis, and, probably, pancreatitis, seems to be justified."

EMBOLISM. THROMBOSIS 27R2

   In 1909, Dr. Rosenow had been able to consistently isolate a "green producing diplococcus of low virulence from the thrombus or blood in each of a number of cases of thrombosis and pulmonary embolism" [09R4] using a special technic which afforded gradients of oxygen pressure [14R12]

   In 1927 Dr. Rosenow was "impelled ... again to study the question" as a result of an unprecedented number of cases of postoperative thrombosis in the Mayo Clinic. He noted that "the occurrence of cases of pulmonary embolism in groups, especially when certain respiratory infections are prevalent, speaks for a microbic etiology of the disease." He again emphasized the use of an oxygen-gradient culture medium, and "the importance of making cultures from goodly amounts of tissue, and with what tenacity they [tissue] hold onto the infecting organism."

   At this time he again isolated an identical diplostreptococcus from the embolus of each of 5 cases of pulmonary embolism; reproduced thrombi experimentally in guinea pigs, rabbits and dogs; and then isolated the same organism from thrombi so produced. The organism was also identified microscopically in all but two of 25 other cases (from which pulmonary emboli and thrombi had been preserved in a 10% solution of formalin). Of the organism, Dr. Rosenow stated: "They were never numerous; prolonged search was often necessary to find them. ... The organism is of low general virulence. ... It rarely causes lesions in the various tissues except those secondary to thrombosis or embolism. The blood of animals was usually sterile or contained relatively few organisms, facts in harmony with the noteworthy lack of, or mild, febrile reaction and the usual

absence of the organism from the blood. ... Experiments have been
successful with each of the four strains and injected and
isolated from thrombi and with one strain isolated from foci of
infection at the apexes of teeth. Such results have not been
obtained in numerous experiments following injection of
morphologically similar organisms from cases other than pulmonary
embolism." Dr. Rosenow suggested "the possibility of a means of
prevention through specific inoculation with a vaccine prepared
from this organism." [27R2]

EPIDEMIOLOGIC ROLE OF FOCI, E.G. TONSILS   27R9 - 593
FOCAL INFECTION SCOPE: DENTISTRY, MEDICINE & SURGERY 27R9
FOCUS-SITE FOR ACQUIRING/MAINTAINING INVASIVE POWER 27R9
   There is much clinical evidence indicating that foci of
infection, as in tonsils, are often directly responsible for
rendering attacks of acute infectious diseases more severe than
they would otherwise be, and for increasing the incidence of
complications, such as in diphtheria and scarlet fever. Foci of
infection in the upper respiratory tract, as in the tonsils, may
also be of epidemiologic importance, as is indicated by the
suddenness with which the diphtheria-carrier state disappears
after tonsillectomy. In fact, the question of focal infection in
its broader sense is as wide in its scope and as difficult of
proper application as is the practice of dentistry, medicine and
surgery, combined.. It cannot be applied by rule of thumb any
more than can the healing art. A focus of infection that for
mechanical or any other reason cannot heal or drain, that is
teeming with organisms, often in mixed culture, must ever be
considered not only as a favorable place for entrance but also as
a good place for bacteria to maintain or acquire high and
particular invasive powers."

FACTORS WHICH INCREASE LIKELIHOOD ELECTIVE LOCALIZATION 27R9
"Exposure, trauma and fatigue of certain structure, improper food
and bad sanitation, lack of sunshine, alcoholism and other
excesses, undoubtedly lower the threshold of local or general
resistance and thus greatly increase the likelihood of elective
localization of bacteria and other infective processes."-594

"'OUNCE OF PREVENTION IS WORTH A POUND OF CURE' ..." 28R7
Rosenow authored the "Focal Infection" section in the 1928
Encyclopedia Brit. [28R7-433]:
   "In this field, more than in others, the maxim 'An ounce of
prevention is worth a pound of cure' holds good. ...
   "Diseases of the heart valves, appendicitis, shingles,
inflammation of the gall bladder and gallstones, diseases of the
kidney and of the nervous system, infection of the roots of
nails, were produced in large part, with germs from infected
teeth or tonsils. ...
   "This method of treatment is not, however to be taken as a
cureall. Many conditions may be too firmly established to be
materially benefitted; others are not due to focal infection; or

the responsible focus may be hard to locate and may easily be missed."

DOSAGE - SMALL PREFERRED 28R10-234
"If the dosage of vaccine is gauged so that the local and constitutional reactions are relatively slight, the tolerance may often be greatly increased, even tenfold, and the patient improves. If the dosage is too large tolerance may not increase but actually diminish, reactions becoming progressively more marked with each succeeding injection, and the patient's condition grow worse." 28R10-234

OL-NACL SUSPENSION OF DIRECT BACTERIA IN VACCINE 29R1
   Dr. Rosenow relates how vaccines are made from either directly from unwashed sedimented bacteria "or at various intervals from those preserved in dense suspension in glycerol, two parts, and saturated NaCl solution, one part."   29R1-506
   The preservation of streptococci in glycerol-NaCl menstruum and preferential use of such streptococci in vaccines was to become standard operating procedure for Dr. Rosenow. [see: 48R2-371, 50R1-120, 45R4-163, 51R4-610, 34R3-407]

SYMPTOMLESS FOCI IMPORTANCE 29R1-506   "The causative streptococcus often was isolated not only from badly infected tonsils but from tonsils that appeared small and normal but which on removal were large and sometimes contained abscesses, from unsuspected remnants of tonsils, and from symptomless roentgenographic-ally positive and negative pulpless teeth, root tips and residual areas which had not been considered previously or which were thought to be harmless."29R1-506

TABLE (Table 2.2, above)
     Foci in:

Diseases:	tonsils	teeth	pulpless teeth
encephalitis	70%	56%	87%
arthritis	51	69	61
torticollis	60	75	76
MS	78	67	89
chronic polio	65	71	92
gastroduod.ulcer	74	74	52
lesions of eye	53	53	50
lesions of skin	74	56	77
prostatitis	63	54	69

FAVORABLE RESULT AFTER BOTH FOCUS REMOVAL AND VACCINE 29R1-510
Rosenow responded to Holman's fraudulent "critical review" in a gentlemanly fashion, and then provided summary data for 358 cases of various diseases, comparing results where vaccines were or not used, and foci were or were not removed 29R1

TABLE (Table 2.4, above)

Vaccine	All foci removed (% improved)	All foci not removed (% improved)
-Used:	61	25
-Not used:	54	21

REMOVAL OF FOCI NECESSARY EVEN WITH SPECIFIC VACCINE   29R1-511
"Since streptococci appear to be a cause of so many diseases, since immunity is of short duration, and since mechanical factors play so large a part in maintaining infection in structures so commonly the seat of foci, even after prolonged use of specific vaccines, mechanical correction or removal, so far as possible, will probably always be necessary even if highly effective specific or other remedial agents are discovered. Recurrence of the previous condition or new localizations are prone to occur unless the predisposing cause, the focus, is eliminated. Likewise, operation will probably always be indicated in many of the chronic systemic lesions, such as chronic indurated ulcer, cholecystitis with gallstones, and appendicitis with fecal stones or constricted lumen from previous attacks.

DOSAGE, ALLERGY   29R1-511
ALLERGY, DOSAGE   29R1-511
   "Considerable evidence has been obtained in this study which suggests that tissues in the cases of various chronic diseases, particularly the diseased tissues, become hypersensitive to the infecting organisms and their toxic products, as indicated by exacerbations which are particularly prone to occur following too strenuous or incomplete removal of foci of infection, and by the reactions which sometimes follow injection of autogenous vaccines, a point stressed by Kolmer. If the dosage of vaccine is gauged so that the local and constitutional reactions are relatively slight the tolerance may often be greatly increased, even tenfold, and the patient improves, a result in accord with that of Wherry and others in bronchial asthma. If the dosage is too large tolerance may not increase but actually diminish, reactions may become progressively more marked with each succeeding injection and the patient's condition grow worse. This narrow limit of effective dosage determined more by the reaction in the patient than by the number of bacteria and the use, without bacteriologic diagnosis, of stock vaccines made from bacteria long cultivated in the laboratory have, we believe, contributed much to the general disrepute into which vaccine therapy has unfortunately fallen."

PHYSICAL CHARACTERISTICS AFFECTING LOCALIZATION   30R1-49-50
As concerns microorganisms: "Some of these are size, formation of clumps, stability of suspension, susceptibility of phagocytosis and electric charges. Other physical characteristics are found in the tissues, i.e., in the capillary bed of certain tissues there is gradation from high to low vascularity and hence from

high to low oxygen tension. This is especially seen in the
valves of the heart, in the periarticular structures, in the
tendon sheaths, and the ciliary body of the eye." 30R1

BACTERIA BEAR NEGATIVE ELECTRICAL CHARGE   30R1-50
  "It has long been known that bacteria bear negative electrical
charges, that is, they are negatively charged colloidal
suspensions, for the motion of the bacterial cells in an external
electrical field is toward the positive electrode. ... We have
measured the electrical charges, that is, the cataphoretic
mobility, of about 5,000 cultures of green-producing streptococci
isolated from material obtained from [various sources]." It was
noted that measurements of 8.0 u/sec was obtained in 88 % of 100
nasopharyngeal cultures from encephalitis; vs. measurements of
10.6u/sec in 69% of 49 cultures from arthritis.

PASSLER'S ROLE 30R6-29
  Dr. Rosenow notes that the importance of chronic low-grade,
often symptomless infections in oral foci "have been emphasized
repeatedly for years by good clinical observers, and by Passler
as early as 1909 ..."

ELECTIVE LOCALIZATION DEFINED 30R6-36
  ... the term "elective localization" is used to designate the
tendency of certain bacteria, especially streptococci, which have
been obtained from various localized regions of infection, from
practically normal mucous membranes (such as the nasopharynx and
gastro-intestinal tract), from systemic lesions, or from the
blood, to localize and produce lesions in animals corresponding
to those in the patients or in the animals from which the
microorganisms were isolated originally. The idea that different
diseases might be due to a single member of the pneumococcus-
streptococcus group which had different elective localizing
power, is basic in this work nd had its birth in my experiments
from 1912 to 1914, in which mutations of pneumococci into
streptococci, and vice versa, were induced. The occurrence ... "
[e.g. see 14R4]

MUTATIONS 30R6-36
DISSOCIATIONS 30R6-36
"The occurrence of similar changes in the streptococcus-
pneumococcus group has been reported since by numerous
investigators [e.g. P. Hadley, J.Infect.Dis., 1927]. The
production of marked changes in cultural characteristics, as well
as in localizing or infecting power of members of this group, has
since been reported by Morgenroth, Schnitzer and Berger.
[Z.f.Immunitat., u. exp. Therap. 43, 169, 1925]. I fulfilled the
pure-line requirement by obtaining cultures derived from single
cells of different members of the group.
  In the work of Morgenroth etal, as in mine, not all strains
yielded to attempts to produce mutations or "dissociations"; a
premutational stage, therefore, seemed necessary. It was found...

VIRULENCE AND ANIMAL PASSAGE
VIRULENCE AND CULTIVATION
VIRULENCE AND LOCALIZATION
   "It was found that as nonvirulent strains of this group became
virulent by successive passage through animals, and highly
virulent strains became less virulent by cultivation on
artificial mediums, the site of localization, with production of
lesions, changed markedly. When the virulence was lowest the
localization was almost wholly in relatively avascular tissue,
such as cardiac valves, joints and tendinous ends of muscles;
when the virulence was moderate, iritis, myositis, ulcer of the
stomach, cholecystitis, and focal lesions of the kidneys were
more prone to develop, and when virulence was high from
successive passage through animals, or when the organism had been
freshly isolated, lesions of the lung and death from bacteraemia
occurred commonly. Striking ...

ELECTIVE LOCALIZATION CONCEIVED 30R6-37
"Striking as these results were, it was not until the unusual
localization in the mucous membrane of the stomach of strains
from several sources occurred, and hemorrhage and ulcer were
produced, that the idea of elective localization took definite
form.
   "Variation in oxygen tension, variation in concentration of
sodium chloride, growth in symbiosis with other bacteria, and
injection into closed cavities in animals commonly called forth
mutational forms of pneumococci and streptococci. Consequently,
it seemed highly probable that similar changes might occur in
various localized but mild inflammatory processes or in foci of
infection in which organisms of this group exist under similarly
varying conditions in large numbers."
   Dr. Rosenow here proceeds to discuss the results of various
elective localization experiments, as discussed above and below;
results from 11,000 animal experiments are summarized in Table
2.1, above (data from 40R3).

RECIPE: GLUCOSE-BRAIN BROTH, FROM "SCRATCH"   30R6-40
   "The glucose-brain broth is prepared by dissolving 8 gm. of
dehydrated bacto-broth in 1000 cc of distilled water, adding 8
gm. of sodium chloride, 2 gm. of chemically pure glucose, and,
after cooling, 10 cc. of Andrade's indicator. It is also
prepared from beef infusion, adding 0.2% glucose in the usual way
and titrating to pH 7.4. Several bacteriologic peptones on the
market have been used with about equally good results. The
glucose-brain agar is prepared from the broth by adding 4 or 5
gm. of powdered agar to each litre, just a sufficient quantity to
cause it to set. The mediums are placed in tubes 20 by 1.5 cm.
To each tube are added three pieces of calf brain or beef brain,
each about 1 cc., and two or three pieces of calcium carbonate in
the form of crushed marble to insure correct reaction. The
column in each tube, after the brain and marble are added, is

about 12 cm. high. The mediums are sterilized for twenty minutes
in the autoclave at a pressure of 17 pounds (7.5 kg.). Growth in
these mediums, kept at 35° to 37° C., usually occurs within
twenty-four hours, and in most instances, especially when the
cultures are from pulpless teeth, begins at the bottom of the
tube and forces its way to the top as oxygen is consumed. This
usually occurs within twenty-four hours in the glucose-brain
broth, whereas, in the glucose-brain agar, growth to the top, or
more often to within 1 cm. of the top, frequently takes from two
to three days. Negative cultures are observed daily for a week
or ten days before they are discarded. Colonies in the agar may
be exceedingly small or may develop only around the pieces of
brain at the bottom and may be easily overlooked, or they may be
so numerous as to give the appearance of a negative culture."
[30R6-40]

IMPORTANCE OF BRAIN IN DEXTROSE-BRAIN BROTH   30R6-40
  "It was found that two or three pieces of brain, approximating
1 cc each, when added, before sterilization, to tall columns (8
to 10 cm.) of glucose broth (0.2% glucose) or agar, contained in
test tubes 1.5cm. in diameter, sufficed, after sterilization, to
decolorize methylene blue in the deeper part of the tubes and to
keep it decolorized for a long time on standing. Moreover, it was
found that anaerobic streptococci, tetanus spores, Bacillus
welchii, and Bacillus fusiformis in mixed cultures, and other
strictly anaerobic organisms, grew readily when inoculated into
the bottom of the tubes containing the pieces of brain. On the
basis of these observations, the brain-containing mediums were
adopted in most subsequent work on elective localization. In
special instances, ascites fluid or serum, or fresh sterile
tissue is added, and the surface is covered with a layer of
petrolatum or paraffin oil."30R6-40

PRESERVATION OF SPECIFICITY, VIABILITY OF ORGANISMS 30R6-42
  "Numerous attempts have been made, with only partial success,
to find a method of culture that might be relied on to retain
elective localizing power and viability for long periods.
Preservation in latent life under reduced oxygen tension in tall
tubes of meat-mash infusion, in shake cultures containing
relatively few colonies in glucose-brain agar or ascites-glucose
agar, on plain-meat-extract-blood-agar slants sealed with a
paraffined cork, in dense suspensions in glycerol (two parts),
and saturated solution of sodium chloride (one part) often have
served to retain viability and elective localizing and other
specific properties for a long time [reference: 29R4]. In
exceptional circumstances this was true for as long as eight
years, when the corresponding strains, grown aerobically, had
lost elective localizing power in the course of several daily
transfers." [reference: 23R6].

IMPROVEMENT AFTER FOCI REMOVED 30R6-54
  "Improvement followed removal of those foci which were proved

to contain the causative organism of the large number of diseases studied with such great regularity in my hands that I have come to consider failure to relieve a given relevant condition as presumptive evidence that the responsible focus or other source has not be found."

FILLED ROOT CANAL NOT PREVENTION OF LATER INFECTION 30R6-56
"Hence, devitalization of teeth and the filling of root canals, as practised in the past, at least in America, should cease. It is to be hoped that efficient methods may be found that will not only sterilize pulpless teeth and periapical tissues that have become infected, but will also prevent subsequent infection, especially of the periapical tissues. The fulfillment of the latter requirement seems almost unattainable, and until this has been accomplished it would seem wiser to remove teeth that have become infected or that require extirpation of the pulp than to retain them at the risk of having them become the source of an insidious infection later. Vital teeth, free from pyorrhea and fillings, should never be extracted except as it becomes necessary for restorative work, but the extraction of pulpless teeth seems to me to be indicated, regardless of the appearance of the roentgenograms. It seems ...

TONSILS - REMOVE IF NO OTHER FOCUS FOUND 30R6-56
"It seems to me also, that the tonsils should be removed regardless of whether they are large or small or whether they are visibly infected or not, unless this is contraindicated for various reasons, in all patients who have serious systemic disease presumed to be of focal origin, and provided no other focus can be found." 30R6-56

STREPTOCOCCI IN DIFFERENT DISEASES: SAME OR NOT?   30R6-58
"It is uncertain whether the streptococci isolated in each of the many diseases studied ... are distinct varieties or modifications of a single strain. ... They all belonged to the pneumococcus-streptococcus group and were much alike in morphology and cultural reaction." [30R6-58]

ULCERATIVE COLITIS   30R9
SERUM SICKNESS, HOW TO AVOID 30R9
  Bargen, JA, EC Rosenow and GFC Fasting, Archives of Internal Medicine, 1039-1047, "Serum treatment for chronic ulcerative colitis" [30R9], discussed the alteration of immune serum so as to avert serum sickness reactions while preserving beneficial attributes. This was accomplished by dilution in ether water which causes the precipitation out of a modified euglobulin containing essential antibodies, which is then preserved in glycerin-salt solution. This antibody euglobulin solution was administered in approximately 200 cases, given deeply in the muscles. Reporting specifically on the first 50 consecutive cases: "Twenty-four patients became free from symptoms; thirteen became from 75-90 percent well, and six were improved at least 50

percent. In only seven cases was there little if any change
following the treatment. These seven cases were either severe,
long-standing cases with extensive involvement of the colon and
destruction, or there were serious complications, such as
multiple polyps or strictures."

"Certain factors seemed to have a bearing on recurrence of
symptoms after patients become clinically well. One of the
significant features seemed to be the failure to remove possible
foci of infection."

Please note that Dr. Rosenow was later able to fully avoid any
potential negative effects of "immune serum" through the
preparation of "thermal antibody", which was successfully
employed therapeutically in a wide range of diseases. (see also
58R1).

OBSERVATIONS WITH RIFE MICROSCOPE 32R5-192

Dr. Rosenow had been invited by Drs. Kendall and Rife to share
their observations of filter-passing forms of Eberthella typhi,
and to examine Rosenow's streptococcus from poliomyelitis, with
an improved model of the Rife microscope.   "The findings under
the Rife microscope of cocci and diplococci in filtrates of
cultures of the streptococcus from poliomyelitis, and in
filtrates of the viruses of poliomyelitis and herpes
encephalitis, not detectable by the ordinary methods of
examination, and which resembled in form and size those found in
the respective cultures, and the absence of minute forms, suggest
that the filterable, inciting agency of these diseases is not
necessarily small, as is universally believed. Indeed, the
filterable, inciting agent may be the non-staining, highly
plastic, hyalin stage of the visible, stainable, cultivable
organism, the streptococcus.

"It is, of course, possible that these unstained, invisible
forms revealed be ordinary methods of examination are not the
inciting agents or 'viruses' of these diseases and that they
represent merely the filterable or other state of the
streptococcus."

CATAPHORETIC VELOCITY VS. ELECTIVE LOCALIZATION [33R7-503]
"It is difficult to conceive of a situation in which the
modification of the state of surface electrification per se, as
indicated by cataphoretic velocities, should determine
specificity or localization." 33R7-503 [It may be offered that
electrical charge/velocity may be indicative of relative weight
of respective organisms, in accord w/Graham's law.]

STREP. ROSENOW DEFINED 34R2-92
"In this as in other papers dealing with streptococci, all
diplococci and all organisms in chains of various length having
the usual form and size of streptococci when grown in liquid
mediums, especially dextrose-brain broth, are considered as
streptococci, irrespective of whether they are soluble in bile,
ferment inulin or produce green, indifferent or hemolytic

colonies on blood-agar plates." 34R2-92

DEXTROSE-BRAIN BROTH MEDIUM   34R3
  --"...cultures made by usual methods ... may yield the easily
cultivable saprophytic organisms, including streptococci, instead
of the highly sensitive, disease-producing strains. ... Special
mediums, such as dextrose-brain broth and dextrose-brain agar,
which afford reduced oxygen tension and other favorable
conditions for growth, are essential in the primary culture in
many diseases to insure isolation of the really causative
streptococci." [34R3]

STREPTOCOCCUS V.S. VIRUS IN COMMON COLD AND INFLUENZA 34R3-403
  "It is becoming more generally recognized, despite the
demonstrated importance of the 'virus' factor, especially in
colds, that the more serious manifestations referable to the
respiratory tract and remote tissues, incident to epidemic colds
and influenza, are due to visible, cultivable organisms, chiefly
streptococci, and more rarely to Bacillus influenzae and
staphylococci. The results of studies on cataphoresis and
virulence [and with vaccines indicate] ... that these
streptococci are more often of primary than of secondary
importance." [34R3, p. 403]

VACCINE PREPARATION DETAILS 34R3, 408
  "In this study the vaccines used for prophylactic and active
immunization against colds and influenza were prepared from the
respective streptococci by adding enough of the dense suspension
in glycerin-salt solution to 0.85 per cent sodium chloride
solution to bring the density to that of the dextrose-brain broth
culture, or approximately 2 billion streptococci per cc. The
suspensions were heated to 75 degrees C for one hour, in vials of
a capacity of 30cc., sealed with perforated screw-caps containing
a rubber disk; the vials were completely immersed in water. For
prophylactic inoculation, 0.3, 0.5 and 1.0 cc. were injected
subcutaneously, a week apart, and then one injection of 1.0 cc
was given once a month throughout the season when colds and
influenza are prevalent. The dosage for children was reduced
according to age. If the reactions proved too severe for
hypersensitive patients the dosage was reduced according to the
degree of reaction, but this was almost never necessary. For
treatment, regardless of the duration or character of the
respiratory manifestation, 0.3 cc of the vaccine was given
subcutaneously as the initial injection; this was followed in 24
hours by 0.5 cc, and a day or 2 later by 1.0 cc subcutaneously,
provided the reactions were not too severe and the patient's
condition was improved or was no worse. In order to facilitate
absorption as much as possible, the area of subcutaneous
injection was massaged immediately, and the patient was
instructed to massage it once or twice daily for three or four
days following injection ... regardless of the degree of local
reaction." [34R3, p. 408]

SYMPTOMLESS FOCI, IMPORTANCE 34R5-721
"Lucas, in an extended study, reported that 319 of 364 patients having symptoms of various diseases, in many of whom inadequate consideration of foci had previously been given, were relieved from symptoms after thorough eradication of foci of infection in the dental area. Streptococci were isolated from nearly all of these foci, which included the remnants of the enamel organ of unerupted teeth. Vaccines, even though specific, have only limited value when given to patients without removal of evident foci."[721] [Lucas, C.D., "Periapical Infection", Dental Cosmos 71: 555-564, June 1929].

RESIDUAL INFECTIONS IN JAWS, ETC. 34R5, 721
  "Simple extraction of pulpless teeth does not always result in eradication of infection in the jaw. it is still too common to find residual areas, pulpless teeth and root tips in the jaws, and symptomless, infected tonsils and tags of tonsils among patients in whom the question of foci was thought to have been adequately considered."

EXACERBATION OF DISEASE WHEN FOCUS REMOVED PROVES CAUSE 34R5
"Exacerbation of disease following removal of certain foci, especially infected teeth..., although not so considered, is as convincing proof of a causal relationship as a spectacular cure would be... ." 34R5

COMMON SITES, FOCAL INFECTION 34R5, 722
  Especially common sites of focal infection were the tonsils or tonsillar tags, teeth, prostate gland, uterine cervix and, much less often, the paranasal sinuses. ... The streptococcus was commonly isolated from symptomless, roentgenographically positive or negative pulpless teeth, root tips, residual areas of infection in the jaw, partially erupted, impacted teeth, and from accumulations of pus beneath deciduous teeth which had not been discovered or considered previously or which were thought to be harmless."

PRACTICALLY ALL PULPLESS TEETH ARE INFECTED 34R5-723
  Dr. Rosenow presents statistics reporting on various workers and involving hundreds of teeth which "reveal that from 80 to 90 percent of adults harbor teeth with filled root canals and that an average of 69.5% of these pulpless teeth show evidence of periapical rarefaction due to infection.
  "By making cultures chiefly in dextrose-brain broth and soft dextrose-brain agar, media affording a gradation of oxygen tension, and aerobic cultures on blood-agar plates, I found that practically all pulpless teeth of persons suffering from various systemic diseases were infected with streptococci, which often were highly sensitive to oxygen and extremely specific in the primary culture."
  Dr. emphasized that this was true of all pulpless teeth, x-ray

negative as well as x-ray positive, and for both apices removed aseptically with the teeth in situ, and for apices of pulpless teeth extracted under sterile precautions.

NUMEROUS RESEARCHERS SHOW PULPLESS TEETH ARE FOCI [34R5-724]
"From these [Rosenow's] and similar results of Meisser, of Austin and Cook, Haden, Price, Lucas, Lehmnann, Rickert, Lyons and Hadley, Rhoads and Dick, and Grumbach, who made a thorough study of the question and cites similar results of other recent workers, it seems justifiable to regard most pulpless teeth as possible foci of infection, whether they show apical changes in the roentgenograms or not."

PULPLESS TEETH CONSTITUTE *LOCUS MINORIS RESISTENTIAE* 34R5-724
   "The marked difference in the bacteriology of pulpless and vital teeth indicates that, with the removal of the pulp, the apex of the root and the periapical tissues constitute a locus minoris resistentiae, and become more easily infected. The problem of rendering pulpless teeth sterile is not only one of sterilizing the canal with antiseptics at the time the infected pulp is removed or when found degenerated from infection, but also to keep them free from infection for years."

ANTISEPTICS IN ROOT CANALS, FAILINGS [34R5-724]
"Sealing antiseptics in the canal and filling it with various impervious materials does not suffice [to keep canal sterile], for I have isolated streptococci from apices of teeth so treated long before, and with the freshly isolated strains have reproduced the disease the patient was suffering from when the distinctive odor, or crystals of the antiseptic, were present at the time within the root canal." [Note that as per contemporary endodontics doyen Samuel Selzer, this is still the case.] [34R5-724]

MS: PASSLER IN 1932, ON FOCI OF INFECTION AND M.S. 34R5-733
   "Passler [H.] of Dresden, in a recent paper [Deutsch. Ztschr. f. Nervenh., 126:225-264, June 1932] emphasized the importance of foci of infection in functional diseases of the nervous system, peripheral neuritis, chronic progressive encephalitis and multiple sclerosis."

ILL EFFECT OF CHRONIC FOCI ON OTHERWISE-SUFFICIENT DIET 34R5
"A diet sufficient to keep the control animals well was inadequate for the dogs who had chronic foci of infection." [presumably this particularly involves or at a minimum holds true for vitamins]-733

SPECIFICITY IS APPARENTLY ACQUIRED IN PATIENT'S TISSUES 34R5
   Dr. Rosenow relates that implicated specific streptococci "repeatedly have been demonstrated to be present in various foci of infection and elsewhere (carrier state) over a period of years, and long after onset of symptoms [of] chronic diseases,

such as arthritis and encephalitis. This is believed to be of
fundamental significance, for it indicates that the patient's
tissues or tissue juices afford the conditions favorable for
streptococci to acquire and maintain particular elective
localizing power and cataphoretic velocity, peculiar to the
disease from which the patient is suffering. ..."-734

FROM GENETIC PREDISPOSITION TO PHYSICAL DISEASE 34R5-734
"Might not the inherited rheumatic diathesis, the neuropathic or
the allergic constitution and other 'diatheses' and
'constitutional predispositions' be expressions in part of a
peculiar interaction between host and parasite, and not
expressions only of an inherited 'weakness' of joint, brain or
other organ, as is usually assumed? The focus furnishes ... .
34R5

RELATION OF FOCI TO HYPERSENSITIVENESS AND TO ALLERGY 34R5
"The focus furnishes a ready source of infecting organisms and
bacterial antigens to which the host reacts variously, depending,
among other factors, on inherited or acquired constitutional
peculiarities. If of allergic tendency, local and general
hypersensitiveness is prone to develop; if of normal
constitution, increased resistance or immunity is probable. The
particular tissue in which local hypersensitiveness develops and
in which allergic manifestations are especially marked is
determined, it would seem, by the specific or elective localizing
power of either or both the bacteria and their antigens or
toxins." 34R5-734

SUDDEN DISAPPEARANCE OF SPECIFICITY EXPLAINED 34R5-738
   Dr. Rosenow emphasized that the puzzling fact, often observed,
of sudden disappearance of specificity, appearance of new
specificity, and certain discrepancies of some workers, may all
be explained by the fact that "consideration of the inherent
property, changeability of streptococci, is basic in studies on
focal infection and elective localization. ...

DEXTROSE-BRAIN BROTH MEDIUM 34R5-738
   "Of great importance is the fact that the medium, dextrose-
brain broth, with which I have obtained the best results in
experiments on elective localization, is by far the best medium
for preserving characteristic [specificity]. Several transplants
in other media, ... even the same dextrose-brain broth, but minus
the brain, often suffice to convert a strain ... which had
elective localizing power, into one ... without this faculty."
[34R5, p. 738]

REMOVAL OF FOCI AS PROPHYLAXIS [34R5-739]
"The still far too common practice of waiting until the disease
is far advanced or until a serious condition such as a hemorrhage
in ulcer or a heart attack in heart disease, has developed, or
until advanced age before evident foci, especially pulpless

teeth, are removed, is deplorable."

PULPLESS TEETH - RECAP OF INFECTED STATUS 34R5-740
"... The majority of pulpless teeth, irrespective of
roentgenographic findings, are infected and hence potential foci
of infection.
   "Devitalization of teeth and the filling of root canals ...
should cease. ... Many who formerly skillfully practised the art
... consider it safer to remove pulpless teeth and to attach
restorations in a way harmless to vital teeth. It is to be hoped
that efficient methods may be found that will not only sterilize
pulpless teeth and periapical tissues that have become infected,
but will also prevent subsequent infection, especially of the
periapical tissues. The fulfillment of the latter requirement
seems almost unattainable, and, until this has been accomplished,
it would seem wiser to remove teeth that have become infected or
that require extirpation of the pulp than to retain them at the
risk of having them become the source of an insidious
incapacitating and perhaps fatal infection.

VITAL TEETH, DO NOT EXTRACT 34R5, 740
"Vital teeth free from pyorrhea and fillings should never be
extracted except as it becomes necessary for restorative work,
but the extraction of pulpless teeth seems to me to be indicated,
quite regardless of the appearance of the roentgenograms."

TONSILS, REMOVE IF NO OTHER FOCI 34R5-740
"It seems to me, also, that tonsils of all patients who have
serious systemic disease presumed to be of focal origin should be
removed, regardless of whether they are large or small or whether
they are visibly infected or not, even in the absence of a
history of recurring attacks, unless this is contraindicated for
various reasons, and provided no other focus can be found."

SYMPTOMLESS RESID. JAW INFECTION 34R5-740
   "Symptomless, residual areas of infection in the jaws, even in
edentulous jaws, often difficult of demonstration and often
unsuspected foci of infection, have yielded the streptococcus
with great regularity, and should be eliminated more often."

STREPTOCOCCUS WITH NO NAME 34R5-741
Dr. Rosenow noted that "none of the many strains that showed
well-marked specificity have been given names [due to uncertainty
over whether they] are distinct varieties or modifications of a
single strain." Implying that the latter is the case, Dr.
Rosenow describes them thusly: "The different strains all
belonged to the pneumococcus-streptococcus group and were much
alike in morphology and cultural reaction. Nearly all produced a
greenish zone of partial hemolysis surrounding small grayish
colonies on horse-blood-agar plates, but qualitative tests showed
them to be low in production of peroxide. A few were indifferent
to blood-agar, and a few produced a narrow zone of clear

hemolysis. The usual fermentation reactions in sugar were variable and of little value in classification from the standpoint of elective localization." 34R5

PULPLESS TEETH ARE INFECTED TEETH [34R5]
"The majority of pulpless teeth, irrespective of roentgenographic findings, are infected and hence potential foci of infection. ... Vital teeth free from pyorrhea and fillings should never be extracted except as it becomes necessary for restorative work".

CHICK EMBRYO MEDIUM RECIPE 35R5-410
"The chick-mash medium consists of finely ground twenty-day incubated eggs, containing almost fully matured live chicks and water. The eggs are passed through a meat-chopper, eggshell and all. To this mash is added from three to seven parts of water. The mixture is placed in the refrigerator for 24 to 48 hours, then transferred to tall tubes or flasks, autoclaved at 17 pounds' pressure for 20 minutes, and then layered with sterile liquid petrolatum."

LIMITATION OF EARLIER WORK ON POLIO DISCUSSED   35R5
   In 1935 Dr. Rosenow [35R5] reported that while symptoms of poliomyelitis had regularly been reproduced by injections of streptococci freshly isolated from polio victims, that "the lesions induced, however, were usually atypical, both in type and distribution."

LIMITATION OF EARLIER POLIO WORK OVERCOME WITH CHICK MASH 35R5
TRANSFORMATIONS: STREPTOCOCCUS TO VIRUS TO STREPTOCOCCUS   35R5
SERIAL DILUTION CULTURE, FIRST TIME USED TO ISOLATE STREP 35R5
   "Each of four [streptococcus] strains has been passed consecutively through the 'streptococcal to virus' phase and through the 'virus to streptococcal' phase three times." The use of "a new medium, autoclaved chick mash", allowed for development of characteristic symptoms and lesions of "natural" virus, and apparent transformation of streptococcal into viral forms. The reverse action involved high dilution: "The dilution of the virus from which these streptococci were isolated was extremely high $(200^{-10 \text{ to } -21})$."
   This was Dr. Rosenow's first use of serial dilution cultures, which he extended to use with inoculum of virus and phage into dextrose-brain mediums [38R5], which method was to become the general practice in subsequent works involving the isolation of streptococci.

L-FORMS PIONEER HEILMAN WAS ROSENOW UNDERSTUDY   37R1
   A 1937 article [37R1] entitled "Newer methods of study and treatment of chronic streptococcal disease", by F.R. Heilman and E.C. Rosenow, incorporates the use of glycerine-salt menstruum to preserve antigenic specificity (citing 29R1) and dextrose-brain broth (citing 30R6). Heilman's work with Rosenow provides a clear link between Rosenow's pioneering efforts on the one hand;

and the modern field of study concerning "l-forms"/cell-wall
deficient forms of bacteria, wherein is found Heilman as a very
early influence.

ANTIGEN IN BLOOD IN ACTIVE STREPTOCOCCAL INFECTIONS 37R1
   "Patients with active streptococcal infections often appear to
have free bacterial antigen in the blood which gives a precipitin
reaction with the specific or related antiserum." [37R1]

ANTIGEN IN BLOOD OF (ENCEPHALITIC) HORSES [37R5-825]
"In a previous paper we have shown that streptococci and
streptococcal antigen are present in the blood and noses of
nearly all horses acutely ill with epidemic encephalomyelitis and
that both promptly disappear from the blood following intravenous
injection of an antiserum prepared in the horse against
streptococci isolated in studies of encephalitis of human
beings." [addressing effects, not cause of diseases]

STREPTOCOCCUS V.S. VIRUS IN COMMON COLD AND INFLUENZA [38R2]
   "... It is becoming increasingly apparent that whatever the
causative role of the viruses of the common cold and influenza
may be, the cultivable organisms, chiefly streptococci or
pneumococci, are the main cause of the symptoms, lesions and
deaths." [38R2, 17]

PURE CULTURE, VERIFICATION 38R2-19
The streptococci incorporated in the vaccines used in this study
were isolated from the nasopharynx or sputum in cases of the
common cold and influenza, respectively. The primary isolations
were made in dextrose-brain broth. If the cataphoretic velocity
was typical, or if the strain caused hemorrhagic edema of the
lungs or bronchopneumonia in rabbits following intracerebral
inoculation, and if platings revealed a pure culture of the
streptococci, subcultures were made in the dextrose-brain broth
in rapid succession three to five times. Large volumes ...

HARVESTING AND PRESERVATION OF STREPTOCOCCI 38R2-19
   "Large volumes of previously warmed, 0.2% dextrose broth were
then inoculated. Each bottle containing 3500 cc received the
entire young culture in one tube of dextrose-brain broth, or
approximately 20cc. As soon as abundant growth had occurred, the
organisms were harvested in a continuous feed centrifuge and the
putty-like mass suspended in glycerin (2 parts) and 25 percent
solution of sodium chloride (1 part). Glass beads were added and
the mixture emulsified by shaking in a shaking machine. The
vaccines ...

VACCINE PREPARATION SUMMARY (COLDS AND INFLUENZA) 38R2-19
   "The vaccines were made as needed, preferably not before one
year after preservation, by diluting the dense suspension with
sodium chloride solution to about the density of a broth culture
(2 billion organisms per cc) and heating to 75 degrees C for one

hour.   Phenol to make 0.2 percent was added as a preservative.
... Routinely, 0.3, 0.5, and 1.0 cc were given subcutaneously a
week apart, and then 1.0 cc once every three or four
weeks..[38R2, p. 19]

ORAL COLD, INFLUENZA VACCINE 38R2-19
  "Impressed by the work of Ross, and Powell, and Rockwell and
van Kirk [J.I., 27 273-353 (1934), 28 475-483] on the results
from vaccination by mouth, we prepared a vaccine for this purpose
by adding one part of a saline suspension, of suitable density,
of the heat-killed streptococci (to which phenol was added to
make 0.2 percent) from the dense suspension in glycerin-salt
solution, to four parts of a concentrated solution of dextrose,
maltose, dextrins and saccharose in the form of Karo syrup, the
final concentration being 20,000,000,000 organisms per cc. This
vaccine is flavored with oil of peppermint and colored pink with
a harmless dye. Vaccines prepared by this method have a number
of advantages. Dosage can readily be changed for particular
needs. Owing to the high concentration of hygroscopic sugars the
bacteria are dehydrated, contaminants cannot grow because of the
absence of free water, and hence refrigeration is not necessary.
 The organisms should retain their specific antigenicity
indefinitely. We have been using this vaccine for the
prevention\on of respiratory infections and in treatment with
seemingly striking results. Five drops are taken directly on the
tongue or are allowed to trickle into the pharynx through the
nostrils while the head is held in a retracted position, or the
vaccine may be taken in water, preferably a half to one hour
before breakfast. For prophylaxis the dosage is increased by
five drops daily, up to twenty drops; then twenty drops are to be
taken once or twice weekly, provided no untoward symptoms
develop. Similar dosages are used for treatment."

VACCINE (COLD AND INFLUENZA), BENEFICIAL RESULTS 38R2-20-1
  Dr. Rosenow exhibits data on nearly 7000 prophylactic and more
than 5000 therapeutic uses of 'cold and influenza' streptococcal
vaccines, in which overall some 90% of patients reportedly
benefitted, most of these "markedly". 38R2-20-1

GLYCERINE SALT MENSTRUUM 38R2
  --"It was found that heat-killed vaccines prepared from
dilutions of the dense suspensions were much less toxic and more
highly antigenic than those prepared directly from cultures and
caused a more rapid, and more favorable, response ... ." [38R2]

APPARENT PHASAL NATURE OF VIRUS-BACTERIA RELATIONSHIP [38R5-70]
"Two schools of thought exist regarding the nature of viruses.
The one considers viruses to be distinct entities, wholly
unrelated to bacteria; the other believes that viruses may be a
phase of the cultivable bacteria associated with virus
diseases."38R5

ISOLATION OF BACTERIA FROM VIRUS AND PHAGE BY SERIAL DILUTION;
SERIAL-DILUTION CULTURE METHODOLOGY; DISCUSSION [38R5-71]
"... I wish now to report the isolation, by a modification of the
methods previously employed [35R5], of streptococci from filtered
and unfiltered viruses and of the respective organisms from
cultures of various bacteria which had been lysed with phage.

   "The extension of the method is the use of serial dilutions of
the inoculum in dextrose-brain agar and dextrose-brain broth.
When this is carried out in multiples of ten, it may be
frequently observed that although little or no growth occurs in
the first or second tube, at still higher dilutions growth is
shown. Absence of growth in the low dilutions may be due, it is
thought, to inhibiting substances in the inoculum which are
rendered inactive by serial dilution."38R5

DEXTROSE-BRAIN BROTH DETAILED RECIPE 38R5-71
   "The mediums were prepared from dehydrated broth or meat
extract and peptone in the usual concentrations, to which 0.2%
dextrose and 0.1% decolorized fuchsin (Andrade's indicator) (and
in the case of agar, 0.25% agar) were added. The reaction was
adjusted to pH 7. Approximately 18cc of the medium was placed in
each of tall tubes (20 x 1.5 cm) and to each tube 2 or 3 pieces
of fresh calf brain, about 3cc in volume, were added before
autoclaving (20 lbs. [9 kg] for 20 minutes). Cultures were made
under sterile conditions, either in a hood equipped with a glass
shield and a copper roof, which radiates heat from the Bunsen
burner, without change of air, and in which the air and the walls
were sterilized with a fine spray of solution (1:1000) of
mercuric chloride or a saturated solution of phenylmercuric
chloride, or in a hot air sterilizer equipped with a glass shield
and in which the air was sterilized by heat. All materials used
in making the cultures and the mediums placed in the hoods were
sterilized immediately before.
   "The agar was melted in the autoclave at several pounds'
pressure and was cooled to about 40 degrees C before inoculations
were made in it. ...".

SERIAL DILUTION CULTURE DETAILS 38R5
   After mixing the contents of the first tube by means of a
pipet, without bubbling air through the medium, 2 cc was
transferred to the next tube, like transfers of 2cc each were
made in succession to 6 other tubes, and then 0.2 cc were
transferred successively to each of 5 additional tubes, so the
last tube represented a dilution of 10^{-20} from the original
inoculum.

SERIAL DILUTION CULTURE RESULTS 38R5
   Dr. Rosenow reported that "although little or no growth occurs
in the first or second tube, at still higher dilutions growth is
shown. Absence of growth in the low dilutions may be due, it is
thought, to inhibiting substances in the inoculum which are
rendered inactive by serial dilution."

Dr. Rosenow exhibits photographs illustrating this phenomenon
in the cases of equine encephalomyelitis virus, horse acute-
encephalomyelitis, and streptococcus isolated from poliomyelitic
virus, after growth of the streptococcus in chick mash medium.
In all three instances there was diffuse or no growth in the
first two tubes, numerous colonies/growth in the third, and
diminishing numbers from then on.

BACTERIAL GROWTH AT VERY HIGH DILUTIONS, E.G. 10^{-20} [38R5-71]
"I wish to state clearly that I am fully aware of the growth to
be expected from mathematical relationship after successive
tenfold dilutions. Nevertheless, growth has been observed in
dilutions which cannot be explained on this basis. The
significance, if any, of this growth is under investigation."

GROWTH, PHAGE-LYSED CULTURE 38R5-73
"Serial dilution cultures in dextrose-brain agar were made in
18 freshly phage-lysed cultures, representing 3 staphylococcus
phages and one each of Bacillus coli, Bacillus aerogenes,
Bacillus subtilis and B. Friedländer A and B. Growth that was
characteristic of the organisms lysed by phage was obtained in 17
of 18 dilution cultures."

BEYOND THE "WELL ESTABLISHED LAWS OF DILUTION" 38R5
GROWTH OF BACTERIA FROM VIRUS AND PHAGE-LYSED CULTURES 38R5
"By use of the serial dilution culture method with a dextrose-
brain agar and dextrose-brain broth it has been found that growth
of bacteria can occur from the so-called bacteria-free viruses
and phage-lysed cultures after these have been submitted to high
dilution. This is true even when low dilutions and cultures in
ordinary mediums remain sterile. The number of colonies in the
dextrose-brain agar was not in proportion to the well established
laws of dilution. Viruses and phage-lysed cultures and cultures
in chick-mash medium of streptococci isolated from viruses often
yielded pure cultures in dilutions so high as to exclude the
possibility of growth from stainable, visible organisms
originally present as such."

RECIPES: DEXTROSE-BRAIN BROTH/DEXTROSE-BRAIN AGAR 39R1
"The media were prepared from dehydrated broth or meat extract
and peptone in the usual concentrations, to which 0.2 percent
dextrose and 0.1 percent decolorized fuchsin (Andrade's
indicator) (and in the case of agar, 0.25 percent agar) were
added. The reaction was adjusted to pH 7.0. Approx. 18cc of the
media were placed in tall tubes (20 x 1.5 cm.) and to each tube
two or three pieces of fresh calf brain, a total of about 3cc in
volume, were added before autoclaving (20 pounds for 20 minutes).
The inoculated mediums are incubated at 35 degrees C. overnight.
If the primary dextrose-brain broth and dextrose-brain agar
tubes are free from gas, and if smears disclose the presence of a
pure culture f large streptococci of uniform size, in short
chains, or a great preponderance of streptococci, the culture may

be considered satisfactory for the preparation of an autogenous
vaccine. The supernatant growth ...

GLYCEROL SALT MENSTRUUM 39R1
STOCK VACCINES; ADVANTAGES 39R1
   "The supernatant growth is centrifuged and the sediment
suspended in the glycerol-salt solution. The growth from 15 cc
of broth is suspended in about 0.1 cc of the menstruum. Larger
amounts of sediment are made more concentrated. The longer these
strains are kept in the glycerol-salt solution the less toxic
the vaccine is and for this reason stock vaccines often are more
useful than autogenous vaccines. These stock vaccines can be
prepared by pooling suspensions that may remain after autogenous
vaccines have been prepared for individual cases.

VACCINES, AUTOGENOUS INSTRUCTIONS 39R1
   "Autogenous vaccines are made by diluting the glycerol-salt
solution suspension in sodium chloride solution to the density of
a dextrose-brain broth culture (approximately 2 billion organisms
per cc) and heating the diluted suspension at 70 or 75 degrees C
for an hour. ...

VACCINE DOSAGE - VARIOUS DISEASES 39R1
In most diseases such as ulcer of the stomach, chronic sinusitis,
encephalitis, spasmodic torticollis, chronic poliomyelitis,
amyotrophic lateral sclerosis and multiple sclerosis, the
respective vaccines are used undiluted, or diluted 1 to 10 in
salt solution to which 0.2 percent phenol was added. For cases of
chronic infectious arthritis, iritis and other diseases of the
eye, chronic myositis, dermatomyositis, neurofibromyositis and
bronchial asthma, the vaccines are diluted routinely 1 to 100,
and for cases of myasthenia gravis, 1 to 1000 or as high as 1 to
100,000. Routinely, for adults 0.1 cc is injected subcutaneously
for the first dose.

VACCINE ADMINISTRATION, REACTIONS 39R1
   It is important that all vaccines be injected immediately
beneath the skin, preferably in the relatively insensitive area
of the arm between biceps and triceps. If an untoward reaction
does not occur the dose is increased by 0.1 cc twice weekly until
1 cc is reached, when 1 cc is given weekly for an indefinite
period, depending on results obtained. The reaction of the
patient, however, should be the chief guide to dosage rather than
the prescribed schedule. the aim should be to keep the dose
small enough that increased tolerance to the vaccine is obtained.
   If this is accomplished clinical improvement usually occurs. If
tolerance is not increased, or if sensitivity to the vaccine is
increased and improvement does not occur, the dose, regardless of
the amount in cc, may be considered to be too large and should be
reduced even a hundred or thousand fold, if need be, and then
gradually increased. If a given dose is followed by favorable
results, this dose may be repeated a number of times before the

amount is increased. Subcutaneous lumps should be avoided. Their occurrence is indicative of increasing sensitivity instead of increased tolerance."

DENTAL CARIES & MODERNIZATION 40R3-260-1
  Dr. Weston A. Price served as honorary chairman of the "Oral Diagnosis and Bacteriology Section for Dental Centenary Celebration (260-1); his introductory comments, preceding a major presentation by Dr. E.C. Rosenow, addressed the subject of the modern diet as cause of the advent of dental caries in primitive races:
  "In my studies among primitive races in various parts of the world ..., I have found many isolated groups where less than one percent of the teeth in a community have been attacked by dental caries. ... [However,] the immunity to dental caries was lost when they changed their nutrition ... to the foods of modern commerce of the white man. White flour and sugar constituted the principal displacing factors. ... The exposure of the dental pulps by caries provided bacterial access to the interior of the fortress and serious systemic involvements developed from focal infection of dental origin."

EXPERIMENTAL EVIDENCE, ETIOLOGICAL ROLE OF PULPLESS TEETH 40R3
"Barnes and Giordano have isolated from [pulpless teeth], after death of the patients, streptococci with which they reproduced in animals the disease from which the patient died. I have had similar results." Dr. Rosenow illustrated with the case of a patient who died of pulmonary embolism, from whom the same "usual green-producing Streptococcus" was isolated from both embolus and a pulpless tooth normal in roentgenogram, which streptococcus from both sources reproduced pulmonary embolism when injected in rabbits and dogs. 40R3-264

PULPLESS TEETH: THE INSOLUBLE PROBLEM OF APICAL ENDS 40R3-265
Specific mention was made of three supporting studies, one in which 89% of 100 pulpless teeth and 4% of vital teeth yielded streptococci, a second in which the number of colonies from the apexes of pulpless teeth was 700 to 1000 times greater than the number obtained from identically treated vital teeth, and a third in which 96% of 1220 root-filled pulpless teeth and 98% of 582 non-root-filled pulpless teeth yielded a growth, chiefly green-producing streptococci.

"BLOOD-BUILDING TISSUES": AIDS? 40R3-271
TRIGEMINAL NEURALGIA, PRESENCE OF FOCI CONSTANT IN 40R3-271
"The lesions most frequently seen in patients referable to focal infection are those of the locomotor system, joints, muscles, tendon sheaths and ligaments. The kidney, skin, heart, stomach, duodenum and eyes are often affected. Less commonly, other organs such as those of the nervous system and blood-building tissues may be involved. Rarely, very unusual localizations of streptococci from dental and other foci of infection such as

onychia occurred as shown by Haden and Jordan, thyroid disease (especially thyroiditis) as shown by Cantero and lesions of the gasserian ganglion produced electively in experiments of my own in cases of trigeminal neuralgia. The removal of foci in instances of trigeminal neuralgia (and in my experience their presence is constant in this condition) obviously should be done as a preventive measure ... ." 40R3-271

EXPERIMENTAL ENCEPHALITIS FROM STREPTOCOCCUS 40R3-271
"Van Kirk and Swanson [J.Dent. Res., Sept. 1935 15, 315-316] produced encephalitis in rabbits by the intravenous injection of streptococci obtained from the pulpless teeth from patients who had encephalitis, an observation corroborative of our own studies." 40R3-271

TOXINS AND STREPTOCOCCI   40R3-271
"... streptococci that manifest elective localizing power have been shown to produce within themselves, and to free in dextrose-brain broth cultures, poisons or toxic products which specifically localize and produce lesions in the same tissues as do the living microorganisms. Specific effects have been produced by the intravenous or intracerebral injection, respectively, of the living streptococci, the dead bacteria or filtrates of active cultures obtained from patients suffering from pyelonephritis, myositis, endocarditis, myocarditis, arthritis, dental neuritis and pulpitis, ulcer of the stomach or duodenum and myasthenia gravis." 40R3-271

SLOWING ACTION OF CONVALESCENT SERUM ON STREPTOCOCCI 40R3-275
[While Rosenow characterized this as "charge-reducing", this might also be viewed as a function of size; i.e., a case may be made for the effect of the serum being one of causing the organisms to agglutinate or otherwise become larger thus slower.] 40R3-275

BEYOND KOCH: ROSENOW'S SIX TYPES PROOF OF ETIOLOGY[40R3-277]
1. IV, other injection in animals [FULFILLED KOCH] (Table 2.1)
2. induction with streptococci of foci in teeth in dogs (see APPENDIX B1: Cook 1931, Jones & Newsom 1932, Welsch per Morse 1977; and APPENDIX A1: 22R3, 23R10, 26R4.
3. cataphoretic studies (see APPENDIX A2: 33R7)
4. diagnostic cutaneous tests w/euglobulin of horse serum (see APPENDIX A1: 52R3, 57R1).
5. precipitation reaction with blood serum and antiserum (see APPENDIX A1: 42R2, p. 342).
6. agglutination tests (see APPENDIX A1: 42R2, p. 352).

INTRAMUSCULAR INJECTION; DOES NOT PRODUCE FOCUS [40R3]
"Injection of bacteria into soft tissues does not suffice to produce a chronic focus from which bacteria and their products are continually disseminated. Prompt healing ... , unless the micro-organisms are highly virulent, usually occurs... ." 40R3

ODOR; BAD BREATH & HEART DISEASE 40R3
  Dr. Rosenow noted that during a visit with a large European
clinic, "the chief himself had been ill in bed suffering from an
unexplained fever for some time prior to my visit. It was
clearly evident that his condition was an example of the very
problem under discussion. His teeth were literally floating in
pockets of pus arising from pyorrhea and his breath was
malodorous. He died several years later, long before he should
have died, from cardiac disease."

ETIOLOGICAL IMPORT. OF NON-VITAL OR DISEASED VITAL TEETH 40R3
    The insidious nature of pulpless teeth: "The [oral] focus
affords ready entrance of bacteria and their toxic products which
may, depending on inherited or acquired predispositions or other
factors, cause infection in remote tissues, general ill effects,
hypersensitiveness or allergy or a combination of some or all of
these in the same persons, or perhaps at times increased
resistance and immunity.
  "The localizing and necrotizing power peculiar to these
organisms (usually streptococci) determines largely the site or
tissues to be affected. ... The common practice of waiting
until the disease is far advanced or until a serious condition,
such as a hemorrhage in ulcer or a cardiac attack in heart
disease, has developed, or until advanced age has occurred before
evident foci, especially pulpless teeth are removed, is most
deplorable." [40R3]

RELATION OF FOCI OF INFECTION TO HYPERSENSITIV. & ALLERGY 40R3
  Dr. Rosenow here reviews the works of several investigators
relating focal infection to allergic states, and bacterial
allergy as a factor in various diseases. "Might not the
inherited rheumatic diathesis, the neuropathic or the allergic
constitution and other 'diatheses' and 'constitutional
predispositions' be expressions in part of a peculiar interaction
between host and invading organism, and not expressions merely of
an inherited 'weakness' of joint, brain or other organ, as is
usually assumed?" 40R3

POLIO - ELECTRON MICROSCOPE, NATURAL & ARTIFICIAL VIRUS [42R1]
  Comparable forms were found in filtrates of both natural
poliomyelitis virus and artificial polio virus derived from
streptococci, and from chick-mash culture of the streptococcus
from poliomyelitis, but not in controls: "Microdiplococci,
sometimes in short chains, of varying size and opacity, were
found in each of the filtrates made of natural poliomyelitis
virus, of poliomyelitic virus derived from streptococci, and of
the chick-mash culture of the streptococcus from poliomyelitis.
Exceedingly small ovoid and diplococcal forms and short chains of
small diplococci, some too small to photograph, were seen. The
smallest forms seen resembling organisms approximated the
postulated size of the virus particle. Some large forms

seemingly were breaking into small diplococci similar to those
seen in certain cultures of the streptococcus." ... p. 101: "The
films directly from the formalinized cultures in dextrose-brain
broth revealed, in addition to the large organisms, numerous
exceedingly small, elongated oval or diplococcal forms projecting
radially from the margins, with few or no free forms. ... The
location, radial orientation, number and uniformity of size and
shape of these 'midget' forms suggest that they are dispersions
of the large organisms and not artifacts. ... this might be a
reason for occurrence of growth ... in [extreme] serial dilution
cultures ..."

DEXTROSE BRAIN BROTH, pH 7.2, 44R1-151
  "The dextrose-brain broth as used in this study consisted of
ordinary 0.2 percent dextrose broth adjusted to pH 7.2, and the
soft dextrose-brain agar also used likewise consisted of 0.2
percent dextrose broth containing 0.2 percent agar, to both of
which approximately one part of pieces of fresh calf brain to six
or seven parts of medium in tall (10 cm.) columns was added
before autoclaving.

SUBMICROSCOPIC IMPLICATION OF SERIAL DILUTION SUCCESS   44R1
  "In the serial dilution cultures transfers were made alternately
in tubes containing 20 cc. of dextrose brain broth and dextrose
brain agar at intervals of 10 to 12 seconds with a nichrome wire
to which there adhered approximately 2 cu mm of liquid, making a
dilution of 1:10,000 at each transfer. The transferring wire was
thoroughly agitated in the mediums at each transfer and was
sterilized only before and after the first transfer. In serial
dilution cultures made in this way the growth of pathogenic
streptococci that occurs at dilutions far beyond what would be
possible from mathematical calculations, considering the
streptococcus as an inert particle, may be due to differential
adhesion to the transferring wire or to dispersion or synthesis
of submicroscopic components of the streptococcus. It has thus
far been impossible to determine the relative importance of these
three factors." [44R1, p. 151]
  [Note: Later work involved sterilization of wire at each
transfer and did not specifically discuss "impossible" aspect]

POLIO; ROSENOW RESPONDS 44R3
  In 1944 Dr. Rosenow specifically addressed the "apparent
inability" of some other investigators [including Sabin and
Olitsky 1936 to confirm his findings concerning the role of a
streptococcus in poliomyelitis, noting that tissue cultures
favorable for the cultivation of viruses "are not suitable for
primary isolations of the highly specific streptococcus ... from
material containing virus. Dr. Rosenow notes and cites the
corroborating results of those who did use his methods
consistently, and asserted "The discrepancies and the claimed
inability of some [including Olitsky etal., JAMA 1929, 92, 1725]
to isolate or demonstrate the streptococcus and to obtain

evidence of its specificity in accord with my results may truly be said to be due to differences in concept leading to inadequate attempts, to differences in methods, to dearth of experiment or to misinterpretation of results.

"By the use of autoclaved dextrose-brain broth and soft dextrose-brain agar in tall tubes [as per Arch Path.. 1938, 26, 70] this same type of streptococcus has since [initial 1916 studies] been isolated consistently from the very tissues, fluids or other material in which virus has been demonstrated most often, such as nasopharynx, tonsils, stool, cerebrospinal fluid, brain and spinal cord. This has been done in altogether 37 widely separated rural or urban epidemics and 7 institutional outbreaks of poliomyelitis, and from cerebrospinal fluid or brain and spinal cord of more than 400 monkeys that had succumbed to poliomyelitis following inoculation of many different strains of virus. ...

"The streptococcus, while of low general virulence, was found to have specific affinity for the anterior horns of the spinal cord on appropriate inoculation, producing as the outstanding manifestation flaccid paralysis in guinea pigs, rabbits and monkeys - a property that is lost promptly on aerobic cultivation, and which was not found of similar streptococci isolated in studies of other diseases.

"Relation of the streptococcus and virus was further indicated during experiments in which viability of streptococcus and virus ran closely parallel for as long as 5 years in glycerolated brain and cord tissue of persons and monkeys that had succumbed to poliomyelitis."

Dr. Rosenow summarized results of treatment by him, co-workers and other physicians, with "poliomyelitis antistreptococcic serum", whereby there were 9.5% deaths out of 2664 total treated; versus 21.3% deaths in 2737 controls, patients not treated with serum during the same epidemics. In followup on 2256 of the surviving patients, 10.4% of 1716 treated patients suffered severe residual paralysis; versus 33% of controls.

"The results of these studies, summarised all too briefly here, indicate that the inciting agent of poliomyelitis represents interrelated phases of the streptococcus and what is now considered virus, that the streptococcus plays the primary role in the causation of the disease, occurrence of epidemics and immunity, and that the virus is the small, filtrable, highly invasive, relatively non-antigenic phase of the streptococcus." [44R3: The Lancet Poliomyelitis, Studies on the inciting agent ...]

This belief that the filtrable phase of the organism was "relatively non-antigenic" is of course brought sharply into question by the apparent use of such phase in the production of prophylactic vaccines by Salk and Sabin a decade later.

HIDDEN FOCI IN X-RAY NEGATIVE VITAL TEETH   [44R8]
Dr. Rosenow provided thorough details of an illustrative case in which "x-ray negative vital teeth having large restorations

were a local and systemic source or focus of infection." [44R8]

VITAL TEETH FREE FROM CARIES ARE STERILE   44R8-329
"Intact vital teeth, free from caries or fillings, which had been removed in a sterile manner, have been shown to be essentially sterile." (3 references given: L.T. Austin and T.J. Cook 1929, A.T. Henrici and T.B. Hartzell 1919, and Ruth Tunnicliff and Carolyn Hammond 1937)   44R8-329

PULPLESS TEETH MUST GO: 8 SUPPORTING REFERENCES [44R8-329]
FILLED, VITAL, ROENTGENO.-NEGATIVE TEETH, INFECTION IN   44R8
   "Pulpless teeth, irrespective of whether they gave roentgenographic evidence of changes, have proved to harbor specific types of streptococci [which] on injection into animals, tend to localize and produce disease resembling that of the patient". 44R8-329

FOUL BREATH RELIEVED BY REMOVAL OF FOCI   44R8-332
   Case report: Following removal of 6 teeth containing small to large fillings, episodes of neuromuscular pains and fatigability, persistent foul breath, and a dull aching pain in the mandible were relieved. 44R8

PREPARATION OF ANTIBODY, WITH ASSIST FROM LINUS PAULING   45R4
   Dr. Rosenow's work on thermal production of antibodies "was stimulated by the production in vitro of pneumococcus antibodies by Pauling and Campbell from specific polysaccharide and beef globulin [Pauling L and Campbell D, 1942, J. Exper. Med. 76:211], and by the demonstration of auto-antigen and auto-antibody in the eggs of keyhole limpets and sea urchins by Tyler [Tyler, A, 1942, West. J. Surg. 50:126.]   [45R4]
Beyond the finding that antibodies may be produced from streptococci by heat, "The appearance of agglutinins in supernatants of suspensions of streptococci that had been heated at body temperature for 10 days and their progressively earlier appearance in greater titer with increasing temperatures may be considered as evidence in favor of treatment of certain diseases or conditions by the artificial application of heat, as is now so frequently done." [45R4]

STREPTOCOCCUS V.S. VIRUS IN COMMON COLD AND INFLUENZA   [45R5]
   Notwithstanding the common presence of virus in acute respiratory infections, Dr. Rosenow noted the likewise common association of organisms of the pneumococcus-streptococcus group with more serious manifestations and death in these diseases. Rosenow asserted that the streptococci are not secondary invaders, but rather that "The data obtained indicate that the streptococci isolated in this study had etiologic relationship to seasonal epidemic respiratory infections, including influenza, the common cold, influenzal bronchopneumonia and so-called virus pneumonia." [45R5] The characterization of streptococcus and virus as two phases of a single organism is discussed elsewhere

(e.g. 34R3; 38R2; 44R3; 53R2).

WATER: OCCURRENCE OF PATHOGENIC STREPTOCOCCI IN 45R7
     In water: Dr. Rosenow found a striking "parallel occurrence
of streptococci in unpotable water and raw water supplies and in
the throats of widely separated ill and well persons during
epidemics" in contrast to "normal types of streptococci remote
from epidemics". The possibility of contaminated water
contributing to an epidemic is discussed. [45R7]

PREP. OF "THERMAL" ANTIBODY 47R1-219
  "The antibodies prepared with heat alone had extreme avidity
for particulate matter and were not filtrable. Those prepared
with H2O2 and heat passed through fritted glass, diatomaceous
earth and Seitz filters with little or no loss of titer. They
were slowly dialyzable through cellophane against running water
and running isotonic solutions of sodium chloride, were
distillable on boiling, and were demonstrable in high titer in
solutions of the dry residue." [47R1, p. 219]
     See also 48R3 for additional details.

MENTAL ILLNESS SERIES - CONTENTS
   Rosenow in 1947-8 [47R2, 48R1, 48R2] published a three-part
series on schizophrenia:
     47R2: I.-Methods and material
    -Results of cultures
    -Results of agglutination and precipitation experiments
     48R1: II. -Effects in animals following inoculation of alpha
streptococci
     -Methods
     -Results of cultures
     -Experiments with rabbits
          "   "   mice
     -Illustrative protocols
     48R2: III.-Cutaneous reactions to intradermal injection of
streptococcal antibody and antigen
     -Methods
     -Results
     -Cutaneous reactions in relation to therapeutic injections of
thermal antibody and to electro-shock

CONFIRMING STUDIES USING SAME METHODS, LIST OF 15 [48R1-125]
--1. Haden RL, Dental Infection and Systemic Diseases, Phila.:
Lea and Febiger, 1928, 165.
--2. Barnes AR & AS Giordano, J.Indiana Med.Ass. 15: 1-7, 1932.
--3. Nickel AC and AR Hufford, Arch.Int.Med. 41: 210-230, 1928;
Nickel AC, Staff Meetings of the Mayo Clinic, Vol. 3 Aug. 8,
1928)232-5; Nickel AC and WW Sager, ibid, Oct. 10, 1928, 297-9.
--4. Cooper ML, Tr.Am.Pediat.Soc. 43:32-33, 1931.
--5. Jarlov, E. and Brinch, O., Hospitalstid 81:80-5, 1938.
--6. Welsh AL, Arch.Derm.&Syph. 30:611-629, 1934.
--7.   "   " , J.Invest.Dermat. 7:7-42, 1946.

--8. Meisser JG & BS Gardner, <u>J.Nat.Dental Assn.</u>19:578-592,1922.
--9. Cook TJ, <u>J.Amer.Dent.A.</u> 18, 2290-2301, 1931
--10. Bernhardt H, <u>Z.f.Klin.Med.</u> 117:158-174, 1931.
--11. Irons EE, etal, <u>J.Inf.Dis.</u> 18:315-334, 1916.
--12. Kelley TH, <u>Ohio State MJ</u> 14:221-223, 1918.
--13. Topley WWC, and HB Weir, <u>J.Path.& Bact.</u> 24:333-346, 1921.
--14. Wilkie DPD, <u>Brit.J.J.</u> 1:481-4, 1928.
--15. Jones NW & SJ Newsom, <u>Arch.Path.</u> 13:392-414, 1932.

TIME OF REACTIONS TO ANTIBODY (IMMED) VS ANTIGEN (SLOWER) 48R2
"The erythema at the site of injection of antibody occurred
almost immediately and reached its maximum in a few minutes,
while the flare to injections of antigen, if it occurred at all,
occurred more slowly and reached its maximum in 5-10 minutes.
Both reactions occurred without itching or formation of
pseudopodia, differing in these respects from reactions due to
injection of histamine or of antigen to which persons are
allergic." 48R2-368

AUTOIMMUNITY AS POSSIBLY INVOLVED IN MS 48R3-291-2
"The evidence adduced indicates that fatalities in the
experimental and naturally occurring disease, in the absence of
living streptococci, may be due to the formation of a
streptococcic neurotoxin having predilection for vital nerve
centers, and to which vital centers become allergic, and perhaps
to the formation of an autogenous sensitizing streptococcal-
nerve-tissue complex which may function in a manner similar to
the wholly foreign adjuvant-nerve-tissue complexes used
successfully by others in the production of 'allergic'
encephalomyelitis." 48R3

ADMINISTRATION OF ANTIBODY FOR POLIOMYELITIS [48R4-274]
   Thermal antibody was prepared from very dense suspensions of
streptococci, approx 1000 billion organisms per ml (or the growth
from 500ml of dextrose broth) in glycerol 2 parts and saturated
NaCl solution 1 part, kept at 10 degrees C.
   "Two types of artificial antibody were used ... . One was
prepared by autoclaving at 17 lbs pressure, NaCl solution
suspensions containing 20 billion streptococci per ml. for 96
hours, the other by autoclaving suspensions containing 10 billion
streptococci per ml. but for 1 to 3 hours after adding 1.5
percent H_2O_2." The former was routinely used for cutaneous test
after being diluted with an equal volume of NaCl solution
containing 0.4% phenol. However, as noted above (47R1) the
antibodies prepared with heat alone had extreme avidity for
particulate matter and were not filtrable, whereas those prepared
with heat and peroxide passed through filters with little or no
loss of titer.
   We may note that in the treatment of acute poliomyelitis, Dr.
Rosenow used relatively large, single applications of large
quantities of antibody, as compared to his work a decade later
with multiple sclerosis, wherein repeated smaller doses were

used:

" ... Only one therapeutic, intramuscular, or subcutaneous injection of artificial antibody was given to each patient. This usually consisted of 2 ml. of the solution of antibody from 5 billion streptococci for children 5 years of age or younger and two additional milliliter for each additional year of age up to 21 years. A truly remarkable diminution of antigen and increase in antibody uniformly occurred in from one to three hours after the injection and remained at low and high level respectively for 24 or 48 hours or longer. control injection of NaCl solution had no apparent effect. ... Of the 26 patients each receiving one therapeutic injection of the 'poliomyelitic' streptococcal antibody, 19 showed clinical improvement ... . No clinical change attributable to the injection of antibody occurred in seven ..." [48R4-274]

PREPARATION OF ANTIBODY FOR CUTANEOUS TESTS, TREATMENT 48R5

"The thermal antibody for cutaneous tests and for treatment was prepared by diluting glycerine-NaCl streptococcal suspensions with isotonic saline to a concentration of 20 billion cells per ml. These cells ... were then autoclaved at 17 lbs for 96 hours. The resulting bacteria-free supernate was diluted with equal volume of sterile isotonic saline solution containing a phenol preservative. Artificial antibody used therapeutically was [also] prepared by autoclaving NaCl-solution suspensions containing 10 billion streptococci per ml., by diluting the respective dense suspensions in glycerol-NaCl-solution 100 fold and autoclaving for three hours [at 17 lbs. pressure; per 54R1] after adding 1.5 percent H_2O_2. [48R5, p. 489]

DESCRIPTION, REINJECTION OF "THERMAL" ANTIBODY   48R5-489

"...The slightly opalescent solution, containing the sharply agglutinated remnants of the organisms thus obtained, was brought to pH 6.8 [7.0 per 54R1], diluted 1 to 5 with NaCl-solution, and from 2 to 10 ml of such dilution were injected subcutaneously or intramuscularly in treatment." [48R5, p. 489]

DEXTROSE-BRAIN BROTH MEDIUM 50R1

--"When grown aerobically in the usual manner on solid mediums and in liquid mediums such as dextrose broth in which acid is produced, specific properties often disappeared promptly, and isolations of respective specific strains in these mediums usually were unsuccessful. [50R1]

CHICK EMBRYO MEDIUM - OLD CULTURES YIELD FILTRABLE AGENTS 50R1

Autoclaved chick embryo infusion was found (a) to "not turn acid from growth of streptococci", (b) "to be highly favorable for rapid growth and maintenance for a very long time of viability of streptococci."; and (c) "As cultures in this medium became old, extremely small and filtrable forms of the streptococci appeared, and in some instances, filtrable transmissible agents resembling in their effects in animals those of the respective viruses were demonstrated. Moreover, on prolonged storage of cultures in this medium at room temperature or in the incubator, changes in agglutinative titer and in virulence were found to occur seasonally in accord with the streptococci isolated in studies of current epidemics of poliomyelitis, encephalitis, and respiratory infection."-117

SUBMICRO. FORMS CHANGE VIRULENCE IN CHICK EMBRYO MEDIUM 50R1
   "When specific strains, isolated in mediums affording a reduced or gradient of oxygen tension were grown in sealed tubes of blood-agar slants, they often remained viable for years due to high concentration of carbon dioxide, retained original serologic properties, but lost animal virulence.
   "When grown for 24 hours at 34 degrees C and then stored in the dark at room temperature in tall columns of autoclaved chick embryo medium layered with oil, the respective streptococci remained viable for years, small filtrable and 'virus' forms sometimes developed, and changes in serologic and localizing properties or virulence occurred in accord with alpha streptococci associated with or the cause of current seasonal epidemics [poliomyelitis, encephalitis, and respiratory infection].
   "Alpha streptococci that possessed properties characteristic of streptococci associated with or the cause of epidemic diseases [were] ... demonstrated not only in persons stricken, contacts and non-contacts during respective epidemics, but also broadly in nature such as in water, milk, flies, mosquitoes, and indoor and outdoor air during epidemics. ...
   "The data adduced indicate that some atmospheric influence in temperate climes may be operative ...
   "The parallelism between the seasonal in vitro changes and those which occurred in human beings and in nature in accord with epidemics reported herewith was so striking ... as to leave little doubt as to the importance ... in pathogenesis and hence control of the respective epidemic diseases."
   In that Rosenow had been able to induce changes in cataphoretic velocity and virulence of streptococci by exposing cultures to high frequency radiation, and others had produced mutations or dissociations in bacteria and viruses on exposure to radiation, this suggested "that the influence causing the changes in streptococci may be some form of radiant energy."

SIMILAR ORGANISM, DIFFERENT DISEASE 50R1
   Dr. Rosenow repeatedly emphasized that the alpha streptococcus isolated by special methods "in studies of epidemic poliomyelitis, encephalitis, hiccup, MS, and respiratory infections ..., while morphologically and culturally indistinguishable, were found highly specific serologically and in localizing and disease-producing properties.[50R1]

CHICK EMBRYO MEDIUM RECIPE 50R1-117
"The chick-embryo medium consisted of the mash (1 part), obtained

by passing through a meat chopper 19-day hatching chick-eggs, including the shell, and distilled water (7 parts)", refrigerated for 24 hours, stirred at intervals, placed in tall columns or bottles and autoclaved at 17-lb. pressure for 20 minutes." 50R1 ["and then layered with sterile liquid petrolatum." (35R5)]

In contrast to cultures preserved in dense glycerine (2-parts)-saturated NaCl solution (1-part), which retained their specificity over periods of years, the chick-embryo-stored cultures assumed characteristics of current epidemics, e.g., polio or influenza and epidemic hiccup as evidenced by experiments with inoculated animals and agglutination tests.

CONTACT, AERIAL INFECTION MAY PLAY MINOR ROLE IN EPIDEMIC 50R3
RADIANT ENERGY CAUSES SEASONAL CHANGE IN STREPTOCOCCI 50R3
NEUROTROPIC (POLIOMYELITIS) VS PNEUMOTROPIC (INFLUENZA) 50R3

The thesis that radiant energy causes seasonal changes in indigenous streptococci which relate to disease epidemics was tested in three long-lasting storage experiments, in which "neurotropic" (from poliomyelitis) and "pneumotropic" (from influenza) streptococci were stored in a mine 5000 feet under limestone and compared with samples stored at ground level where they would be exposed to solar radiation and also in a lead-lined safe where they would not. Dr. Rosenow found that the samples exposed to radiation changed properties seasonally, as indicated by measurements of cataphoretic velocity, but that samples shielded from solar radiation did not change.

"It is postulated that the seasonal changes which occurred at ground level in these organisms and therefore presumably in persons and in nature during respective epidemics were due to a physical agent, radiant energy, which probably comes from the sun, capable of passing through thin sheets of glass and metal but not through one inch of lead and hence not due to the highly penetrating cosmic radiation. ...

"If such influence be really operative in nature the seasonal incidence of epidemics, especially epidemics such as influenza and poliomyelitis that often occur almost simultaneously over vast and isolated regions, becomes more inexplicable in that such epidemics arise owing to seasonal changes in temperate climates in streptococci indigenous in the subjects and in nature and that aerial and contact infection may play a minor role. Active and passive immunization with respective harmless specific vaccines, antigens, antiserums, or thermal antibody in advance of or abreast with anticipated seasonal recurrent epidemics may prove necessary in addition to the usual measures now directed for their control." [50R3]

PARALLEL PRODUCTION: ALTERED STREPTOCOCCI/FILTRABLE FORMS 51R2

Dr. Rosenow also reported the genesis of the respective pneumotropic and neurotropic filtrable phases "from a streptococcus initially having high pneumotropic virulence, as isolated from outdoor air in winter during a severe epidemic of influenza", which was transformed into a streptococcus having high neurotropic virulence" as isolated six months later in summer from a chick-embryo culture that had been stored in the dark at room temperature".

The data indicated that seasonal epidemics of respiratory infections in winter and nervous system diseases in summer "may be attributable in part to changes in the indigenous streptococcal flora in the throats and respiratory tracts of human beings and in outdoor air, which for reasons still obscure tends to acquire pneumotropic properties in temperate climates in winter and neurotropic properties in summer and to dissociate into respective filtrable phases or viruses."

PHASAL NATURE OF STREPTOCOCCUS, VIRUS; SUPPORTING STUDIES 51R3

"... The experimental production of dwarf and filtrable forms from staphylococci and B. proteus by Tulasne (Nature 161:316,1948; 164:887-7, 1949), the observations on the importance of a non-hemolytic streptococcus in atypical or virus pneumonia (by L Thomas etal., J.Clin.Investig.,24:227, 1945], and the climatic changes of races of Achillea (Clausen J, etal, Carnegie Inst. Publ. 581, 1948) are in accord with such concept." [that virus and streptococcus are phases of the same organism in poliomyelitis] [51R3]

AIR: SPREAD OF VIRULENT STREPT. IN 51R3

In air: Dr. Rosenow reported that "The parallelism in cultural characteristics, type of virulence or elective localizing and agglutinative properties of the streptococci isolated seasonally from outdoor air and those isolated from persons ill during respective epidemics was most striking." ... "Their virulence, with few exceptions, was less than corresponding streptococci isolated from persons ill during current epidemics but was roughly proportional to the severity of current infections especially infections of the respiratory tract." He offers "that the respective streptococci in outdoor air may in part be derived from 'human' sources", and may in any case "be responsible in part for the widespread occurrence of epidemics" of these diseases. [51R3]

PENICILLIN, SULFADIAZINE FAIL IN EPIDEMIC INFLUENZA 51R4-609

Dr. Rosenow noted a lack of effect of penicillin, streptomycin or aureomycin on nonhemolytic streptococci and staphylococcus aureus in cases of epidemic influenza, i.e., "In the case of penicillin, 200,000 u/ml. of solution had less bactericidal action on the 'pneumotropic' non-hemolytic streptococci and on staphylococcus aureus than 0.2 units per ml of solution had on D. pneumoniae nd hemolytic streptococci."

SERIAL DILUTION METHOD [51R4, p. 616]

--"... the wire used in making the serial dilutions was sterilized in a Bunsen flame between transfers. Streptococci outgrew Gram-negative gas-forming bacilli and Gram-positive bacilli and micrococci in low serial dilutions in dextrose-brain broth, and pure cultures of streptococci nearly always grew at the end-point of growth. Non-hemolytic streptococci usually grew in this medium at dilutions of 10^{-5} and sometimes at 10^{-9} even after standard pasteurization. This indicated that the streptococci concerned were highly resistant to heat." [51R4,616]

COMPULSIVE VIOLENCE AS DISEASE 51R5
   In 1951 Dr. Rosenow offered "evidence that highly specific neurotropic toxins or poisons produced by a non-apparent type of streptococcal infection in nasopharynx or elsewhere may be responsible for the abnormal compulsions that characterize the behavior and acts of criminally inclined persons."
   "The idea that a specific type of streptococcal infection or intoxication might in some way be causative of morbid or perverted compulsions in human beings criminally inclined did not occur to us until an unexpected reaction occurred to the control antibody in the following experiment: It was found that highly nervous prisoners who had intercurrent respiratory infection, ulcer of the stomach, myositis or arthritis reacted specifically to the respective streptococcal thermal antibodies and reacted more to the 'neurotropic' streptococcal thermal antibody prepared from streptococci isolated in studies of chronic encephalitis injected as a control than did persons from outside who were ill with these same diseases but who were normal in behavior and other respects. It was this clue that led to a study of criminals from a bacteriologic standpoint."
   "The streptococcus isolated, while morphologically and culturally similar to streptococci present normally in nasopharynx of well persons and persons having other diseases, was found to possess certain specific properties. On isolation from the end point of growth of serial dilution cultures in dextrose-brain broth it tended to localize in the brain of mice on intravenous injection. On cerebral inoculation it produced in significant incidence changes in behavior which in some respects simulated those characteristic of incorrigible prisoners.
   "... These consisted of severe tremors and excitation, hyperirritability, dashing about wildly, jumping up at the wall of the cage at repeated intervals, burying the head in bedding on the floor or under other mice and dashing over the huddle of more normal mice. Others walked slowly about in a dazed manner."
   "... Moreover, reactions to antibody in prisoners were greater in winter than in summer, paralleling the seasonal incidence of admissions to the Ohio Penitentiary and the seasonal incidence of crime according to the FBI.
   "... The studies reported previously in Sydenham's chorea, epidemic hiccup, spasmodic torticollis, respiratory arrhythmia, persistent sneezing and convulsion, idiopathic epilepsy and schizophrenia and those summarized herein - all conditions characterized by distinctive abnormal behavior patterns - are in accord with the thesis that bacterial infection or intoxication may cause changes in behavior referable to the central nervous system. But these studies go a step farther, for they indicate

that the infections and consequent intoxications are due to
respective highly specific but closely related types of
nonhemolytic streptococci."

Dr. Rosenow concluded with the suggestion "that passive and
active immunization with specific streptococcal antibody and
antigen may prove of value in diagnosis, treatment and prevention
of recurrences of this deplorable state." [51R5]

CRIMINALITY-REACTIONS TO ANTIBODY VS. F.B.I., OHIO STATS-51R5-431
"... reactions to [specific, incorrigible-related antibody in
prisoners were greater in winter than in summer, paralleling the
seasonal incidence of admissions to the Ohio Penitentiary and the
seasonal incidence of crime according to the F.B.I."

VIOLENT CRIMINALITY DUE IN PART TO INFECTION 51R5-432
"The data adduced are tentatively considered to indicate (1) that
incorrigibility, morbid compulsions and other abnormal
behaviorisms which characterize this group of criminally-inclined
persons may be due in part to a specific neurotropic type of
streptococcal infection or intoxication, (2) that cutaneous
reactions to thermal antibodies are diagnostic of such infection
or intoxication" and thus might be used for monitoring or parole
considerations, and "(3) that passive and active immunization
with specific streptococcal antibody and antigen may prove of
value in diagnosis, treatment and prevention of recurrences of
this deplorable state."51R5

SERUM TREATMENT FOR POLIO 52R1-396
Herein Dr. Rosenow discussed previous work involving
antistreptococcic serum prepared in horses, which had been used
somewhat successfully to treat poliomyelitis. In a group of
monkeys inoculated with the virus of the disease, 36 per cent of
those receiving the serum before inoculation died of the disease;
of the control group, 82 percent. In a series of poliomyelitis
patients treated with the serum the mortality rate was 8 per
cent; in a control series, 21 per cent. In a series treated in
all stages of the disease by the author, 10 per cent died; of
those who did not receive the serum, 25 per cent. However, this
serum deteriorates rapidly in storage.

Fortunately, "studies on the production in vitro of antibody
from streptococci and other bacteria have resulted in the
development of non-sensitizing and more stable solutions of heat-
treated antibody from streptococci isolated in studies of a
number of diseases including epidemic poliomyelitis. ... which
appears to prevent paralysis and otherwise mitigate poliomyelitis
and to provide immunization from the disease."

TROPISM: DEAD STREPTOCOCCI VS PHARMAC. ACTION OF DRUGS 52R1
In an attempt to determine the cause of elective localization
of streptococci from poliomyelitis v.s. arthritis, "large numbers
of streptococci of these types were killed by heat and injected
intracerebrally in parallel manner into rhesus monkeys and
rabbits. The results were remarkable. The streptococcus of

poliomyelitis remained in the cerebrospinal fluid and spinal cord, producing great weakness or flaccid paralysis, but no lesions were produced in the muscles or joints ... . The streptococcus of arthritis disappeared promptly from the cerebrospinal fluid and appeared in large numbers in the knee joint fluid ... .   The cause of these examples of specificity or tropism in the dead streptococci is considered similar to or identical with that involved in the well-recognized specific pharmacological action of drugs, chemicals and bacterial toxins."

 Four of the monkeys that had received the dead streptococci of poliomyelitis and two that had received the dead streptococci of arthritis were inoculated intranasally with highly potent poliomyelitis 10 days later. The former four remained well; the latter two developed typical poliomyelitis. [52R1, 398]

 "The clinical and pathologic features of the poliomyelitis caused by the experimentally developed virus were indistinguishable from those caused by the natural virus. Monkeys that recovered from poliomyelitis produced with the experimental virus were found to be immune to natural virus, and vice versa ... "; etc. [52R1, 399]

VIRUS VS FILTRABLE AGENT IN HERPES ZOSTER, MUMPS, ENCEPH. 52R1
 "Proof now appears complete that the virus of poliomyelitis is particulate, spherical or elongated, and grouped in diploid or in short filamentous chain formation, as evidenced in electron micrographs by Loring, Schwerdt and Marton [Physical Rev., 65:354, 1944, "Studies ... of the MV strain..."] and, most convincingly, by Reagan Schenck and Brueckner. [J. Infec. Dis. 86:295-296, 1950, "Morphological observations ... of the Brunhilde strain ..."] The observations of these investigators further strongly suggest that the virus and the streptococcus are related. The recent reports by others of electron micrographs of particles of various sizes, spherical or ovoid and in diploid or short chain formation, in the viruses of herpes zoster, mumps, encephalitis and influenza - the treatment of which remains an unsolved problem - may be taken to indicate that the viruses of these diseases may likewise be related to the respective specific streptococci which the author has isolated by special methods in these diseases and with which the lesions characteristic of the diseases have been reproduced or closely simulated." 52R1-400

ANTIBODY ADMINISTRATION - SUBCUTANEOUS OR INTRAMUSCULAR [52R1]
 It is noted that Dr. Rosenow referred to both intramuscular and subcutaneous administration of antibody in his later articles, in the cases of polio, multiple sclerosis, epilepsy and schizophrenia, and not distinguish between the two types of injection:
     Polio: "... Subcutaneous or intramuscular injection of [thermal (artificial)] antibody in therapeutic amounts in persons with poliomyelitis causes abrupt diminution of antigen and increase in antibody (as determined by reaction to intradermal injections of antibody and antigen); the treatment appears to

prevent paralysis and otherwise affect favorably the clinical course of the disease and, prophylactically used, to prevent transmission within family groups." [52R1 p. 400]

BECOMING OF AGE AT MAYO 52R2-244
"Owing to my becoming of age, these [epilepsy, dementia pr.] and other studies were unavoidably interrupted." 52R2

EPILEPSY, SCHIZOPHRENIA
   Rosenow in 1952 [52R2] (South Dakota M.J., Sept.) reported that a pregnant mouse, which received repeated intracerebral inoculation of the suspected pathogen from a case of epilepsy had remained well, but one of 4 offspring died in an apparent gran mal seizure several weeks after birth. "This occurrence was first considered as perhaps an example of hereditary epilepsy ... a pure culture of the d[suspected pathogenic alpha] streptococcus was isolated from the brain in serial dilution cultures in dextrose-brain broth. The streptococcus from the end point of growth produced spasms in 19 and convulsions in 16 of 22 mice that were repeatedly inoculated intranasally."
   Rosenow [52R2], p. 243, "The recovery from symptoms in nervous states or psychoses following the removal of infected teeth [from which neurotropic alpha streptococci were isolated, which on inoculation in rabbits caused extreme excitation; and the favorable results from the use of vaccines prepared from neurotropic alpha streptococci] were taken to indicate that a specific type of streptococcus might be causative of schizophrenia."
   Rosenow [52R2], p. 245, contrasts reactions of rabbits injected with material from schizophrenia vs. rabbits injected with material from epilepsy, with greater hyperirritability in the former and more convulsions in the latter; and reactions of mice injected with material from epilepsy exhibited greater incidence of convulsions than mice injected with material from well controls (material taken directly from nasopharynx, tonsils, infected teeth or dextrose-brain-broth cultures).

Table A2 [52R2]:
Rabbits injected w/material from:

	Schizophrenia	Idiopathic Epilepsy
No. of Rabbits -	77	106
Hyperirritability	87%	25%
Convulsions	3%	34%

Mice injected with material from:

	Epilepsy	Well-control
No. of Mice	130	44
Convulsions	69%	2%

EPILEPSY, SCHIZOPHRENIA
   Rosenow [52R2] p. 245, "Convincing evidence that specific types

of alpha streptococci may in fact be causative of both epilepsy and schizophrenia have now been obtained during extensive studies at Longview Hospital [Cincinnati Ohio].

p. 248, Rosenow found an increase of specific antibodies and decrease of corresponding antigen in both schizophrenia following electroshock therapy and in epilepsy following spontaneous gran mal seizures, indicating "that preformed so-called sessile antibodies are mobilized during the course of the violent reactions." Dr. Rosenow notes that this raises the possibility that an "inherited constitution affords the very conditions favorable for alpha streptococci normally present in the throat and elsewhere of human beings to acquire specific affinity for structures in the brain..."

SCHIZOPHRENIA - ELECTROSCHOCK AND STREPTOCOCCI 52R2
Effects of electroshock: "The prompt increase of respective specific streptococcal antibodies and a decrease of corresponding antigen in schizophrenia following electrically induced convulsion during electro-shock treatment and in idiopathic epilepsy following spontaneously occurring grand mal seizures indicate the presence of specific types of subclinical streptococcal infections and that preformed, so-called sessile antibodies are mobilized during the course of the violent reactions." [52R2, 248]

STREPTOCOCCI AND NEUROTOXINS 52R2
p. 262, conclusions:
Streptococci, neurotoxins and schizophrenia: "the consistent isolation of alpha streptococci in studies of idiopathic epilepsy and schizophrenia, the reproduction in important respects of the disease pictures in animals, the proof of their serologic specificity by the special methods employed, and the data obtained in these studies indicate: (1) that persons suffering from epilepsy and from schizophrenia harbor in nasopharynx, in pulpless teeth, and sometimes in their blood, specific types of alpha streptococci of low general but high and specific 'neurotropic' virulence; (2) that the streptococci produce neurotoxins which have predilection for certain structures in the brain and thus may play a role in pathogenesis and (3) that attempts to combat such inapparent infections specifically by passive and active immunization with the respective antigens and antibodies are indicated in addition to present-day methods of prevention and cure."[52R2]

We are reminded of JC Hurley's recent work [Lancet, 1993 May 1, 341(8853):1133-5] indicating endotoxins encountered in sepsis may merely comprise markers for transition to wall-deficient bacterial a smaller phase, thus it is tempting to speculate that this may also be so in the case of presumed "neurotoxins".

VIRUS COMPARED TO FILTRABLE AGENT IN POLIO 52R3-304
CHICK EMBRYO INFUSION: SMALL FORMS APPEAR IN OLD CULTURES [52R3]
"Numerous attempts to produce the virus from the streptococcus

always resulted in failure until [as early as 1935: see also
35R5] a medium, chick-embryo infusion, was discovered which does
not turn acid from growth of streptococci. ... Small forms
appeared in old cultures, and upon appropriate intracerebral
inoculation of such cultures and of filtrates into mice and
monkeys typical poliomyelitis developed after successive brain to
brain passage including strains of streptococci from sources
wholly remote from poliomyelitis. Monkeys that recovered from
paralytic poliomyelitis produced with natural virus resisted
natural and the experimental virus and vice versa."

GLYCERINE SALT MENSTRUUM [52R3, p. 306]
     Glycerine-salt menstruum: "The specificity of the
respective freshly isolated streptococci was preserved by placing
the centrifuged organisms from young 0.2 percent dextrose broth
cultures in very dense suspension (1,000 billion streptococci or
the growth from 500 ml of dextrose broth per ml kept at 5 to 10
degrees C) of glycerin, 2 parts and saturated NaCl solution, 1
part. [52R3, p. 306]

PREPARATION OF ANTIBODY AND ANTIGEN FOR CUTANEOUS TESTS 52R3
   "The solutions of antibody used for the detection of specific
streptococcal antigen in skin or blood were prepared routinely by
diluting the dense glycerol-NaCl suspensions 50 fold or to 20
billion per ml in isotonic NaCl solution autoclaving for 96 hours
at 17 lbs pressure and diluting with an equal volume of NaCl
solution containing 0.4% phenol.
   "The corresponding solutions of antigen used for the detection
of streptococcal antibody were prepared by diluting the dense
glycerol-NaCl solution suspension 100 fold or to 10 billion per
ml, heating at 65 or 70 degrees C for one hour and adding 0.2%
phenol as a preservative. The tests were made with the
respective supernatant bacteria-free NaCl solutions as antibody
and as antigen. [52R3, p. 306]

ANTIBODY ADMINISTRATION - SUBCUTANEOUS OR INTRAMUSCULAR 52R3
     Polio, multiple sclerosis, epilepsy, schizophrenia: "It has
been found in previous studies that subcutaneous or intramuscular
injection of respective thermal streptococcal antibody in
therapeutic amounts is followed by a prompt improvement in
symptoms and a diminution in specific streptococcal antigen and
an abrupt increase in antibody titer in skin or blood of persons
having influenza or other respiratory infections, poliomyelitis,
multiple sclerosis, and epilepsy and schizophrenia. ...
   "The antibody solution injected subcutaneously was prepared by
autoclaving at 17 lbs pressure, a suspension of NaCl solution
containing 10 billion streptococci per ml isolated in studies of
poliomyelitis for 3 hours after adding 1.5% hydrogen peroxide
(initial) bringing the pH to 6.5 with a concentrated solution of
NaOH and diluting the supernatant with an equal volume of NaCl
solution containing 0.4% phenol. Two or three ml of the solution
of antibody and of NaCl solution in controls depending on the age

of patients were injected subcutaneously immediately after the primary intradermal tests had been made ... [52R3 p. 309]

CUTANEOUS TEST RESULTS SUPPORT ROLE OF STREPTO. IN POLIO 52R3
  "The results obtained from the use of poliomyelitis streptococcal thermal antibody and of antigen in cutaneous tests are so precise as to support further the thesis (1) that a specific type of streptococcus, in some way, is causative of epidemic poliomyelitis and thus makes more explicable the occurrence of epidemics almost simultaneously over vast and isolated regions in summer for it has been found that the streptococcus normally present in the nasopharynx of human beings tends to acquire neurotropic properties in summer in temperate climates, (2) that the streptococcus and the virus are related and (3) that immunity according to age may be due in part to an inapparent infection in summer by the neurotropic streptococcus and perhaps by the related virus. The streptococcus appears to be the large cultivable, toxicogenic, antigenic phase and a source of the virus and the virus - the small highly invasive relatively non-antigenic phase." [52R3 p. 309-310]

STREPTOCOCCI SOURCE OF TOXINS, EPILEPSY AND SCHIZOPHRENIA 53R1
  "The results in animals support the view generally held that the seizures in epilepsy and certain symptoms in the psychoses, including schizophrenia, are of toxic origin and that the respective specific neurotoxins may in fact be derived from specific types of streptococci. Furthermore, the studies suggest that the tissues for which the 'neurotoxin' or streptococci have predilection may become hypersensitive or allergic so that extremely small amounts of the 'neurotoxin', too small to be detected by chemical methods or small numbers of the streptococci, suffice to produce the respective characteristic symptoms. [53R1]

ANIMALS AND HUMANS: SIMILAR TISSUES AND INTUITION [53R1, 422]
  In 1953 Dr. Rosenow shared some rather remarkable overview observations on the physiology and mentality of laboratory animals: "The results obtained in these studies in a way transcend the importance of streptococci and their specific toxins in the causation of disease for they indicate how much alike the functions and underlying organic constitution of the respective tissues of experimental animals and that of human beings are. From long observation of inoculated and well animals, much evidence has been found to indicate that their intuitive and acquired responses to external stimuli and stresses of life are also similar, as indicated especially by the following observations in the behavior of white mice. They practice sanitation and immunization seemingly by intuition. With 10 or 12 in a cage (10 x 12 x 10") they normally sleep in a huddle, often 2 or 3 deep, as far away as possible from the area where excreta are deposited. The mice that become ill are not allowed in the huddle or they voluntarily remain apart and are

not molested while life lasts. But after death, the well mice if cannibalistic almost invariably eat the diseased organ, such as pneumonic lungs produced by cerebral and/or nasal inoculation of 'pneumotropic' streptococcus or virus of influenza. In sharp contrast if death was due to encephalitis following inoculation of the streptococcus or virus of encephalitis, they remove the skull and eat the diseased brain."
   "I humbly present the results of these studies in deep appreciation of the thrills which I have had as ideas which have come to me were substantiated by experiments of trial and error."
   [53R1, 422]

DEXTROSE-BRAIN BROTH MEDIUM; GLYCERINE-SALT MENSTRUUM 53R2
   Dextrose-brain broth: "The virulent nonhemolytic streptococci in dextrose-brain broth outgrew the nonvirulent variants in young cultures. The use of this medium for primary isolations and for rapidly repeated subcultures for inoculation of animals and the preservation of antigenic specificity in the glycerin and sodium chloride solution menstruum for serologic studies and for the preparation of vaccines was found essential."
[53R2, p.612]

PREP. OF "THERMAL" ANTIBODY 53R2-615
   "... When suspensions in sodium chloride solution containing 20 billion streptococci per ml prepared from dilutions of the dense glycerin-sodium chloride solution suspension are autoclaved at 17 lb. of pressure for 96 hours, the organisms disintegrate; the remnants become sharply agglutinated and brownish in color, and substances resembling the natural antibody suitable for diagnostic cutaneous tests and treatment appear in the supernatant sodium chloride solution." [53R2, p.615]

VIRUS COMPARED TO FILTRABLE AGENT IN INFLUENZA 53R2 - 620
   Influenza: Dr. Rosenow summarized results of comparisons between the natural influenza virus and filtrable agents produced experimentally from the streptococcus isolated from persons with influenza, including the action of respective convalescent serums, immunization of mice, production of pneumonitis, agglutination experiments, and electron microscopy, concluding "The Streptococcus appears to be the toxicogenic, antigenic phase and the virus the relatively non toxicogenic nonantigenic, but highly invasive phase." [53R2:p.620-1; see also 45R6]

PRESERVATION OF VIABILITY OF STREPTOCOCCI IN TRANSIT 54R1
   p. 196: "Cotton, wrapped on flexible aluminum wire and bent to a suitable angle, was used to make nasopharyngeal swabbings, without touching the tongue ... . The swabs which had adsorbed the material were immediately replaced in narrow test tubes and several drops of a glycerine-NaCl menstruum were added to prevent growth of contaminating bacteria and to preserve viability and specificity during airplane transit [from Reno NV to Cincinnati OH].

PREPARATION OF "THERMAL" ANTIBODY [54R1, p. 197
"... Thermal antibody used in treatment was ... prepared by
autoclaving for 3 hours at 17 lbs. pressure the NaCl solution
suspensions containing 10 billion streptococci per ml.
[representing a 100-fold dilution; per 48R5] from the respective
dense suspensions in glycerine-NaCl solution after adding 1.5 per
cent hydrogen peroxide [H2O2], bringing the reaction to pH 7.0
with sodium hydroxide." [54R1, p. 196]

CONTINUING THERAPY FOR SEVERELY PARALYZED POLIO VICTIMS [54R1]
"... it is suggested that the administration of the poliomyelitis
streptococcal thermal antibody used with favorable results in the
treatment of acute epidemic poliomyelitis be extended to persons
having severe paralytic poliomyelitis long after onset and who
according to the cutaneous tests have antigen in excessive titer
and, according to cutaneous and agglutinative tests, have
antibody in deficient titer."-204

VIRUS COMPARED TO FILTRABLE AGENT IN POLIO [54R1, 204-5]
   Polio: "The results of combined studies of the filtrable
virus and the specific type of streptococcus in both epidemic and
experimental poliomyelitis indicate that what has been considered
as the virus is but the small filtrable, mildly antigenic but
highly invasive phase of the specific type of the non-filtrable,
highly toxicogenic, antigenic, neurotropic alpha streptococcus.
Exceedingly small spheres, ovoids and diplococcal forms sometimes
in small chains have been demonstrated in unstained films in
filtrates of the virus with the electron microscope ... [and] as
many as 40 of such forms in radial formation in the capsular
substance of the streptococcus suggestive of extrusions as grown
in dextrose brain broth have been demonstrated after special
staining with the electron microscope. That these minute
diplococci are capable of growing into the mature streptococcus
under favorable conditions may be the explanation as to why
growth of streptococci in serial dilution cultures in dextrose
brain broth often occurs in dilutions far greater than what would
be possible from the mathematical calculations of the number of
mature forms revealed by the light microscope.

STREPTOCOCCUS CULTURED FROM FILTRATES OF POLIO VIRUS [54R1]
  "In attempts to determine whether the small diplococcal forms
which have been demonstrated in filtrates of poliomyelitis virus
represent in fact the filtrable phase of the streptococcus and
not a separate entity, rhesus monkeys were inoculated
intracerebrally with filtrates of the virus and cultures were
made in dextrose brain broth from such filtrates and from the
spinal fluid. Pure cultures of the streptococcus were isolated
from the filtrates in significant incidence in dextrose brain
broth and no growth occurred in conventional mediums. The spinal
fluid was found free from cells and bacteria and cultures were
negative before and during the quiescent period of incubation but

as fever, tremors and staccato voice developed, but not yet
paralysis, the streptococcus became readily demonstrable in
appropriately stained films of the spinal fluid and was isolated
in pure culture. This important finding has apparently been
missed by investigators who have studied poliomyelitis from the
purely virus standpoint. then in the inoculated monkeys as in
epidemic poliomyelitis, the streptococcus disappeared from the
spinal fluid as paralysis developed, but was isolated
consistently from and demonstrated in the lesions of the spinal
cord after death.

   "It appears therefore that the primary infection in nasopharynx
and perhaps in the intestinal tract in epidemic poliomyelitis is
streptococcal in accord with the predominant occurrence of
epidemics in summer when the streptococcus normally present in
human beings and in nature tends to acquire neurotropic or
poliomyelitis properties in temperate climates. As such
infection occurs, the 'virus' or filtrable, highly invasive phase
of the streptococcus may develop and which because extremely
small penetrates the blood-brain-barrier where in turn it reverts
in part into the highly toxicogenic, antigenic streptococcal
phase as fever and symptoms of poliomyelitis develop.
...
   "... the virus has in fact been produced experimentally from
the streptococcus and shown to be the small, filtrable, highly
invasive, relatively non-antigenic phase of the much larger,
highly toxicogenic, antigenic, neurotropic streptococcus." [54R1,
204-5]

POLIOMYELITIS VACCINE; SUCCESSFUL PROPHYLAXIS [54R1-205]
   Poliomyelitis streptococcal vaccine and thermal antibody have
been used successfully for the prevention of poliomyelitis in
family groups [Rappaport B, Journal-Lancet 68:395-7; Quart.
Bull., Northwestern U. Med. School, Chicago, 1954, 28:57], and
monkeys have been immunized against inoculation of highly
virulent virus with vaccine prepared from the poliomyelitis type
of streptococcus [Proc. Staff Meet., Mayo Clinic, 13:328-330.]"

SERIAL DILUTION METHOD [55R1]
     Serial dilution method: "Separation of staphylococci, E.
coli and saprophytic streptococci from the specifically virulent
streptococci in nasopharyngeal swabbings was accomplished in
serial dilution cultures in dextrose-brain broth using a nicrome
wire at steps of 10-2, 10-6 and 10-10 in which the specifically
virulent streptococci outgrow the avirulent streptococci,
staphylococci and E. coli." [55R1]

SCAVENGER ORGANS: LIVER, SPLEEN AND KIDNEY 55R1-242
   Regarding a number of diseases, including glaucoma, epilepsy,
MS., epidemic poliomyelitis and coronary heart disease: "The
number of colonies and percentage incidence of isolation of the
streptococcus from the liver, spleen and kidney without evidence
of lesions were uniformly high regardless of the source of the

streptococcus, indicating it would seem a protective scavenger-
like function of these organs."

REMARKABLE INCREASE IN VIRULENCE IN MIXED CULTURES   [55R1]
   In 1955 Dr. Rosenow noted that a "remarkable elective or
specific localization occurred in organs of mice corresponding to
those chiefly involved in patients from whom the streptococcus
was isolated from the nasopharynx ..."
   However, when 14 specific strains were mixed and stored at 10
degrees C for 71 days in glycerin-NaCl solution, and then grown
in dextrose-brain broth and injected intravenously in laboratory
mice, not only had characteristic specificities disappeared, but
also "the number of streptococci and percentage incidence of
isolations from the different organs of mice were almost without
exception far greater than what would be expected ... [comprising
a] remarkable increase in localizing property or 'virulence'".
Moreover, results indicated that "each streptococcus that
remained viable in the stored composite glycerine-NaCl solution
suspension had acquired the diverse localizing properties
characteristic of the 14 respective specific strains. ... Most
remarkable of all are the facts (1) that the changes in the
composite mixture of the specific types of streptococci occurred
at a temperature of 10 degrees C and other conditions that
precluded growth, (2) that the newly acquired properties were
transmissible as the streptococci grew in subculture in the
dextrose brain broth, and (3) that such changes never occurred
under comparable conditions of storage of specific strains
separately."
   "The maintenance almost indefinitely of respective
specificities on storage separately of specific strains of alpha
streptococci as partially dehydrated in the glycerol-NaCl
solution menstruum nd the phenomenal increase in organotropic
localization on additional identical storage of composite
mixtures of respective specific strains of streptococci is new,
truly remarkable and fundamental, for it indicates the importance
of environmental conditions for the acquisition and maintenance
of respective specifies of the ever-present alpha streptococci
in human beings. The importance of determining specifities
inherent or acquired of alpha type streptococci in studies on
etiology such as these is obvious." [55R1, p. 246]

CHLORPROMAZINE CONTRAINDICATED AS SCHIZOPHRENIA THERAPY [55R2]
"The agglutinative titer for the streptococcus [of schizophrenia]
of the blood serum of schizophrenics receiving chlorpromazine
unfortunately has been found far lower and of the urine
significantly greater than in comparable schizophrenics not
receiving chlorpromazine. ... The administration of
chlorpromazine and serpasil in the treatment of schizophrenics
was found to cause a reduction instead of a hoped for increase in
the agglutinative titer of the serum of schizophrenics for the
streptococcus isolated in studies of schizophrenia. ... from the
immunological standpoint [the use of chlorpromazine to treat

schizophrenia] is contraindicated, for it does not eliminate the basic cause, the specific neurotropic streptococcus, nor does it neutralize the specific toxicogenic streptococcal antigen."55R2-330

STREPTOCOCCUS IN NASOPHARYNX, SOMETIMES BLOOD IN SCHIZO.[55R2]
These and previous studies indicate that "... schizophrenia and related mental disorders ... are due to a specific type of non hemolytic neurotropic streptococcal infection or intoxication. ... The streptococcus of schizophrenia has a low, general virulence but is highly neurotropic in that it localizes electively in the brain of persons stricken and in animals on intravenous injection. In keeping with this low general virulence, the general health is maintained, and stimulation of the formation of antibody is minimal; hence the disease process tends to continue unabated. ... It is realized how contrary to current psychiatric tenets the concept that schizophrenia and related mental disorders can possibly be due to an infectious process, but the results of bacteriologic studies by the special methods used indicate that such is nevertheless the case."55R2-328

INJECTION OF ANTIBODY AND ANTIGEN FOR CUTANEOUS TESTS [55R2]
   The tests for circulating antigen or antibody were made by injecting approx. .03 ml of respective antibody or antigen solutions intradermally into the skin of the volar aspect of the forearm. [55R2]

VACCINE PREPARATION SUMMARY 55R2
   Streptococcal thermal antibody solutions and vaccines were prepared routinely from the streptococci in the dense glycerol saturated NaCl solution suspensions. The vaccine represented suspensions in NaCl solution of 2 billion streptococci per ml. and heated at 70 degrees C for one hour. ... [55R2]

CUTANEOUS TEST RESULTS - MS AND OTHER DISEASES [57R1]
Erythematous cutaneous reactions (sq. cm.) in persons having MS to the intradermal injection of thermal antibody-indicating antigen and of antigen-indicating antibody prepared respectively from streptococci isolated from the nasopharynxes of persons who had MS, neuroses, and arthritis (see Table 8.1; and full reprinted article in APPENDIX D3):
   "Cutaneous erythematous reactions indicating antibody (5.75 and 6.25 sq. cm.) were significantly less in persons not receiving such therapeutic injections than in persons receiving such treatment (7.86 sq.cm.). ...
   "It will be seen that the immediate erythematous reactions to the intradermal injection of streptococcic antibody (taken to indicate specific circulating streptococcic antigen in patients not receiving antibody or vaccine therapeutically) were far greater (7.31, 8.07, and 9.63 sq. cm.), respectively, than in persons receiving therapeutic injections of antibody and vaccine

(3.15 sq.cm.)..

"Erythematous reactions following intradermal injection of control antibody solutions were uniformly minimal, but in each of the three groups having multiple sclerosis reactions were greater to injections of 'neurotropic' (8126) streptococcic thermal antibody than to corresponding injections of "arthrotropic" (8134) antibody prepared respectively from streptococci isolated in studies of diseases of the nervous system and arthritis."

MS: THERAPEUTIC ADMIN. OF VACCINE & ANTIBODY, DOSE [57R1-783]
"Since such injections were harmless and had to be repeated over long periods, some members of the family of a nurse was instructed to give the injections."

MS: PREFERABILITY OF AUTOGENOUS VACCINE AND ANTIBODY [57R1]
"Clinical response to the subcutaneous therapeutic injection of heterologous streptococcic vaccine ant thermal antibody solutions, while favorable, was usually not as great nor as constant as it was to the autogenous preparations." 57R1-784

ADMINISTRATION OF VACCINE AND ANTIBODY (FOR M.S.) [57R1]
"One-tenth milliliter of the autogenous or stock vaccine containing 200,000,000 streptococci per milliliter isolated from the nasopharynxes of persons who had multiple sclerosis was injected subcutaneously for the first injection. This dose was increased by 0.1 ml. twice weekly up to the amount of 1 ml. Then 1 ml. was injected each week for an indefinite period, provided local and constitutional reactions were minimal and provided favorable clinical effects occurred.
"One-half milliliter of the stock or autogenous [multiple sclerosis] thermal streptococcic antibody from 10 billion streptococci per milliliter was injected separately subcutaneously, but at the same time or more often, if favorable results ensued. This dose was increased to 2 ml. and was given twice weekly or daily, provided local reactions at the point of injection were minimal or negative and provided clinical results were favorable." [57R1]

EXPLANATION OF DESIGNATION OF THERMAL ANTIBODY [58R1-756]
"It was postulated that the formation of both natural and artificial antibody might be due to oxidation of antigen. Accordingly, suspensions of streptococci in NaCl solution were subjected to the oxidative action of prolonged heat (96 hours) without hydrogen peroxide and for but three hours on adding 1.5% hydrogen peroxide to the autoclave. As this was done specific agglutinins and other antibodies developed which had respective curative action on subcutaneous injection in therapeutic dosage in respective persons ill." 58R1
" ... The material in the supernatant of NaCl solution suspensions of streptococci and other bacteria, after the application of prolonged heat in the autoclave and the application of heat for a far shorter period on the addition of

1.5% of the oxidizing agent, hydrogen peroxide, are designated as 'antibody' because (1) the supernatant of respective solutions agglutinated specifically the organisms from which they were prepared, (2) they precipitated specifically the respective dissolved antigens and (3) had curative action in the treatment of diseases in which they were causative, in a manner similar to convalescent serum and the serum of horses hyperimmunized with the streptococcus."

CANCER, LEUKEMIA; AGGLUTINATION TITERS FOR STREPTOCOCCI [58R1]
   "In keeping with the concept generally held that leukemia is 'cancer' of the blood are the fairly comparable crosswise agglutinative titers for the respective streptococci isolated in leukemia (69 and 63%) and carcinoma (50 and 81% respectively." 58R1

DIVERSE SPECIFICITIES OF STREPTOCOCCI ACQUIRED IN HOSTS [58R1]
"Evidence ... indicates that the diverse specifities of nonhemolytic streptococci ... is acquired in the respective hosts, rather than being due to streptococci from diverse extraneous sources, such as from milk and other foods or from air or water supplies." 58R1-760

ISOLATION AND PRODUCTION OF STREPTOCOCCI   [58R1]
   The following particularly detailed account of Dr. Rosenow's methodology is to be found in his last published article:
   "Serial dilution cultures at steps of 10^{-1}, 10^{-6}, and 10^{-10} were made of nasopharyngeal swabbings, with cotton-wrapped aluminum wire swabs, of the nasopharynx of persons having diverse chronic disease. The material thus obtained was inoculated into tall (8-10 cm.) columns of 0.2 percent dextrose broth adjusted to pH 7.0, to which pieces of fresh calf or beef brain were added, comprising approximately one part of brain substance to six or seven parts of broth, and autoclaved at 17 pounds' pressure for 20 minutes.
   "Cultures were made in this freshly prepared medium directly or soon after sterilization, but after prolonged storage the test tubes containing the tall columns of medium were heated in a boiling water bath for 15 minutes to remove absorbed oxygen."
   "The nasopharyngeal swabbings were obtained without touching the tongue. The material on the swabs was washed off in 2 ml. of NaCl solution, and then a tube of dextrose-brain broth was inoculated with the swab, representing an estimated dilution of the material swabbed of 10^{-2}. Two serial transfers were then made, with a nicrome wire, the length of the column of dextrose brain-broth sterilized in a Bunsen flame at each step, representing dilutions of inocula of 10^{-6} and 10^{-10} respectively. Growths after incubation at 35 degrees C. for 18 to 24 hours, at a dilution of 10^{-2}, consisted of predominating numbers of gram-staining, short-chained streptococci and, usually, of moderate numbers of gram-staining micrococci and sometimes also gram-negative, gas-producing bacilli. Growth at the dilution of 10^{-6}

usually consisted of a pure culture of short-chained, alpha-type streptococci. Growths usually did not occur at dilutions of 10^{-10}, but if positive such growth consisted of a pure culture of streptococci.

One milliliter of pure cultures from such end points of growth in dextrose-brain broth were inoculated into [previously warmed, per 54R1] 200 ml. or gallon lots of 0.2 percent dextrose broth, and the streptococci, thus grown at 35 degrees C. for 18 hours in the smaller lots, were harvested in a cup-type centrifuge. Pure cultures of streptococci in the gallon lots of 0.2 percent dextrose broth were harvested in the revolving bowl of the Sharples super-centrifuge. The sedimented streptococci from the cup-type centrifuge were in turn suspended in dense suspension of an estimated 200 billion streptococci per milliliter, and those from the larger lots from the bowl of the super centrifuge at 1000 billion per milliliter of two parts of chemically pure glycerol and one part of saturated NaCl solution and stored in the dark in the refrigerator at 10 degrees C. Some of the streptococci in this menstruum remained viable for months. All remained gram-positive and antigenically specific for many months on storage at 10 degrees C. Such storage made it readily possible to maintain serologic and other specific properties of streptococci as isolated in diverse diseases.[58R1]

SIMILAR ORGANISM, DIFFERENT DISEASE 58R1

--"The streptococci isolated in dextrose-brain broth from nasopharyngeal swabbings of persons having diverse diseases were much alike in size, chain formation and staining reactions. All were gram-positive and none produced zones of clear hemolysis on blood-agar, but instead, small colonies surrounded by a narrow green or indifferent zone were formed. The freshly isolated strains from nasopharyngeal swabbings of persons who had diverse acute or chronic disease on intravenous injection into mice and rabbits, localized and produced lesions "electively" in the organ or organs corresponding to those involved in patients from whom the streptococci were isolated."[58R1]

PREPARATION OF "THERMAL" ANTIBODY 58R1

"... Thermal antibody solutions ... were prepared by autoclaving the respective specific and control NaCl solution suspensions containing 20 billion streptococci per milliliter for 96 hours, and diluting the supernatant of such autoclaved suspensions with an equal volume of NaCl solution and adding 0.2 percent phenol as a preservative."[58R1]

APPENDIX A2: E.C. ROSENOW BIBLIOGRAPHY

02R1: Rosenow, E.C., On the association of stone and tumor of the urinary bladder, with report of a case. Am. Jour. Med. Sc. 123:634-642, 1902.

03R1: Rosenow, E.C., Blood cultures in lobar pneumonia and agglutination of the pneumococcus, Tr. Chicago Path. Soc. 5:265-274, 1903; Medicine 9:435-440, 1903.

03R2: Rosenow, E.C., Further studies in pneumonia. Abstract. Tr. Chicago Path. Soc. 6:80-82, 1903-1904.

04R1: Rosenow, E.C., Studies in pneumonia and pneumococcus infections. Jour. Infect. Dis. 1:280-312, 1904.

04R2: Rosenow, E.C., Streptococci in air of operating room and wards during an epidemic of tonsillitis. Am. Jour. Obst. 50:762-768, 1904.

05R1: Rosenow, E.C., The Blood in Lobar Pneumonia, with remarks concerning treatment, JAMA 44:871-873, (March 18) 1905, 871-3.

06R1: Rosenow, E.C., The role of phagocytosis in the pneumococcidal action of pneumonic blood. Jour. Infect. Dis. 3:683-700, 1906.

07R1: Rosenow, E.C., Human pneumococcal opsonin and the anti-opsonic substance in virulent pneumococci. Jour. Infect. Dis. 4: 285-296, 1907; Tr. Chicago Path. Soc. 7: 55-66, 1907-1908,

07R2: Rosenow, E.C., Phagocytic Immunity and the Therapeutic Injection of Dead Bacteria in Endocarditis. Tr. Chicago Path. Soc. 7:169-174, 1907-1908; Jour. Am. Med. Assn. 51 (1908), 1571-1572.

08R1: Rosenow, E.C., Virulence of pneumococci in relation to phagocytosis. Abstract, Science 27:657, 1908.

08R2: Rosenow, E.C., Virulent pneumococci, opsonin, and phagocytosis. Illinois Med. Jour. 13: '3-19. 1908.

08R3: Rosenow, E.C., "A Review of Anaphylaxis, with Especial Reference to Immunity", Science XXVII (Apr. 24, 1908), 643-4.

09R1: Rosenow, E.C., Immunological observations in ulcerative cystitis caused by pseudodiphtheria bacillus. Jour. Infect. Dis. 6:296-303, 1909.

09R2: Rosenow, E.C., Immunological and experimental studies on pneumococcus and staphylococcus endocarditis (~chronic septic endocarditis"). Jour. Infect. Dis. 6:245-281, 1909.

09R3: Rosenow, E.C., Phagocytic immunity and the therapeutic injection of dead bacteria in endocarditis. Preliminary report. Illinois Med. Jour. 15:263-267, 1909.

09R4: Rosenow, E.C., Primary portal thrombosis. Arch. Int. Med, 3:232-248, 1909. (With D, D. Lewis.)

09R5: Rosenow, E.C., A simple method of keeping frozen various specimens. Tr. Chicago Path. Soc. 8:283, 1909-1912.

09R6: Rosenow, E.C., On the mechanism of the production of infectious endocarditis. Tr. Chicago Path. Soc. 8:344, 1909-1912.

09R7: Rosenow, E.C., A new stain for bacterial capsules

with special reference to pneumococci. Tr. Chicago Path. Soc. 8: 144-145, 1909-1912; Jour. Am. Med, Assn. 61:418-419, 1911; Jour. Infect. Dis. 9:1-8, 1911.

09R8: Rosenow, E.C., A case of pyemia due to an anaerobic bacillus. Tr. Chicago Path. Soc. 8: 240-242, 1909-1912. (With A. D. Bevan.)

09R9: Rosenow, E.C., The toxic material from various bacteria. Tr. Chicago Path. Soc. 8:248-250, 1909-1912.

10R1: Rosenow, E.C., A study of pneumococci from cases of infectious endocarditis. Jour. Infect. Dis. 7:411-428, 1910.

10R2: Rosenow, E.C., Immunological studies in chronic pneumococcus endocarditis. Jour. Infect. Dis. 7:429-456, 1910.

10R3: Rosenow, E.C., "The Autolysis of Pneumococci and the Effect of the Injection of Autolyzed Pneumococci", JAMA 54 (June 11, 1910), 1943-5.

10R4: Rosenow, E.C., Autogenous vaccine therapy in endocarditis. Jour.

Am. Med. Assn. 55:1719-1720, 1910.

11R1: Rosenow, E.C., Anaphylaxis and the toxic substance from virulent pneumococci. Jour. Am. Med. Assn. 57:285, 1911.

11R2: Rosenow, E.C., Pneumococcus anaphylaxis and immunity. Jour. Infect. Dis. 9:190-211, 1911.

11R3: Rosenow, E.C., A bacteriological and cellular study of the lung exudate during life in lobar pneumonia. Jour. Infect. Dis. 8:500-503, 1911.

12R1: Rosenow, E.C., Pyemia due to an anaerobic polymorphic bacillus, probably bacillus fusiformis. Jour. Infect. Dis. 10:1-6, 1912. (With Ruth Tunnicliff.)

12R2: Rosenow, E.C., An epidemic of sore throat due to a peculiar streptococcus. Jour. Am. Med. Assn. 58:773, 1912. (With D. J. Davis.)

12R3: Rosenow, E.C., Immunity in and the specific treatment of pneumonia. Illinois Med. Jour. 21:425-430, 1912.

12R4: Rosenow, E.C., Further studies of the toxic substances obtainable from

pneumococci. Jour. Infect. Dis. 11:94-108, 1912.

12R5: Rosenow, E.C., Further immunological studies in chronic pneumococcus endocarditis. New York State Jour. Med. 12:441-445, 1912.

12R6: Rosenow, E.C., On the nature of the toxic substance from pneumococci. Jour. Infect. Dis. 11:235-242, 1912.

12R7: Rosenow, E.C., On the toxicity of broth, of pneumococcus broth culture filtrates, and on the nature of the proteolytic enzyme obtainable from pneumococci. Jour. Infect. Dis. 11:286-293, 1912.

12R8: Rosenow, E.C., Experimental infectious endocarditis. Jour. Infect. Dis. 11:210-224, 1912.

12R9: Rosenow, E.C., Immunization in pneumococcus infections. Jour. Am. Med. Assn. 59:795-796, 1912.

12R10: Rosenow, E.C., The action on dogs of the toxic substance btainable from virulent pneumococci and pneumonic lungs: Jour. Infect. Dis. 11:480-495, 1912. (With A. Arkin.)

12R11: Rosenow, E.C., The vaccine treatment of some unusual infections, with report of cases. Illinois Med. Jour. 22:676-680, 1912.

12R12: Rosenow, E.C., A study of streptococci from milk and from epidemic sore throat, and the effect of milk on streptococci. Jour. Infect. Dis. 11:338-346 1912.

12R13: Rosenow, E.C., 496 = 12R10?

13R1: Rosenow, E.C., The etiology of articular and muscular rheumatism. JAMA 60:1223-1224, 1913.

13R2: Rosenow, E.C., Studies on the transmutation of pneumococci and streptococci. Tr. Chicago Path. Soc. 9:61-63, 1913.

13R3: Rosenow, E.C., On the mechanism of intoxication in pneumococcus anaphylaxis and in pneumococcus infections. Tr. XV Internat. Cong. Hyg. and Demog., Washington, 1912, 2:338-341, 1913.

13R4: Rosenow, E.C., The myocardial lesions of rabbits inoculated with streptococcus viridans. Lancet 2:1692, 1913. (With

C. Coombs.)

13R5: Rosenow, E.C., Treatment of pneumonia with partially autolyzed pneumococci. JAMA 59:2203--2240, 1913. (With L. Hektoen.)

13R6: Rosenow, E.C., The etiology and vaccine treatment of Hodgkin's disease. Jour. Am. Med. Assn. 61:2122-2123, 1913. (With F. Billings.)

13R7: Rosenow, E.C., The production of ulcer of the stomach by injection of streptococci. JAMA 59 1947-1950, 1913.

13R8: Rosenow E.C., in discussion following : Mayo, Charles H., "The Relation of Local Foci of Infection to General Systemic Conditions", Dental Rev. XXVII (1913), 281-297], p. 321.

14R1: Rosenow, E.C., Mouth infection as a source of systemic disease. Jour. Am. Med. Assn. 63: 2026-2027, 1914.

14R2: Rosenow, E.C., Relation of and the lesion produced by various forms of streptococci with special reference to arthritis. Abstract. Illinois Med. Jour. 25:11-14, 1914.

14R3: Rosenow, E.C., The etiology and

specific treatment of rheumatism. In: Forchheimer's Therapeutics of Internal Diseases, New York, D. Appleton and Co., 1914, Vol 5, Pp 509-516.

14R4: Rosenow, E.C., Transmutations within the streptococcus-pneumococcus group. Jour. Infect. Dis. 14:1-32, 1914.

14R5: Rosenow, E.C., Studies in endocarditis and rheumatism. Journal-Lancet 24:1-4, 1914.

14R6: Rosenow, E.C., Wechselseitige Mutation von Pneumokokken und Streptokokken. Centralbl. f. Bakteriol. 73:284-287, 1914.

14R7: Rosenow, E.C., Lesions produced by various streptococci; endocarditis and rheumatism. New York Med. Jour. 99:270-272, 1914.

14R8: Rosenow, E.C., The etiology of acute rheumatism, articular and muscular. Jour. Infect. Dis. 14:61-80. 1914.

14R9: Rosenow, E.C., Etiology of arthritis deformans: preliminary note. Jour. Am. Med. Assn. 62:1146-1147, 1914.

14R10: Rosenow, E.C., Eine einfache Methode

für das Anfertigen von Gewebskulturen. Centralbl. f. Bakteriol., I abt., Jena, 74:366-368, 1914.

14R11: Rosenow, E.C., Preliminary note on the etiology of arthritis deformans. Tr. Chicago Path. Soc. 9: 115-118, 1914.

14R12: Rosenow, E.C., The newer bacteriology of various infections as determined by special methods (provides insights into development of Rosenow's methodology; includes reference to Hodgkins), JAMA LXIII (Sept. 12, 1914), 903-908.

14R13: Rosenow, E.C., Bacteriology of cholecystitis and its production by injection of streptococci. Jour. Am. Med. Assn. 63:1835-1836, 1914.

15R1: Rosenow, E.C., Local infection due to intravascular dissemination of bacteria: the association of diphtheroid bacilli with various disease conditions. Surg., Gynec., and Obst. 20:403-405, 1915.

15R2: Rosenow, E.C., Relation of focal infection to and the bacteriology of arthritis. Lancet Clinic 113:32-34, 1915.

15R3: Rosenow, E.C., The bacteriology of appendicitis and its production by intravenous injection of streptococci and colon bacilli. Jour. Infect. Dis. 16:240-268, 1915.

15R4: Rosenow, E.C., The etiology and experimental production of erythema nodosum. Jour. Infect. Dis. 16:367-384, 1915.

15R5: Rosenow, E.C., The etiology and experimental production of herpes zoster. Preliminary note. Jour. Am. Med. Assn. 64:1968, 1915; Jour. Infect. Dis. 18:477-500, 1916. (With S. Oftedal.)

15R6: Rosenow, E.C., On an epidemic of sore throat and the virulence of streptococci isolated from the milk. Jour. Infect. Dis. 18:69-71, 1915. (With V. H. Moon.)

15R7: Rosenow, E.C., The bacteriology of ulcer of the stomach and duodenum in man. Jour. Infect. Dis. 17:219-226, 1915. (With A. H. Sanford.)

15R8: Rosenow, E.C., Pathogenesis of spontaneous and experimental appendicitis, ulcer of the stomach, and cholecystitis. Jour. Indiana State Med. Assn. 8:458-460, 1915.

15R9: Rosenow, E.C., Elective localization of streptococci. Jour. Am. Med. Assn. 65:1687-1691, 1915

15R10: Rosenow, E.C., Iritis and other ocular lesions on intravenous injection of streptococci. Jour. Infect. Dis. 17:403-408, 1915.

15R11: Rosenow, E.C., "The vaccine treatment of various infections", Wisc. M. J. xiii (1914-1915), 260-1

16R1: Rosenow, E.C., Treatment of lobar pneumonia with autolyzed extracts of pneumococci. Jour. Am. Med. Assn. 67:1929-1930, 1916. (With F. H. Falls.)

16R2: Rosenow, E.C., Elective localization of the streptococcus from a case of pulpitis, dental neuritis, and myositis. Jour. Immunol. 1:363-381, 1916.

16R3: Rosenow, E.C., The etiology of cholecystitis and gallstones and their production by the intravenous injection of bacteria. Jour. Infect. Dis.

19:527-556, 1916.

16R4: Rosenow, E.C., The etiology of epidemic poliomyelitis. Preliminary note. Jour. Am. Med. Assn. 67:1202-1205, 1916; New York Med. J., (4 Nov. 1916) 918. (With E. B. Towne and G. W. Wheeler.)

16R5: Rosenow, E.C., The bacteriology and experimental production of ovaritis. Jour. Am. Med. Assn. 66:1175-1180, 1916. (With C. H. Davis.)

16R6: An epidemic of appendicitis and parotitis probably due to streptococci contained in dairy products. Jour. Infect. Dis. 18:383-390, 1916. (With Stella I. Dunlap.)

16R7: Rosenow, E.C., Elective localization of bacteria in diseases (of the nervous system. Jour. Am. Med. Assn. 67:662-665, 1916.

16R8: Rosenow, E.C., The causation of gastric and duodenal ulcer by streptococci. Jour. Infect. Dis. 19:333-384, 1916.

16R9: Rosenow, E.C., The Etiology of Epidemic Poliomyelitis (see 16R4)

17R1: Rosenow, E.C., An epidemic of septic sore throat due to milk. Jour. Am. Med. Assn. 68: 1305-1307, 1917. (With C. L. v.Hess.)

17R2: Rosenow, E.C., Observations on immunity of monkeys to experimental poliomyelitis. Jour. Am. Med. Assn. 68:280-282 (Jan. 27) 1917. (With E. B. Towne and G. W. Wheeler.)

17R3: Rosenow, E.C., Bacteriological observations in experimental poliomyelitis of monkeys. Jour. Med. Res. 31:175-186, 1917. (With E. B. Towne.)

17R4: Rosenow, E.C., The production of an antipoliomyelitis serum in horses. Jour. Am. Med. Assn. 69:261-265, 1917.

17R5: Rosenow, E.C., The relation of dental infection to systemic disease. Dental Cosmos 59: 485-491, 1917.

17R6: Rosenow, E.C., The treatment of epidemic poliomyelitis with immune horse serum. Preliminary report. Jour. Am. Med. Assn. 69:1074-1075, 1917.

17R7: Rosenow, E.C., Results of studies on epidemic poliomyelitis. Am. Jour. Pub. Health 7:994-998, 1917.

18R1: Rosenow, E.C., Partially autolyzed pneumococci in the treatment of lobar pneumonia. Results in two hundred cases. Jour. Am. Med. Assn. 70:759-763, 1918.

18R2: Rosenow, E.C., The etiology of epidemic poliomyelitis. Jour. Infect. Dis. 22:281-312, 1918. (With G. W. Wheeler.)

18R3: Rosenow, E.C., The elective localization of streptococci from epidemic poliomyelitis. Jour. Infect. Dis. 22:313-344, 1918. (With E. B. Towne and C. L. v.Hess.)

18R4: Rosenow, E.C., Agglutination of the pleomorphic streptococcus isolated from epidemic poliomyelitis by immune serum. Jour. Infect. Dis. 22:345-378, 1918. (With Hazel Gray.)

18R5: Rosenow, E.C., Report on the treatment of fifty-eight cases of epidemic poliomyelitis with immune horse serum. Jour. Infect. Dis. 22:379-426, 1918.

18R6: Rosenow, E.C., Treatment of acute poliomyelitis with immune horse serum. Further studies. Jour. Am. Med. Assn. 71:433-437, 1918.

18R8: Rosenow, E.C., The pathogenesis of focal infection. Jour. Nat. Dental Assn. 5:113-124, 1918.

18R9: Rosenow, E.C., The etiology and treatment of acute poliomyelitis. Journal-Lancet 38:624-625, 1918.

19J1: Tehon, L.R., Autogenous, formulas for use in standardizing autogenous vaccines, JAMA 73: 1063, Oct. 4, 1919

19R1: Rosenow, E.C., Prophylactic inoculation against respiratory infections during the present pandemic of influenza. Preliminary report. Jour. Am. Med. Assn. 72:31-34, 1919.

19R2: Rosenow, E.C., Studies in influenza and pneumonia. II. The experimental production of symptoms and lesions simulating those of influenza with streptococci isolated during the present pandemic. III. The occurrence of a pandemic strain of streptococcus during the pandemic of influenza. Jour. Am. Med. Assn. 72: 1604-1609, 1919.

19R3: Rosenow, E.C., A method for the preparation of prophylactic and autogenous lipovaccines. Jour. Am. Med. Assn. 73:87-91, 1919. (With A. E. Osterberg.)

19R4: Rosenow, E.C., Study X. The etiology and treatment of acute poliomyelitis. Minnesota Med. 2:253-256, 1919.

19R5: Rosenow, E.C., Studies in influenza and pneumonia. IV. Further results of prophylactic inoculation. Jour. Am. Med. Assn. 73:396-401, 1919. (With B. F. Sturdivant.)

19R6: Rosenow, E.C., Studies on elective localization. Focal infection with special reference to oral sepsis. Jour. Dental Res. 1:205-267, 1919.

19R7: Rosenow, E.C., Studies in influenza. Minnesota Med. 2:423-424, 1919.

20R1: Rosenow, E.C., Studies in influenza and pneumonia. V. Observations on the bacteriology and certain clinical features of influenza and influenzal pneumonia. VI. The leukocytic reaction in influenza and influenzal pneumonia. VII. A study of the effects following the injection of bacteria found in influenza in normal throats, in simple nasopharyngitis, and in lobar pneumonia. VIII. Experiments on the etiology of "gastrointestinal" influenza. IX. Changes in the green-producing streptococcus induced by successive animal passage and their significance in epidemic influenza. X. The immunologic properties of the green-producing streptococci from influenza. XI. Therapeutic effects of a monovalent antistreptococcus serum in influenza and influenzal pneumonia. Jour. Infect. Dis. 26:469-622, 1920.

20R2: Rosenow, E.C., Etiology of and prophylactic inoculation in influenza. Illinois Med. Jour. 37:153-155, 1920; Wisconsin Med. Jour. 18:370-371, 1919-1920; Jour. Iowa State Med. Soc. 10:335-337, 1920.

21R1: Rosenow, E.C., Diaphragmatic spasms in animals produced with a streptococcus from epidemic hiccup. Preliminary report. Jour. Am. Med. Assn. 76:1745-1747, 1921.

21R2: Rosenow, E.C., Focal infection and elective localization of bacteria in appendicitis, ulcer of the stomach, cholecystitis, and pancreatitis. Surg., Gynec., and Obst. 33:19-26, 1921

21R3: Rosenow, E.C., Treatment of acute poliomyelitis with immune horse serum. Summary of results. Jour. Am. Med. Assn. 57:588-590, 1921.

21R4: Rosenow, E.C., Treatment of poliomyelitis with immune horse serum by various physicians. Minnesota Med. 4 588-593, 1921.

21R5: Rosenow, E.C., Focal infection and elective localization in the etiology of myositis. Arch. Int. Med. 28:274-311, 1921. (With Winifred Ashby.)

21R6: Rosenow, E.C., Results of experimental studies on focal infection and elective localization. Med. Clin. N. Amer. 5:573-592, 1921.

21R7: Rosenow, E.C., Elective localization and focal infection from oral sepsis. Can. Jour. Med. and

Surg. 50:34-43, 1921.

22R1: Rosenow, E.C., Nephritis and urinary calculi following the experimental production of chronic foci of infection. Preliminary report. Jour. Am. Med. Assn. 78: 266-267, 1922. (With J. G. Meisser.)

22R2: Rosenow, E.C., Experimental studies on the etiology of encephalitis. Report of findings in one case. Jour. Am. Med. Assn. 79:443-448, 1922.

22R3: Rosenow, E.C., Elective localization of bacteria following various methods of inoculation. and the production of nephritis by devitalization and infection of teeth in dogs. Jour. Lab. and Clin. Med. 7:707-722, 1922. (With J. G. Meisser.)

22R4: Rosenow, E.C., Experimental studies in the etiology of epidemic encephalitis, epidemic hiccup, spasmodic torticollis, and allied conditions. Northwest Med. 21:329-331. 1922.

22R5: Rosenow, E.C., Three cases of acute encephalitis treated with specific serum. Jour. Am. Med. Assn. 79:2068-2071, 1922. (With H. F.

Helmholz.)

23R1: Rosenow, E.C., The etiology of spontaneous ulcer of the stomach in domestic animals. Jour. Infect. Dis. 32:384-399, 1923.

23R2: Rosenow, E.C., Microscopic demonstration of bacteria in the lesions of epidemic lethargic encephalitis. Jour. Infect. Dis. 32:144-152, 1923. (With G. H. Jackson, Jr.)

23R3: Rosenow, E.C., The production of spasms of the diaphragm in animals with a streptococcus from cases of epidemic hiccup. Jour. Infect. Dis. 32:41-71, 1923.

23R4: Rosenow, E.C., The production of spasms of the diaphragm in animals by living cultures, filtrates, and the dead streptococcus from cases of epidemic hiccup. Jour. Infect. Dis. 32:72-94, 1923.

23R5: Rosenow, E.C., Experimental observations on the etiology of chorea. Am. Jour. Dis. Child. 26:223-241, 1923.

23R6: Rosenow, E.C., The specificity of the streptococcus of gastroduodenal ulcer and certain factors determining its localization. Jour. Infect. Dis. 33:248-268, 1923.

23R7: Rosenow, E.C., Changes in streptococcus from encephalitis, induced experimentally, and their significance in pathogenesis of epidemic encephalitis and influenza. Jour. Infect. Dis. 33:531-556, 1923.

23R8: Rosenow, E.C., Elective localization of the streptococcus-pneumococcus group as a factor in the production of disease. Ann Clin. Med. 1:211-230, 1923.

23R9: Rosenow, E.C., Specific serum treatment of epidemic (lethargic) encephalitis. Further results. Jour. Am. Med. Assn. 80:1583-1588, 1923.

23R10: Rosenow, E.C., The production of urinary calculi by the devitalization and infection of teeth in dogs with streptococci from cases of nephrolithiasis. Arch. Int. Med. 31:807-829, 1923. (With J. G. Meisser.)

24R1: Rosenow, E.C., Streptococci in the etiology of epidemic encephalitis, spasmodic torticollis,

respiratory arrhythmia, and chorea. Journal-Lancet 44:479-481, 1924.

24R2: Rosenow, E.C., Experimental and clinical studies on focal infection and elective localization: newer findings and their significance. Jour. Am. Dent. Assn. 11:963-982, 1924; Dental Sum. 44:954-966; 1026-1041, 1924.

24R3: Rosenow, E.C., A precipitin reaction in epidemic poliomyelitis. Proc. Soc. Exper. Biol. and Med. 22:155-156, 1924.

24R4: Rosenow, E.C., Further studies on the etiology of epidemic hiccup. Proc. Soc. Exper. Biol. and Med. 22:187-188, 1924.

24R5: Rosenow, E.C., Experimental studies indicating an infectious etiology of spasmodic torticollis. Jour Nerv. and Ment. Dis. 59:1-30, 1924.

24R6: Rosenow, E.C., Experiments on the etiology of respiratory arrhythmias following epidemic encephalitis. Arch. Neurol. and Psychiat. 11:155-178, 1924.

24R7: Rosenow, E.C., Specificity of streptococci in the etiology of diseases of the nervous system. Jour. Am. Med. Assn. 82:449-453, 1924.

24R8: Rosenow, E.C., Streptococci in relation to the etiology of epidemic encephalitis: experimental results in eighty-one cases. Jour. Infect. Dis. 34:329-389, 1924.

25R1: Rosenow, E.C., A precipitating and neutralizing antistreptococcus (scarlatinal) horse serum. Proc. Soc. Exper. Biol. and Med. 22:189-193, 1924; Jour. Infect. Dis. 36:525-537, 1925

25R2: Rosenow, E.C., A specific precipitin reaction in epidemic poliomyelitis. Jour. Am. Med. Assn. 84:429-432, 1925.

26R1: Rosenow, E.C., The production of urinary calculi by the devitalization and infection of teeth in dogs with streptococci from cases of nephrolithiasis. Jour. Iowa State Med. Soc. 15:297-301, 1925, Illinois Med. Jour. 49:28-33, 1926.

26R2: Rosenow, E.C., The precipitin reaction in the diagnosis of scarlet fever and allied hemolytic streptococcus infections. Jour. Am. Med. Assn. 86:9-14, 1926.

26R3: Rosenow, E.C., Further studies on the etiology of epidemic hiccup (singultus) and its relation to encephalitis. Arch. Neurol. and Psychiat. 15:712-734, 1926.

26R4: Rosenow, E.C., Neuromyelo-encephalitis during and following an epidemic of hiccup: diverse localization of streptococci. Arch. Neurol. and Psychiat. 16:21-36, 1926.

26R5: Rosenow, E.C., Further studies of the poliomyelitis precipitin reaction. Jour. Infect. Dis. 38:532-540, 1926.

26R7: Rosenow, E.C., Studies on poliomyelitis: résumé and newer findings. Minnesota Med. 9:231-235, 1926.

26R8: Rosenow, E.C., A skin reaction in poliomyelitis. Jour. Infect. Dis. 38:529-531, 1926.

26R9: Rosenow, E.C., The precipitin reaction in the identification of scarlatinal hemolytic streptococcus infections: further

results. Jour. Infect. Dis. 39:141-144, 1926.

27R1: Rosenow, E.C., The treatment of acute poliomyelitis with poliomyelitis antistreptococcus serum: results during 1921 to 1925. Am. Jour. Dis. Child. 33:27-49, 1927. (With A. C. Nickel.)

27R2: Rosenow, E.C., A bacteriologic study of cases of pulmonary embolism. Jour. Infect. Dis. 40:389-398, 1927.

27R3: Rosenow, E.C., Thrombosis of the cerebellar and vertebral arteries associated with intermittent hiccup: observations in a fatal case. Arch. Neurol. and Psychiat. 8:348-356, 1927.

27R4: Rosenow, E.C., Changing conceptions concerning oral sepsis. Jour. Am. Dent. Assn. 14:117-124,1927.

27R5: Rosenow, E.C., Oral sepsis in its relationship to focal infection and elective localization. Jour. Am. Dent. Assn. 14:1417-1438, 1927.

27R6: Rosenow, E.C., The air your patients breathe. A practical method for humidifying and partially sterilizing

the air of artificially heated buildings. Hosp. Prog. 8:483-487, 1927. 27R7: Rosenow, E.C., Bacteriologic observations on periodic ophthalmia in horses. Preliminary report. Jour. Am. Vet. Med. Assn. 71:378-383, 1927.

27R8: Rosenow, E.C., Focal infection and elective localization in the pathogenesis of diseases of the eye. Ann. Otol., Rhinol., and Laryngol. 36:883-895, 1927.

27R9: Rosenow, E.C., Changing concepts concerning oral sepsis. Kentucky M. J., Oct. 1927, 592-597.

28R1: Rosenow, E.C., Elective localization of bacteria in the animal body. In: E. O. Jordan and I. S. Falk, The Newer Knowledge of Bacteriology and Immunology, Chicago, University of Chicago Press, 1928, pp. 576-589.

28R2: Rosenow, E.C., Bacteriologic studies on the etiology of periodic ophthalmia in the horse. Jour. Am. Vet. Med. Assn. 72:419-458, 1928.

28R3: Rosenow, E.C., Localization in animals of

streptococci from cases of epidemic hiccup, encephalitis, spasmodic torticollis, and chorea. Arch. Neurol. and Psychiat. 19:424-436, 1928; abstract J.A.M.A., April 28, 1928, 1407.

28R4: Rosenow, E.C., Serum treatment of poliomyelitis. Nebraska State Med. Jour. 13:283-286, 1928.

28R5: Rosenow, E.C., Periodic ophthalmia in solipeds and its relation to uveitis in man. Jour. Am. Med. Assn. 91:621-627, 1928. (With F. P. Lewis.)

28R6: Rosenow, E.C., Streptococci in the spinal fluid in acute epidemic poliomyelitis: preliminary report. Jour. Am. Med. Assn. 91:1594-1595, 1928.

28R7: Rosenow, E.C., Focal infection. In: Encyclopedia Britannica, ed. 14, New York, 1928, vol 9, p 433.

28R8: Rosenow, E.C., Filtration experiments with the streptococcus isolated from the spinal fluid in epidemic poliomyelitis, Staff Meetings of the Mayo Clinic, Oct. 31, 1928, 310-311.

28R9: Rosenow, E.C., in Nickel, A.C., Resultts in various diseases from elimination of foci of infection and use of vaccines prepared from streptococci having elective localizing power, Staff Meetings of the Mayo Clinic, Aug. 8, 1928.

29R1: Rosenow, E.C., Results in various diseases from elimination of foci of infection and use of vaccines prepared from streptococci having elective localizing power. Jour. Lab. and Clin. Med. 14:504-512, 1929.

29R2: Rosenow, E.C., Observations on the cause and prevention of influenza and influenzal pneumonia. Minnesota Med. 12:366-368, 1929.

29R3: Rosenow, E.C., A simple method for finding any particular object in a microscopic slide preparation. Science 70:219-220, 1929.

29R4: Rosenow, E.C., Serologic specificity of streptococci having elective localizing power as isolated in the study of various diseases of man. Jour. Infect. Dis. 45:331-359.

30R1: Rosenow, E.C. and L. B. Jensen, Cataphoretic mobility and elective localization of arthritic and neurotrophic streptococci. Proc. Staff Meetings of Mayo Clinic 5:49-51 (Feb. 19) 1930.

30R2: Rosenow, E.C., Elective localization and cataphoretic potential of streptococci. Proc. Soc. Exper. Biol. and Med. 27:442-444 (Feb.) 1930. (With L. B. Jensen.)

30R3: Rosenow, E.C., Streptococci in the lesions of experimental poliomyelitis in monkeys. Proc. Soc. Exper. Biol. and Med. 27:444-445 (Feb.) 1930.

30R4: Rosenow, E.C., Poliomyelitis with antistreptococcus serum. Further studies on the bacteriology and on the serum treatment. Jour. Am. Med. Assn. 94:777-784 (March 15) 1930.

30R5: Rosenow, E.C., Elective localization of streptococci. Brit. Med. Jour. 1:1100-1101 (June 14) 1930; Dental Rec. 50:349-351 (July) 1930.

30R6: Rosenow, E.C., Focal infection and elective localization. Internat. Clin. 2:

29-64 (June) 1930.

30R7: Rosenow, E.C., Studi clinici e sperimentali sui focolai d'infezione e sulla localizzazione elettiva degli streptococchi. Stomatol. 28:637-643 (Aug.) 1930.

30R8: Rosenow, E.C., Studies on an institutional epidemic of poliomyelitis. Proc. Staff Meetings of Mayo Clinic 5:376 378 (Dec. 23 and 30) 1930.

30R9: Rosenow, E.C., Serum treatment for chronic ulcerative colitis. Arch. Int. Med. 46:1039-1047 (Dec.) 1930. (With J. A. Bargen and (G. F. C. Fasting.)

30R10: Rosenow, E.C., Herdinfektion und elektive Lokalisation. Verhhandl. d. deutsch. Gesellsch. f. inn. Med. 42:408-438, 1930.

30R11: Rosenow, E.C., Streptokokken in der Ätiologie von epidemischem Singultus und spastischer Torticollis. Arch. f. Psychiat. 92:445-460, 1930.

30R12: Rosenow, E.C., Streptococci in the etiology of diseases of the nervous system. Vol. 1,

Microbiologie, Generale Medicale, Veterinaire et Agricole, 1930.

31R1: Rosenow, E.C., Zusammenfassung der Forschungsergebnisse über Fokalinfektion und elektive Lokalisation. Med. Klin. 27:325-326 (Feb. 27) 1931.

31R2: Rosenow, E.C., The relation of streptococci to the filtrable virus of epizootic encephalitis of foxes. Jour. Infect. Dis. 48:304-334 (March) 1931.

31R3: Rosenow, E.C., Focal infection and elective localization of streptococci in causation of disease: summary of results. Acta Rheumatol. 3:3-4 (May) 1931.

31R4: Rosenow, E.C., Klinische und experimentelle Untersuchungen über elektive Localisation von Streptokokken. Schweiz med. Wchnschr. 61:633-637 (July 4) 1931.

31R5: Rosenow, E.C., Cataphoretic mobility and neurotropic virulence of streptococci isolated in the course of an institutional outbreak of poliomyelitis. Proc. Staff Meetings of Mayo Clinic 6:466-468 (Aug. 5) 1931.

31R6: Rosenow, E.C., Further observations on a skin test for susceptibility to poliomyelitis. Abstract. Am. Jour. Path. 7:546 (Sept.) 1931.

32R1: Rosenow, E.C., Electrophoretic potential of streptococci as isolated in studies of encephalitis and other diseases of the nervous system. Proc. Staff Proceedings of Mayo Clinic 7:25-27 (Jan. 20) 1932.

32R2: Rosenow, E.C., Elective localization in determining the etiology of chronic uveitis. Am. Jour. Ophth. 15: 1-18 (Jan.) 1932. (With A. C. Nickel.)

32R3: Rosenow, E.C., An institutional outbreak of poliomyelitis apparently due to Streptococcus in milk. Jour. Infect. Dis. 50:377-475 (May-June) 1932.

32R4: Rosenow, E.C., Observations on filter-passing forms of Eberthella typhi (Bacillus typhosus) and of the streptococcus from poliomyelitis. Proc. Staff Proceedings of Mayo Clinic 7:408-413 (July 13) 1932.

32R5: Rosenow, E.C., Observations with the

Rife microscope of filter-passing forms of microorganisms. Science 76:192-193 (Aug.26) 1932.

32R6: Rosenow, E.C., A simple method for humidifying and partially sterilizing the air of heated buildings. Am. Jour. Hyg. 16:566-581 (Sept.) 1932.

32R7: Rosenow, E.C., A specific reaction of convalescent serum on the streptococcus isolated in studies of poliomyelitis. Jour. Immunol. 23:455-464 (Dec.) 1932.

32R8: Rosenow, E.C., Elective localization and cataphoretic velocity of streptococci as isolated in cases of encephalitis and other diseases of the nervous system. In: Infections of the Central Nervous System, Baltimore, Williams and Wilkins Co., vol. 12, 1932, pp. 208-261.

32R9: Rosenow, E.C., Elective localization and cataphoretic potential of Streptococcus viridans and serum treatment of subacute bacterial endocarditis. In: Libman Anniversary Volumes, New York, International Press, 1932, vol. 3, pp.989 1001.

33R1: Rosenow, E.C., Cataphoretic velocity and virulence of streptococci isolated from the nasopharynx of the same person while well and during attacks of epidemic gastro-enteritis, of sore throat and of influenza. Proc. Staff Meetings of Mayo Clinic 8:6-14 (Jan. 4) 1933.

33R2: Rosenow, E.C., Cataphoretic velocity of streptococci as isolated in studies of arthritis. Arch. Int. Med. 51:327-345 (March) 1933.

33R3: Rosenow, E.C., Cataphoretic velocity of streptococci isolated in cases of encephalitis and of other diseases of the nervous system. Jour. Infect. Dis. 52:167-184 (March-April) 1933. (With L. B. Jensen.)

33R4: Rosenow, E.C., Acute poliomyelitis. Studies of streptococci isolated from throats and raw milk in relation to one epidemic. Jour. Pediat. 2:568-593 (May) 1933. (With H. M. Rozendaah and E. T. Thorsness.)

33R5: Rosenow, E.C., The experimental reproduction of persistent sneezing and convulsions with streptococci isolated respectively from one

case each of persistent sneezing and postinfluenzal convulsion Proc. Staff Meetings of Mayo Clinic 8:380-384 (June 21) 1933.

33R6: Rosenow, E.C., Seasonal changes in the cataphoretic velocity and virulence of streptococci as isolated from well persons, from persons having epidemic or other diseases, and from raw milk. Jour. Infect. Dis. 53: 1-11 (July-August) 1933

33R7: Rosenow, E.C., The high frequency field as an agent in changing the cataphoretic velocity and the localization of streptococci. Proc. Staff Meetings of Mayo Clinic 8:500-502 (Aug. 16) 1933. (With Charles Sheard and C. B. Pratt.)

33R8: Rosenow, E.C., The relation of streptococci to the present epidemic of encephalitis. Bull. St. Louis Med. Soc. 28:69-70 (Oct. 13) 1933. Abstr. in Proc. Staff Meetings of Mayo Clinic 8:559-563 (Sept. 13) 1933.

33R9: Rosenow, E.C., Isolation of streptococci in a study of the epidemic of encephalitis in St. Louis. Preliminary report.

Proc. Soc. Exper. Biol. and Med. 31: 285-286 (Nov.) 1933.

34R1: Rosenow, E.C., Cataphoretic velocity and virulence of streptococci isolated from throats of human beings, from raw milk, flies, water, sewage, and air during epidemics of the common autumnal cold. Am. Jour. Hygiene 19:1-21 (Jan.) 1934.

34R2: Rosenow, E.C., Cataphoretic time and velocity of streptococci and pneumococci. Studies on organisms isolated in cases of the common cold, influenza, bronchopneumonia, and lobar pneumonia. Jour. Infect. Dis. 54:91-122 (Jan.-Feb.) 1934.

34R3: Rosenow, E.C., Cataphoresis as a control of specificity of streptococcal vaccines. Influenzal streptococcus vaccine in the prevention and treatment of infections of the respiratory tract. Jour. Immunol. 26:401-433 (May) 1934.

34R4: Rosenow, E.C., Observations on the epidemic of polio-encephalitis in Los Angeles, 1934. Proc. Staff Meetings of Mayo Clinic 9:443-451

(July 25) 1934. (With F. R. Heilman and C. H. Pettet.)

34R5: Rosenow, E.C., Studies on focal infection, elective localization and cataphoretic velocity of streptococci. Dental Cosmos 76:721-744 (July) 1934; Brit. Jour. Dent. Sc. 79:175-183 (Oct.) 1934.

34R6: Rosenow, E.C., Observations in the epidemic of acute anterior poliomyelitis in Havana, 1934. Proc. Staff Meetings of Mayo Clinic 9:613-616 (Oct. 10) 1934.

35R1: Rosenow, E.C., A method of staining microorganisms and their capsular substance, and its application to streptococci and to filtrates of the viruses and spinal fluids in poliomyelitis and encephalitis. Proc. Staff Meetings of the Mayo Clinic 10:115-121 (Feb. 20) 1935.

35R2: Rosenow, E.C., Specificity of streptococci isolated in studies of diseases of the nervous system: experimental reproduction of persistent sneezing and convulsions. Jour. Nerv. and Ment. Dis. 81:138-160

(Feb.) 1935.

35R3: Rosenow, E.C., The electrophoretic characteristics of streptococci. II. The effects of intravenous injection into rabbits of strains of streptococci which have been exposed to the high frequency field. Protoplasma 23:24-33 (March) 1935. (With C. B. Pratt and Charles Sheard.)

35R4: Rosenow, E.C., Cataphoretic velocity and localization of streptococci isolated from infected teeth of persons having systemic disease. Jour. Dent. Res. 15:123-138 (April) 1935

35R5: Rosenow, E.C., The relation of streptococci to the viruses of poliomyelitis and encephalitis: preliminary report. Proc. Staff Meetings of Mayo Clinic 10:410-414 (June 26) 1935.

35R6: Rosenow, E.C., Elective localization and cataphoretic velocity of streptococci isolated from pulpless teeth and other foci of infection: summary of results. Jour. New York Acad. Dent. 2:92-98 (Sept.) 1935.

36R1: Rosenow, E.C.,

Cataphoretic velocity and localization of streptococci isolated from infected teeth of persons having systemic disease. Jour. Am. Dent. Assn. 23:35-46 (Jan.) 1936.

36R2: Rosenow, E.C., Etiology of muscular spasms during general anesthesia. Am. Jour. Surg. 34:474-485 (Dec.) 1936. (With R. M. Tovell.)

36R3: Rosenow, E.C., Serologic studies with streptococci isolated in cases of myasthenia gravis. Proc. Soc. Exper. Biol. and Med. 34:477-480, 1936. (With F. R. Heilman.)

36R4: Rosenow, E.C., Bacteriologic studies in myasthenia gravis. Proc. Soc. Exper. Biol. and Med. 34:419-425, 1936. (With.F. R. Heilman.)

37R1: Heilman, F.R., and Rosenow, E.C., Newer methods of study and treatment of chronic streptococcal disease. Proc. Staff Meet., Mayo Clin. 12: 252-256, April 21, 1937.

37R2: Rosenow, E.C., Precipitin and cutaneous streptococcal antibody-antigen reactions in poliomyelitis, Proc. Staff Meet., Mayo Clin. 12: 531-535,

Aug. 25, 1937.

37R3: Rosenow, E.C., Studies on relation of Streptococci to etiology of equine encephalomyelitis; preliminary report, Proc. Staff Meet., Mayo Clin. 12: 631-636, Oct. 6, 1937 (with C. F. Schlotthauer).

37R4: Rosenow, E.C., Bacteriologic and serologic studies in epidemic of poliomyelitis in Kentucky, 1935, Kentucky M.J. 35: 437-446, Sept., 1937 (with L.H. South and A.T. McCormack).

37R5: Rosenow, E.C., Further studies on relation of Streptococci to epidemic equine encephalomyelitis: treatment and prophylaxis, Proc. Staff Meet., Mayo Clin. 12: 825-830, Dec. 29, 1937 (with C. F. Schlotthauer).

38R1: Rosenow, E.C., Protection of monkeys (Macacus rhesus) against experimental poliomyelitis with vaccine and antiserum prepared with Streptococcus from poliomyelitis: preliminary report, Proc. Staff Meet., Mayo Clin. 13: 328-330, May 25, 1938.

38R2: Rosenow, E.C.,

Streptococcal vaccines in prevention and treatment of respiratory infections; clinical and experimental study, Am. J. Clin. Path. 8: 17-27, Jan. 1938 (with F. R. Heilman).

38R3: Rosenow, E.C., Mutation of poliomyelitis virus into encephalitis virus, Proc. Staff Meet., Mayo Clin. 13: 371-377, June 15, 1938.

38R4: Rosenow, E.C., Focal infection and elective localization; review and newer findings, Tr. Indiana Acad. Ophth. & Otorlaryng. 22: 80-81, 1938.
38R5: Rosenow, E.C., Isolation of bacteria from virus and phage by serial dilution method, Arch. Path. 26: 70-76, July 1938.

39R1: Rosenow, E.C., Experimental and clinical studies on relation of Streptococci to various diseases, Illinois M.J. 75: 28-38, Jan. 1939.

39R2: Rosenow, E.C., Early diagnosis and treatment of poliomyelitis with poliomyelitis antistreptococcic serum, Illinois M. J. 76: 144-149, Aug. 1939.

39R3: Rosenow, E.C., Failure of sulfapyridine to protect against experimental (virus) poliomyelitis, Proc. Staff Meet., Mayo Clin. 14: 490-495, Aug. 2, 1939.

39R4: Rosenow, E.C., Application of cutaneous test in relation to acute sporadic and epidemic poliomyelitis, 1939, Proc. Staff Meet., Mayo Clin. 114: 734-736, Nov. 15, 1939.

39R5: Rosenow, E.C., Recurring encephalomeningoradiculitis with fibromyositis following poliomyelitis; bacteriologic study of 64 cases, Arch. Int. Med. 64: 1197-1221, Dec. 1939.

40R1: Rosenow, E.C., Further results in treatment of acute poliomyelitis with antistreptococcic serum (1928-1937), Minnesota Med. 23: 161-164, March 1940; JAMA 114 (June 1, 1940), 2253.

40R2: Rosenow, E.C., Specific streptococcal antibody-antigen reactions of skin and serum of monkeys during attacks of experimental poliomyelitis, Proc. Staff Meet., Mayo

Clin. 15: 382-384, June 12, 1940.

40R3: Rosenow, E.C., Focal infection and elective localization in relation to systemic disease; review and results of further studies, Proceedings, Dental Centenary Celebration, Maryland State Dental Association, 1940, pp. 261-282, 1940.

41R1: Rosenow, E.C., Epidemic poliomyelitis, recurrent encephalomeningoradiculitis and fibromyositis in relation to Streptococci obtained from water supply, Arch. Int. Med. 67: 531-545, March 1941.

41R2: Rosenow, E.C., studies on etiology and serum treatment of encephalitis during epidemic in North Dakota and Minnesota, 1941, Proc. Staff Meet., Mayo Clin. 16: 587-588, Sept. 10, 1941 (with H. W. Caldwell).

42R1: Rosenow, E.C., Microdiplococci in filtrates of natural and experimental poliomyelitic virus compared under electron and light microscopes, Proc. Staff Meet., Mayo Clin. 17: 99-106, Feb. 18, 1942.

42R2: Rosenow, E.C., Demonstration of association of specifically different alpha streptococci with various diseases, and methods for preparation and use of specific antiserums and vaccines in diagnosis and treatment, Am. J. Clin. Path. 12: 339-356, July 1942.

42R3: Rosenow, E.C., Relation of neurotropic streptococci to encephalitis and encephalitic virus, Proc. Staff Meet., Mayo Clin. 17: 551-560, Nov. 4, 1942.

42R4: Rosenow, E.C., Studies on etiology and serum treatment of encephalitis during epidemic in North Dakota and Minnesota (1941), Ann. Int. Med. 17: 474-485, Sept. 1942 (with H.W. Caldwell).

42R5: Rosenow, E.C., Etiology and serum treatment of persistent epidemic and postoperative hiccup, J. Lab. & Clin. Med. 28: 277-289, Dec. 1942.

42R6: Rosenow, E.C., Infantile paralysis; inciting agent and specific serum treatment, Scient. Monthly 55: 495-507, Dec. 1942.

43R1: Rosenow, E.C.,

Isolation of specific types of streptococci and virus from stool in studies of epidemic poliomyelitis and encephalitis, and production of virus from "poliomyelitic" streptococci, Proc. Staff Meet., Mayo Clin. 18: 5-16, Jan. 13, 1943.

43R2: Rosenow, E.C., Diagnostic cutaneous reaction in acute poliomyelitis, Proc. Staff Meet., Mayo Clin. 18: 118-128, April 21, 1943.

43R3: Rosenow, E.C., Streptococcic antibody antigen reactions of serum and skin of monkeys during attacks of experimental poliomyelitis, Proc. Staff Meet., Mayo Clin. 18: 205-216, June 30, 1943.

43R4: Rosenow, E.C., Studies on diagnosis and treatment of epidemic and experimental poliomyelitis with poliomyelitis anti-streptococcic serum; summary of results, Minnesota Med. 26: 890-895, Oct. 1943; abstr., Proc. Staff Meet., Mayo Clin. 18: 403-408, Oct. 20, 1943.

43R5: Rosenow, E.C., Epidemic encephalitis in North Dakota nd Minnesota 1941; studies on etiology, epidemiology and serum treatment, Journal-Lancet 63: 247-257, Aug. 1943 (with H.W. aldwell).

43R6: Rosenow, E.C., Studies on the relation of a neurotropic streptococcus and virus to epizootic encephalitis of wild ducks, Cornell Veterinarian 33: 277-304, 1943.

44R1: Rosenow, E.C., Production of filtrable infectious agent from alpha streptococci, Am. J. Clin. Path. 14: 150-167, March 1944.

44R2: Rosenow, E.C., Poliomyelitis; relation of neurotropic streptococci to epidemic and experimental poliomyelitis and poliomyelitic virus, diagnostic serologic tests and serum treatment, Internat. Bull. Econ. M. Research and Pub. Hyg. A44: 9-83, 1944.

44R3: Rosenow, E.C., Poliomyelitis; studies on inciting agent and specific serum treatment, Lancet 1: 491-493, April 15, 1944.

44R4: Rosenow, E.C., Isolation from milk supplies of specific types of green-producing (alpha) streptococci and their thermal death point in milk, Minnesota Med. 27: 469, June; 550, July 1944.

44R5: Rosenow, E.C., Specific streptococcal antibody-antigen reactions in poliomyelitis; preliminary report, Proc. Staff Meet., Mayo Clin. 19: 444-448, Aug. 23 1944.

44R6: Rosenow, E.C., Studies on virus nature of infectious agent obtained from 4 strains of "neurotropic" alpha streptococci, J. Nerv. and Ment. Dis. 100: 229-262, Sept. 1944.

44R7: Rosenow, E.C., Filterable infectious agent obtained from alpha streptococci isolated in studies of case of poliomyelitis, Am. J. Clin. Path. 14: 519-533, Oct. 1944.

44R8: Rosenow, E.C., Infection in filed, vital, roentgenographically negative teeth, Cincinnati J. Med. 25: 329-339, Oct. 1944.

44R9: Rosenow, E.C., Studies on relation of pneumotropic streptococci to influenza virus, Science 100: 434-435,

150   REFERENCE MANUAL ROSENOW ET AL - SHShakman

Nov. 10 1944.

44R10: Rosenow, E.C., Infectious gastro-enteritis; epidemiologic and laboratory study, Am. J. Digest. Dis. 11: 381-391, Dec. 1944.

45R1: Rosenow, E.C., Specific types of alpha streptococci and streptococcal precipitinogen in air in relation to epidemic infections of respiratory tract and nervous system, Journal-Lancet 65: 108-122, March 1945.

45R2: Rosenow, E.C., Further studies on specific streptococcal antibody-antigen reactions in poliomyelitis, Am. J. Clin. Path. 15: 135-151, April 1945.

45R3: Rosenow, E.C., Further studies on muscular spasms during general anesthesia. Experimental results with neurotropic streptococci from nasopharynges of patients, Anesthesiology 6: 12-31, Jan. 1945 (with L.H. Mousel and J.S. Lundy).

45R4: Rosenow, E.C., Production in vitro of substances resembling antibodies from bacteria, J. Infect. Dis. 76: 163-178, May-June 1945.

45R5: Rosenow, E.C., Studies on etiologic relation of Streptococci to acute epidemic respiratory infections, Am. J. Clin. Path. 15: 319-333, Aug. 1945.

45R6: Rosenow, E.C., Studies on relation of pneumotropic streptococci to influenza virus, Am. J. Clin. Path. 15: 362-380, Sept. 1945.

45R7: Rosenow, E.C., Specific types of alpha streptococci and streptococcal antigen in unpotable water and water supplies, Am. J. Clin. Path. 15: 513-528, Nov. 1945.

46R1: Welsh, Ashton L., "Specificity of Streptococci Isolated from Patients with Skin Diseases: Studies on Pemphigus, Dermatitis Herpetiformis, Lupus Erythematosus and Erythema Multiforme", J. Investigative Dermatology 7: 7-42 (1946).

47R1: Rosenow, E.C., Studies on nature of antibodies produced in vitro from bacteria with hydrogen peroxide and heat, J. Immunol. 55: 219-232, March 1947.

47R2: Rosenow, E.C., Bacteriologic, etiologic, and serologic studies in epilepsy and schizophrenia, Postgrad. Med. 2: 346-357, Nov. 1947.

48R1: Rosenow, E.C., Bacteriologic, etiologic, and serologic studies in epilepsy and schizophrenia; effects in animals following inoculation of alpha streptococci, Postgrad. Med. 124-136, Feb. 1948.

48R2: Rosenow, E.C., Bacteriologic, etiologic, and serologic studies in epilepsy and schizophrenia; cutaneous reactions to intradermal injection of streptococcal antibody and antigen, Postgrad. Med. 3: 367-376, May 1948.

48R3: Rosenow, E.C., Bacteriologic studies of multiple sclerosis, Ann. Allergy 6: 271-292, May-June 1948.

48R4: Rosenow, E.C., Study of 1946 poliomyelitis epidemic by new bacteriologic methods, Journal Lancet 68: 265-277, July 1948.

48R5: Rosenow, E.C., Diagnostic cutaneous reactions to intradermal injection of natural and artificial antibody and of antigen prepared from streptococci isolated in studies of diverse diseases, Ann. Allergy 6: 485-496, Sept.-Oct. 1948.

49R1: Rosenow, E.C., Bacteriologic studies by new methods of major epidemic of poliomyelitis, 1947, Journal Lancet 69: 47-55, Feb. 1949.

50R1: Rosenow, E.C., Seasonal changes of streptococci isolated in studies of poliomyelitis, encephalitis and respiratory infection, Postgrad. Med. 7: 117-123, Feb. 1950.

50R2: Rosenow, E.C., Streptococci and diplostreptococci and respective "viruses" in etiology and epidemiology of epidemic respiratory infections and infectious gastroenteritis, Am. J. Digest. Dis. 17: 261-270, Aug. 1950.

50R3: Rosenow, E.C., Radiant energy as probable cause of seasonal changes in specificity of nonhemolytic streptococci, Postgrad. Med. 8: 290-292, Oct. 1950.

51R1: Rosenow, E.C., Streptococci, diplostreptococci and respective filtrable agents from outdoor air during epidemics of respiratory infections and infectious gastroenteritis, Am. J. Digest. dis. 18: 155-163, May 1951.

51R2: Rosenow, E.C., Parallel production of altered infectivity of Streptococcus and related filtrable agents isolated from outdoor air, J. Aviation Med. 22: 225-243, June 1951.

51R3: Rosenow, E.C., Streptococci from outdoor air in relation to seasonal occurrence of infections involving respiratory tract and nervous system respectively, J. Aviation Med. 11: 235-243, June 51.

51R4: Rosenow, E.C., Nonhemolytic streptococci in relation to epidemic of influenza; diagnostic cutaneous tests and specific treatment, A.M.A. Arch. Otolaryng. 54: 609-619, Dec. 1951.

51R5: Rosenow, E.C., Influence of streptococcal infections on compulsive behavior of criminals, Postgrad. Med. 10: 423-432, Nov. 1951 (with O. F. Rosenow).

52R1: Rosenow, E.C., Relation of Streptococcus to epidemic poliomyelitis; studies in etiology, diagnosis and specific treatment, California Med. 76: 396-401, June 1952.

52R2: Rosenow, E.C., Bacteriological studies in idiopathic epilepsy and schizophrenia, South Dakota J. Med. and Pharm. 5: 243-248; 262; 272, Sept. 1952.

52R3: Rosenow, E.C., Specific streptococcal antigen and thermal antibody in prevention, diagnosis and treatment of epidemic poliomyelitis, South Dakota J. Med. and Pharm. 5: 304-310; 328, Nov. 1952.

53R1: Rosenow, E.C., Streptococci in etiology of diverse diseases, including diseases of nervous system, J. Nerv. and Ment. Dis. 117: 415-428, May 1953.

53R2: Rosenow, E.C., Diagnostic cutaneous reactions, specific prevention and treatment in epidemic respiratory infections, A.M.A. Arch. Otolaryng. 58: 609-622, Nov. 1953.

54R1: Rosenow, E.C., Further immunological and clinical studies on importance of neurotropic streptococcus in

etiology of epidemic   123-4.
poliomyelitis and its
relation to natural
virus, J. Nerv. and
Ment. dis. 120:
196-206, Sept.-Oct.
1954.

55R1: Rosenow, E.C.,
Specific types of
alpha streptococci in
etiology and
streptococcal thermal
antibody in diagnosis
and treatment of
diverse diseases, J.
Nerv. and Ment. Dis.
122: 238-247, Sept.
1955.

55R2: Rosenow, E.C.,
Bacteriological
studies on etiology
and chlorpromazine
treatment of
schizophrenia and
related mental
disorders, J. Nerv.
and Ment. Dis. 122:
321-331, Oct. 1955.

57R1: Rosenow, E.C.,
Studies on the
etiology and specific
treatment of multiple
sclerosis, Ohio M.M.,
53(7), July 1957, p.
783-5.

58R1: Rosenow, E.C.,
Studies on specific
prevention and
treatment of diverse
diseases shown due to
specific types of
nonhemolytic
streptococci, Am.
Practitioner and
Digest of Treatment
(Philadelphia), 9(5),
May 1958, p. 755-761.

66R1: Rosenow obit.,
Am. J. of Clin. Path.
46 (July 1966),

APPENDIX B1: FOCAL INFECTION CHRONOLOGY -- ANNOTATED EXCERPTS

The Focal Infection Concept in the 7th Century BC; three accounts:

MEDICAL TIMES 854 (Aug. 1968):
 - "How old is the theory of focal infection? Very old indeed. The physician to King Ashurbanipal of Assyria (669-626 BC) is supposed to have prescribed the extraction of the royal teeth to cure pains afflicting the king in distant parts of his body."

Francke, 1974:
 - "In Niniveh, the capital of ancient Assyria on the eastern bank of the river Tigris, there was found a cuneiform table whose text deals with a king who lived 700 years before Christ and says, 'The pains in his head, arms and feet are caused by his teeth and they must be removed.'"

E.H. Hatton in G.V. Black, 1936:
- "The oldest known record of the extraction of teeth for the purpose of curing systemic disease is found in a letter of a court physician, Arad-Nana, to his king, some 2600 years ago. ...
    "'Continually the king has been asking why Arad-Nana has not made clear his disease and cured him. Now Arad has sent a sealed letter which he hopes they will read before the King. He will make prescription; let the ceremonies be carried out by a seer; let them bathe the King and straightway the fever will depart from the face of the King; let them apply to him oil two or three times. There is infection in the pus; let them bring licorice before the King, as they have done twice already; let them rub it in vigorously, then he will come and give further instructions. At once the strength of the King will revive, in the midst of the full tide to the King he will bring. The King shall place on his neck the salve Arad will send; on the appointed day let the King be anointed. Arad will speak the truth with the King, as the King demanded; the pain in his sides, and his feet has come from his teeth, and they must be extracted from his face.'
[translation by A.T. Olmsted of U. of Chicago]
    "This tablet is one of a large number which were discovered in the ruins of Nineveh and Ashur, capitals of Ancient Assyria. The time is between B.C. 648 and B.C. 626. The King referred to is probably the one named Aanapper in Ezra 4:10."

Hippocrates
   The father of medicine as we know it, Hippocrates of Cos, related how "Many were attacked by erysipelas all over the body, when the exciting cause was a trivial accident or injury."[127]

   It is noted also that Hippocrates regarded epilepsy, "the disease called the sacred" as a common disease, which "arises from causes as the others, namely those things that enter and quit the body ..." [360]; such a view is consistent with Dr.

Rosenow's demonstration of a bacterial cause.

Further we find Hippocrates discussing the seasonality of diseases [300], a subject elevated to considerations of correlations between solar radiation and bacterial mutations by Dr. Rosenow. Hippocrates specifically mentioned many diseases shown by Rosenow to be related to bacteria, e.g., maniacal, epilepsy, bloody flux, coryza, hoarseness, cough, arthritis, sciatica [300]

EIGHTEENTH CENTURY - Benjamin Rush

Benjamin Rush (1745-1813), a signer of the Declaration of Independence, was a Philadelphia physician and the foremost medical man of his time. He also, in 1774, had co-founded the first anti-slavery society in America. He had received his medical education at Cullen at Edinburgh, and was an excellent clinician and writer. [Encyclopedia Britannica 1943; McManus 1963, p. 104]

Rush: "I have been made happy by discovering that I have only added to the observations of other physicians, in pointing out a connection between the extraction of decayed and diseased teeth and the cure of general diseases. ... I am disposed to believe that [the teeth] are often the unsuspected causes of general, and particularly of nervous diseases." Rush specifically mentioned rheumatism, dyspepsia, epilepsy, headache, vertigo, intermitting fevers and consumption as examples of diseases which had apparently been cured when infected teeth were extracted. [Rush 1818, in Duke 1918]]

It is noted that, as per his own statement, Rush's position was neither original nor exclusive to him. His endorsement, rather, indicates a general acknowledgement by physicians of the era of the relationship between diseased teeth and systemic disease.

NINETEENTH CENTURY

Several authors through the 19th century addressed the subject of infected teeth as the cause of various eye diseases; in 1915 A.D. Black compiled a list of 41 such articles, including 22 written from 1839 to 1900. Following is an alphabetical index of subjects covered in these 41 articles (see APPENDIX B2 for citations):
Eye disease from oral infection, in articles, 1842-1915, per A.D. Black 1915:
    --accomodation - Black 1915, Power 1884, Stevens 1901, McConachie 1903, Allport 1904, Wood's Amer. Ency. ... 1915
    --amaurosis - Black 1915, Koecker 1842, Watson 1851, Hogg 1857, Hancock 1859, Salter 1862, Kempton 1862, DeWitt 1868, Alexander 1869, Delestre 1869, Fruhauf 1873, Lardier 1875, Sirletti 1878, Marshall 1883, Power 1884, Stevens 1901, Allport 1904, La Stomato. 1906, Tribbles 1914, Dutrow 1915, Ibershoff 1915, Wood's Amer. Ency. ... 1915
    --amblyopia - Black 1915, Power 1884, Stevens 1901, McConachie 1903, Allport 1904, Wood's Amer. Ency. ... 1915

--blepharospasm - Power 1884, Ibershoff 1915, Wood's Amer. Ency. ... 1915
--cataract - McConachie 1903, Goulden 1911
--chronic ophthalmia - Blanc 1871, Allport 1904
--conjunctivitis - Power 1884, McConachie 1903, Allport 1904, Goulden 1911, Wood's Amer. Ency. ... 1915, Black 1915a
--corneal inflammations - Power 1884, Wood's Amer. Ency. ... 1915
--exophthalmos - Power 1884, Allport 1904, Wood's Amer. Ency. ... 1915
--extra-ocular muscles, spasms or paralysis - Stevens 1901, Goulden 1911, Wood's Amer. Ency. ... 1915
--fatigue - MacWhinnie 1913
--focal infection and - Black 1915
--glaucoma - Power 1884, Allport 1904, Wood's Amer. Ency. ... 1915
--hypermetropia - Goulden 1911
--iridocyclitis - Goulden 1911, Tribbles 1914, Wood's Amer. Ency. ... 1915
--iritis - Allport 1904, Beaumont 1913, Wood's Amer. Ency. ... 1915
    -scleritis - McConachie 1903, Allport 1904
--lagophthalmus - Power 1884, Hutchinson 1886, Allport 1904
--mydriasis - Power 1884, McConachie 1903, Wood's Amer. Ency. ... 1915
--myosis - Wood's Amer. Ency. ... 1915
--neuralgia - Dental News Letter 1847, TMerritt 1911, MacWhinnie 1913, Tribbles 1914, Dutrow 1915, Ibershoff 1915, Wood's Amer. Ency. 1915
--optic neuritis - McConachie 1903, Allport 1904
--orbital abscess - Stevens 1901, Wood's Amer. Ency. 1915
--phlyctenular ophthalmia - Power 1884, Allport 1904, Goulden 1911
--ptosis - St. Bartholomew's 1881, Allport 1904
--sclerotitis - Hutchinson 1886, Stevens 1901, McConachie 1903
--strabismus - Power 1884, Wood's Amer.Ency.1915

TRIFACIAL NEURALGI   Flint 1868
  Flint, 1868, on trifacial neuralgia, "formerly called 'tic douloureux'... . An occasional cause of this condition is caries of the teeth. It is by no means frequently referable to this cause, but that it is so occasionally cannot be doubted."
    Austin Flint, M.D., 1812-1886, 36th President of the AMA
    (1884)

FOCUS OF INFECTION, MOUTH AS   Miller 1891
  In 1891 W. D. Miller presented details of the more general influence of dental infections, describing the human mouth as a focus of infection.
  Hatton (in GV Black) 1936 credits W.D. Miller in 1891 with first use of the term "focus of infection" with reference to

conditions in the mouth. Miller is noted as having mentioned septicemia, pyemia, meningitis, encephalitis, brain abscess, disturbances of the alimentary tract, diseases of the lung, croupous pneumonia, lymphadenitis, infectious anginae and maxillary sinus disease.

ORAL SEPSIS   William Hunter 1899
   Unquestionably the major influence behind the virtual explosion of awareness of the impact of dental infections on overall health was the work of William Hunter of England, primarily from 1899-1911.
   As early as 1899 Hunter discussed dental diseases in relation to general diseases, particularly infectious gastritis. Hunter 1899 referred to the problem of the constant swallowing of pus: "... in pus organisms are so virulent as those grown in connection with necrotizing bone." Therefore, he concluded, oral sepsis is "particularly virulent" as it involves teeth. Hunter thought the matter important "not only in relation to gastritis, but in relation to the whole group of infections caused by pus organisms - local, for example, as tonsillitis, glandular swellings, middle ear supprations, maxillary abscesses; general, for example, ulcerative endocarditis, empyemata, meningitis, nephritis, osteomyelitis and other septic conditions." Hunter proposed the removal of all "useless stumps of necrosed tooth or fang: and daily sterilizing by boiling of every tooth plate worn.

OPTIC NEURITIS McConachie 1903
   McConachie 1903 [McConachie, A.D., *Dental Cosmos*, 1903, p. 941, "Reflex Neuroses of Dental Origins as Manifest in Eye, Ear, Nose and Throat Diseases."], p. 942, speaking to a Maryland State Dental Association and D.C. Dental Society meeting on "the subject assigned me: 'Reflex Neuroses of Dental Origin as Manifest in Eye, Ear, Nose, and Throat Diseases', noted that "Many observers have published records of affections of the eye attributed to decaying or decayed teeth."

OPTIC NEURITIS Allport 1904
   Frank Allport [*Dental Review* 18 (April 15, 1904), #4, Chicago, Ill., U.S.A., "The Relation of Odontology to Opthamology and Otology.", 305-315], discussed mouth disease as relates to sight and hearing.
   p. 306-7, "No argument is necessary to convince you and me that diseases of the teeth and mouth may produce pathological changes in the organs of sight and hearing... . We know it because we have seen it over and over again ... [however] it is much to be regretted that opthamologists and otologists are prone to carelessly neglect the prolific etiologic influence of the mouth.
   "In the *Annals of Ophthamology and Otology* for October 1895, Foucher of Montreal reports a case of a man 50 years of age, who had a decayed, aching and broken molar tooth. He developed a kerato-scleritis and conjunctivitis, together with herpatic eruptions on the cornea, and a little above the eyebrow along the

sensitive branches of the ascending frontal nerve. The tooth was
extracted and permanent relief was obtained.

"Foucher also reports another case of a girl aged 21 years, who
had an irritable third molar, accompained by great pain in the
eye and optic neuritis, with total suppression of vision. The
tooth was extracted and a speedy cure followed. ...

p. 313, "F.W. Marlow, of Syracuse, N.Y., reports a case in the
Annals of Ophthamology for January 1897, of a young lady aged 25
years, who had an alveolar abscess of the first bicuspid of the
lower left jaw which was opened and cured. It proceeded from an
infected root canal. She developed pain in the eye and optic
neuritis with great blurring of vision and subsequently entirely
recovered."

MENTAL ILLNESS AND IMPACTED/INFECTED TEETH Upson 1908
Upson, Henry S., *Insomnia and Nerve Strain*, G.P. Putnam's Sons,
N.Y. and London, The Knickerbocker Press 1908.
Upson 1908, pp. 13-44, provides descriptions of 25 illustrative
cases of neuroses and psychoses, seventeen of which were cured
following the extraction of infected or impacted teeth.

IMPACTED INCISOR/BICUSPID TEETH, & MENTAL ILLNESS Upson 1908
Such impacted teeth discussed were generally molars, but some
cases mentioned other teeth. One patient's teeth "showed no
lesions with the exception of a number of cavities, one of which
affected the pulp chamber. Convalescence began before his dental
work was finished ... ." [p. 13] A patient with severe hysteria
and screaming attacks, following the removal of an impacted lower
third molar tooth and an abscessed upper incisor, "has since been
perfectly well." [p. 31] Another patient's "right upper first
bicuspid tooth was found badly impacted and was drawn. For a
week or ten days he was unmanageable, but then began to quiet
down, slept well, and has gone on to a progressive recovery." [p.
32] A physician with acute mania was found to have a badly
impacted first bicuspid tooth, which was extracted. "For a week
or ten days he was unmanageable, but then began to quiet down,
slept well, and has gone on to a progressive recovery."

TEETH MOST IMPORTANT CAUSE OF MENTAL DERANGEMENT Upson 1908
Upson 1908, p. 131-2, concludes: "Of the viscera responsible
for the more obscure cases of nervous and mental derangement I
have no hesitation in designating the teeth as the most
important. ...

ABSCESS WHEN TEETH FAIL TO DEVELOP/TEMP.TOOTH Upson 1908
JAW IMPACTIONS, ABSCESSES Upson 1908
Upson 1908, 132, "The two most important lesions, impaction and
abscess ... usually ... can only be discovered by skiagraph.
Impactions may be in any region of the jaw. They may be
indicated with some probability by a gap where the missing tooth
should be, but such a gap is by no means conclusive. An
extraction may have been made and forgotten, or teeth fail to

develop, leaving a gap or a temporary tooth persistent sometimes for years."

FRANK BILLINGS COINS TERM "FOCAL INFECTION" Billings 1909
   Francke 1974 noted that several writers in the early 20th century contributed variously to the genesis and popularity of the focal infection concept. For example, Gürich of Germany is said to have "confirmed a focal connection between tonsilitis and rheumatoid arthritis. ... his compatriot Passler drew attention to a causal relation between a series of septic states of ill-health and infected teeth and tonsils." [Francke 1974] In the U.S., the most prominent voice at the time addressing the importance if dental infections was that of Frank Billings.

      Frank Billings was elected (55th) President of the American Medical Association in 1902, and according to Fishbein 1947 "was from that time on to be one of the most important officers in the building of the Association." [p.224] "All those who were privileged to hear his presidential address on "Medical Education" at the dNew Orleans session in 1903, recognized that it ushered in a new epoch in American medical education."
      Hirsch 1966 notes that Dr. Billings had "motivated studies on the relationship of focal infection to systemic diseases. ... Dr. Billings regarded the invitation to deliver the Lane Lectures on focal infection [as relates to systemic disease] at the Leland Stanford Jr. Medical School in San Francisco, September 20-24, 1915, as his greatest honor."
      Although Sir Almroth Wright had previously referred to foci of infection, Frank Billings is generally credited with coining the term "focal infection" with reference to the primary role of diseases of the mouth as causing disease elsewhere in the body. Following this, early in 1913 Charles H. Mayo spoke of "diseases secondary to local infections"

INFECTIOUS ENDOCARDITIS Billings 1909
   p. 411-412, reported that Rosenow had isolated a pneumococcus, which had many of the morphological characteristics of the streptococci, in several cases of endocarditis.
   Billings 1909, p. 414, regarding the source of infection in cases of infectious endocarditis:
   "There can be no doubt whatever that simple local infection, like tonsillitis, as well as abscesses of the aural cavities, infections of the postnasal space of the antra, and so forth, may be the port of entry."

OSLER ON ORAL FOCAL INFECTION Osler 1909
   Sir William Osler (1849-1919) was generally considered the foremost physician of his time. In 1909, even prior to Hunter's major publication and resultant publicity in 1911, and through 1918 (see OSLER 1918, below), Osler was among the many who

referred to Hunter on the subject of the importance of oral focal infection:

"To William Hunter, of Charing Cross Hospital, is due the credit of insisting upon the importance of the mouth as the chief channel of entrance of the pyogenic organisms, and as itself the seat of septic processes. Necrosed teeth, pyorrhoea alveolaris, gingivitis, alveolar abscess, etc., are present in a great many people. A systemic infection may follow or the general health may be lowered by the continuous production of pus. In extensive pyorrhoes alveolaris the daily amount of pus must be considerable, and there can be no question that it has a debilitating influence on the general health and is sometimes associated with a moderate anaemia and with a pasty complexion. Hunter describes septic gastritis and septic enteritis as common sequences; indeed, he regards appendicular, pleuritic, gall-bladder and pyelitic inflammations as forms of "medical sepsis" due largely to infection from the mouth. One form of pernicious anaemia -- infective haemolytic anaemia -- he believes to be due to oral sepsis, or an infective glossitis. Of the 20 cases of pernicious anaemia which I had under observation in 1904, phorrhoea alveolaris was present in more than half, but not one presented the infective glossitis. Certain types of nephritis are also believed to be due to oral infection."

"There is no question of the importance of the subject, and we should insist upon scrupulous cleanliness of the mouth and teeth, particularly clearing away the tartar and the pockets of pus." [Osler 1909, p. 440]

We may note that pernicious anemia, as early as the works of Hunter, throughout the career of Rosenow, and again in the current medical literature has been linked to infected teeth; pernicious anemia is also one of the conditions whose difficult etiology was fodder for purveyors of the "autoimmune disease" craze of recent memory. [see FOCAL UPDATE; AUTOIMMUNITY]

ORAL SEPSIS   Hunter 1911
Particularly well-publicized were his 1911 statements which he described a number of cases of (apparently septic) anemia, associated with a variety of diseases, which were corrected upon the removal of diseased teeth or teeth roots:

"In my clinical experience septic infection is without exception the most prevalent infection operating in medicine, and a most important and prevalent cause and complication of many medical diseases. ... the chief seat of that sepsis is in the mouth, and the sepsis itself [causes] various conditions of ill health with which it is associated ... vis, the general ill health, dirty, sallow complexion, the indigestions, the gastric and intestinal troubles, the anemias which resist treatment, the tonsillitic, pharyngeal, and glandular troubles of children, the chronic rheumatisms, obscure fevers and blood poisonings, etc." [*Lancet*, Jan 14, 1911, reprinted in J. J. Herschfeld, *Bull. Hist. Dent.* 33:35-45 (1985)]

A MASOLEUM OF GOLD OVER A MASS OF SEPSIS Hunter 1911 [*Lancet*, Jan 14, 1911, *Dent. Brief* 16 (1911)]

"My clinical experience satisfies me that if oral sepsis (and naso-pharyngeal) could be successfully excluded, the other channels by which "medical sepsis" gains entrance into the body might almost be ignored." (DENT. BRIEF 16, 1911, 853)

"Gold fillings, gold caps, gold crowns, fixed dentures, built in, on and around diseased tooth roots, form a veritable masoleum of gold over a mass of sepsis to which there is no parallel in the whole realm of medicine or surgery. The whole constitutes a perfect gold trap of sepsis of which the patient is proud and which no persuasion will induce him to part with. ...

"... The worst cases of anaemia, gastritis, colitis of all kinds and degrees, of obscure fever of unknown origin, or purpura, or nervous disturbances of all kinds, ranging from mental depression up to actual lesions of the cord, or chronic rheumatic infection, of kidney disease, are those which owe their origin to, or are gravely complicated by, the oral sepsis produced in private patients by these gold traps of sepsis." [p. 853] ...

"... The sepsis hereby produced is particularly severe and hurtful in its effects. For it is dammed up in the bone and in the periosteum, and cannot be got rid of by any antiseptic measures which the patient or the doctor can carryout. Moreover, it is painless, and its septic effects therefore go on steadily accumulating in inttensity without drawing attention to their seat of origin.

"Such are the fruits of this baneful so-called "conservative dentistry." The title would be a fitting one if the teeth were a series of ivory pegs planted in stone sockets. But the teeth being what they are - - namely, highly developed pieces of bone tissue, possessing, I would point out, a richer blood and nerve-supply than any piece of tissue of the same size in the whole body -- and planted in sockets of bone with the closest vascular relations to the bone and the soft tissues of the periosteum and the gums, the title that would best describe the dentistry here referred to would be that of "septic dentistry." (p. 854)

... a feature of the septic infection in the gums, the teeth or in the sockets of the teeth is that it is infection in contact with diseased bone, and its virulence is intensely aggravated by this fact. For no septic infection is more intensely virulent than that connected with diseased bone.

In his accounting of cases, Hunter discusses the direct question of diseased teeth and results obtained from their removal. Thus septic gastritis, septic colitis, septic anemia, gastric ulcer, erysipelas and ulcerative stomatitis, and possibly nephritis, were found to be caused by (and cured by removal of) oral sepsis, primarily necrosed tooth roots, septic teeth, and in one case a suppration of the frontal sinus. [p. 856-8]

ARTHRITIS Billings 1912

Billings 1912 and 1913 presented papers on focal infection as a causative factor in chronic arthritis.

Billings 1912, p. 484

"There is nothing new in the principle involved in the subject of the paper. It has long been known that acute rheumatic joint-infections are the result frequently of a primary infection of the faucial tonsils, or tissues about them. Pneumonia is doubtless the frequent result of the sudden change of a non-virulent to virulent type of pneumococcus whose common habitat is the upper respiratory passages in city dwellers. It has been shown that a common source of infection in epidemic cerebrospinial meningitis is the nasal mucous surfaces. Acute endocarditis also has its source, in many instances, from faucial tonsils."

NEPHRITIS Billings 1912
CARDIOVASCULAR DISEASE Billings 1912
NEURITIS Billings 1912
MYOSITIS Billings 1912

p. 485, lists as "results of focal infection, chronic arthritis, nephritis, cardiovascular degenerations, and chronic neuritis and myalgia (myositis).

p. 486: "Ordinary tonsillectomy leaves an abundance of lymphoid tissue which may be sealed over by the operative scar and leaves a worse condition than that for which the operation was made. ... in that foci of infection are frequently walled in."

p. 495, "... the streptococcus obtained in almost pure culture from many of the patients, when inoculated into animals, produced an acute arthritis ... [and] from the dead animals' tissues the streptococcus has been again obtained in cultures."

p 496 "It is also true that the cultures from the tonsils of patients who had no evidence of systemic infection contained the streptococcus practically identical with those patients who had systemic disease."

p. 497: "I think there can be no doubt that the insidious, slow, degenerative processes which occur in many patients who arrive at the meridian of life are due to slow intoxications from chronic focal infections variously located. ... The result of the removal of these infections has been most astounding in many instances."

p. 498 "... When the focal infection, wheresoever it may be located, seems to be related to the systemic disease, radical measures should be instituted to remove it. When this is done, those general measures which long have been recognized as essential to the well-being of an individual [e.g. proper hygenic management in diet, exercise, free excretion through the bowels, kidney, skin etc.] should be instituted so that nothing will be left undone which may restore an invalid to health."

ARTHRITIS Billings 1913

p. 819, confirmed his 1912 findings, that focal disease, usually located in the head, and most commonly a chronic streptococcus focus of the faucial tonsils, seemed to be a cause of systemic infection, especially arthritis deformans, as well as a chronic myositis and usually also some evidence of chronic neuritis.

in a study involving 70 chronic arthritis patients, Billings noted: "In this work the chronic focus of infection has been located in the faucial tonsils, dental alveoli or jaw, the antra of the head, and in the seminal vesicles and prostate gland.

"Rationally one may find the septic focus in any circumscribed streptococcus abscess, possibly a chronic appendicitis, chronic cholecystitis, etc. ...

MYOSITIS Billings 1913

"The study of these patients shows that an individual who suffers from what may be called a true arthritis deformans presents not only an arthritis ..., but also a chronic myositis ... which causes shortening of the muscular fibers. ... Most of these patients present evidence of chronic neuritis or perineuritis of single or multiple nerves, at some point in the course of the disease. ...

"There can also be no doubt that faulty metabolism modifies the whole morbid process. If one considers the results of the treatment carried out in this investigation it would seem that the faulty metabolism is not a primary factor etiologically. Nevertheless it is an important factor in the progress of the disease and also in its treatment.

"The severe trophic disturbances which occur in the joints (cartilage, bone, etc.), the appendages of the skin (nails, hair, sweat glands), are difficult to explain. ... Probably the primary cause is the tissue reaction to the bacterial toxin, and this specifically excites a proliferative or degenerative local metabolism with the characteristic morbid anatomy. ... There is ... a strain of the streptococcus which will specifically produce in the inoculated rabbit morbid anatomic lesions, which resemble the morbid joint changes in arthritis deformans in man."

ROLE OF THE KILLER STREPTOCOCCUS Billings 1913

p. 820: "The dominant organism found in abscesses and sealed crypts of the faucial tonsil are Streptococcus viridans and Streptococcus hemolyticus (pyogenes). The S. viridans is usually a surface growth, while the S. hemolyticus is frequently found in pure culture in the deeper infected tissues. In acute rheumatism the bacteria obtained from joint exudate and rheumatic nodes have been studied by Dr. E.C.Rosenow, fellow of the Memorial Institute for Infectious Diseases, cooperating with us. He has found that organisms from rheumatism appear to occupy a position between S. viridans and S. hemolyticus. They are more virulent than the former and less virulent than the latter. Three types of organisms have been isolated from rheumatism. One type produces green on blood-agar and forms very long chains. The second type produces a narrow zone of hemolysis on blood-agar from the beginning or after several generations and forms short chains. The third type produces a grayish-brown colony without affecting perceptively the blood in the media and appears as a diplococcus in short chains and as single cocci. By varying the condition of growth, these types may be changed quite readily, one into the other. the most distinct cultural features are their production of a very high acid reaction in dextrose broth and abundant growth at low temperature."

TRANSMUTATIONS, STREPTOCOCCI TO PNEUMONOCOCCI Billings 1913
   "Three of the strains from arthritis have been converted into typical pneumococci. Reverse transmutations may [also] be made ... by varying the culture mediums, oxygen tension, etc. The strains of streptococci studied from various patients are undoubtedly the same as those described by Poynton and Payne and Beattie as the micrococcus rheumaticus. The results of clinical studies and animal experimentation by Poynton, Payne, Walker, Beattie, Yates, Cole and others have been of great value in establishing the cause of acute articular rheumatism. Confusion has existed in the minds of many because the organisms described by the different investigators did not coincide.
   "The results of the work of Rosenow seem to adjust the differences, for his experiments show that the same organisms may be changed by cultural methods so that they may in medium show progressive phases of transmutation. The range of transmutation is from a type of streptococcus to the pneumococcus. Furthermore, at different stages of the transmutation he has, at will, produced in the inoculated rabbit, supprative arthritis, or at another phase multiple proliferating arthritis, endocarditis, pericarditis and myocarditis, or at another phase myositis of some of the general skeletal muscles, at another phase a virulent type which produces arthritis with proliferative and degenerative joint lesions, and at another phase typical pneumonia. These experiments probably clear up this difference in results and the varying types of streptococci described by many investigators."

AUTOGENOUS VACCINES Billings 1913
   p. 821, advocates autogenous vaccines after rest and improvement of hygiene:
   "There is value in vaccine therapy, but to obtain benefit from vaccines, they should be rationally used. To use vaccines, simple or mixed, in the treatment of a patient, without first ascertaining the nature of the disease, and if infectious, the kind of invading organism, is unscientific, reprehensible and wrong. When the mixed vaccines of the filtrate of culture-broth of countless organisms are used, it is like the shotgun prescription of our ancestors of the profession. ... [These] are usually without benefit to the patient with arthritis deformans and often result harmfully to the health or life of the invalid.

THERAPEUTIC REGIMEN: FOCUS,ENVIRONMENT,VACCINE Billings 1913

p. 822 "The treatment and management [of arthritis deformans] must comprise: (1) removal of the cause and (2) improvement of the immunity by rest, personal hygiene, including good food, pure air and sunshine, rational calesthenics and physical culture, moral support and a cheerful environment. Autogenous vaccine may be added to still further improve immunity"

SURGICAL WONDER - CHARLES HORACE MAYO Mayo 1913

Charles Horace Mayo was the younger son of William Worral Mayo, graduated from Chicago Medical College in 1898 (later merged into Northwestern University Medical School). Mayo was considered a "surgical wonder". [Encyclopedia Britannica] "Dr. Charles" served as the 70th President of the AMA (1917).

SYSTEMIC INFECTIONS Mayo 1913
CARCINOMA Mayo 1913
LEUCOPLAKIA Mayo 1913
ARTHRITIS,ETC Mayo 1913

Early in 1913 Charles H. Mayo spoke of "diseases secondary to local infections". Within the context of focal infection, Mayo made specific mention of transplants, aging, autointoxication, osteomyelitis (282-4), and "embolic bacterial origin" (291); mentioned in subsequent discussions were influenza, arthritis, (318) systemic infections, carcinoma, leucoplakia (p. 314), furunculosis, appendicitis, rheumatism (326).

"From the time of birth, ... and even before animal life continues alone, its destruction is prevented only through maintaining a vigorous conflict against bacteria and protozoa. ... This destructive invasion changes the arteries, the function of the heart, etc., and finally, after making life uncomfortable, brings on a premature old age, due to an exhaustion of nutritive supplies, to a weakening and devitalizing of defenses, until the army of phagocytes retire defeated by death, the conqueror of all things." (283)

BLOOD MAY CONTAIN MANY LIVING BACTERIA Mayo 1913

"... the blood may contain many living bacteria, e.g., pneumococci, streptococci and staphylococci and various bacilli. ... [which] may produce either very great or very little effect as externally manifested." (p. 285)

"That scourge of the human race, pyorrhea, accounts for an enormous amount of blood infection." (p. 286)

Mayo cites experiments which "seem to furnish evidence first that a large proportion of patients with stomach trouble have infected oral cavities and, second, that this infection is in direct relation to the formation of a peptid-splitting enzyme in the saliva." (p. 288)

"Hale White, Osler, Billings and many other noted internists have written on the subject of systemic diseases arising from infections of the mouth." ... (p, 290)

APPENDICITIS Mayo 1913
TONSILS Mayo 1913
RHEUMATISM Mayo 1913
   "... Poynton and Paine [*Lancet* Oct. 28, 1911, 1189] report a
case of appendicitis which, upon removal, gave a pure culture of
the same strain as that cultured from a diseased tonsil removed
at the same time, These streptodiplococci were injected into
rabbits, causing arthritis, and the fluid removed from the
arthritis again gave a pure culture.

BLOOD - PNEUMOCOCCUS IN PNEUMONIA Mayo 1913
   "Rosenow found positive blood cultures of pneumococcus in 132
out of 145 cases of pneumonia."(p. 291) [*J. Infect. Dis.* i
(1904), 280-312]
   "In 1887 Mantel said he believed that rheumatism came from
diseased tonsils. Since then many observers have proved the
truth of his hypothesis. Frank Billings recently reported some
cases of multiple arthritis in which the fluid withdrawn from the
joint gave the same strain of streptococcus grown from pus
removed from the tonsil. Removal of the tonsils cured the
rheumatism."(p. 292)
   Mayo 1913-293 refers to Kobrack (1907) finding of "bacteriemia
to be a very significant diagnostic evidence of sinus thrombosis
in the middle ear and mastoid diseases. They may be present in
the blood in varying degrees for days or 2 or 3 weeks before
other positive indications call for operation."
   "Wright states ... that no one recovers from bacterial disease
unless it be by production of protective substances in his own
body."(p. 293)

ACQUIRED IMMUNITY FROM SMALLPOX Mayo 1913
   "We seem to have a heritage of acquired immunity from ages of
vaccinating against smallpox and the disease is now far less
virulent." (p. 293)
   p. 295, states Wright and Douglas showed that vaccines and
serums act "by raising the opsonic index, thus aiding yet leaving
the blood to fight its own battles."

LAMENTING THE DISAPPEARANCE OF THE FAMILY DOCTOR Mayo 1913
   p. 295, "The old family practitioner has almost entirely
disappeared."
   p. 295, "In obscure maladies and cases of puzzling diagnosis
their immediate or past presence - however remote - in the system
can in most cases be told by the reactions of the skin or of the
blood in the body or in a test tube in the presence of proper
sera."

DANGER OF EXTRACTION Davis in Mayo 1913
   Davis, D.J., in discussion following Mayo 1913:, p. 323
   "I have seen a number of cases in which death has resulted in
young healthy persons - I do not mean old people - from
infections of the mouth, that followed within a week or so the

extraction of a tooth for an alveolar abscess that was in a state
of acute excitement."

PREDICTION: COMING FOCAL INFECTION FAD   Herrick in Mayo 1913
   Herrick, James B., in discussion following Mayo 1913, cites
instances of focal infection in tonsils and teeth, 310.
   "For years William Hunter has contended that pernicious anemia
was due to oral sepsis, ... infection, as he believes, with a ...
peculiar form of streptococcus."p. 311
   "May I add just a word of caution? It is an easy thing for one
to become a fadist. It is easy to follow a fashion and jump to
the conclusion that practically all of our obscure diseases may
be and are due to small foci of infection. There may be, as the
result of a fad, a too wholesale cutting out of tonsils and
pulling of teeth. ... While we should recognize that there is
truth in this important lesson as to focal infections, we must
not in extravagant manner think this accounts for all our chronic
diseases." p. 312

CARCINOMA   Lewis in Mayo 1913
   Lewis, Dean D., in discussion following Mayo 1913, p. 318
   "As yet we are absolutely powerless against carcinomas, and the
only thing we can do is exercise good prophylaxis. We have
recognized for years that the little pigmented moles may at any
time become serious lesions, and an insignificant lesion may
cause the death of the patient by metastatic infection."

CHRONIC FATIGUE SYNDROME? Moorehead in Mayo 1913
   Moorehead 1913 [Frederick B., in Discussion, Mayo 1913a]
   "We have no doubt that many cases in which no focus of
infection or resulting lesion can be demonstrated, where the
patient is physically "below par" might very properly be charged
to a long standing lo grade toxemia."

EMBOLIC PROCESS - INFECTIOUS ENDOCARDITIS Rosenow in Mayo 1913
   Rosenow E.C., in discussion following Mayo 1913, p. 321
   Dr. Rosenow discusses the operative mechanism of infectious
endocarditis: "It is an infective process. The bacteria
probably gain entrance into the body through the tonsil or from
some pyorrheal condition of the teeth, or from abscesses, and
plug the fine capillaries of the heart valves. In these little
capillaries lies the greater susceptibility of infection of the
young heart valve or sclerosed valve. ... One other reason which
enables this organism to grow is the fact that it grows in long
chains and in clumps. It is this characteristic manner of growth
and the mechanical protection in the fine capillaries which
enables this non-virulent organism in a strict sense to produce
this disease."

DEGENERATIVE CHANGES OF OLD AGE - TOXINS Mayo 1913b
   p. 370 "Metchnikoff [*Ann. d. l'inst. Pasteur*, xii, 1898]
states that the toxins produced by the intestinal flora of the

large bowel are the cause of much of the vascular and
degenerative changes of old age."
   p. 371, refers to Hale White, Osler, and billings; discusses
correlations of diseased tonsils with appendicitis, rheumatism,
arthritis, osteomyelitis, hyperthyroidism.

VIRULENCE OF MIXED CULTURES Mayo 1913b
   p. 373, advocates "Wright's vaccines prepared from the
bacterial cultures taken from the patient himself (autogenous
vaccines"." Mayo recommends mixed cultures because "many
bacteria grow well in mixed cultures while some are only thus
rendered virulent."

ARTHRITIS, COMPLEMENT FIXATION Hastings 1914
   Hastings 1914, in a study of complement fixation tests of
arthritis concludes, "p. 71, " ... Streptococcus viridans is the
probable causative agent of the disease in many cases of
arthritis deformans. Probably 40 percent and more of cases of
arthritis deformans should be considered as chronic infective
deforming arthritis."

EYE DISEASES A.D. Black 1915
   Black 1915 lists the following optic conditions as caused by,
and often cured by correction of, diseases of the teeth:
accomodation, amaurosis, amblyopia, blepharospasm, cataract,
chronic opthalmia, conjunctivitis, corneal inflammations,
exophthalmos, extra-ocular muscle spasm or paralysis, fatigue,
glaucoma, hypermetropia, iridocyclitis, iritis, kerato-scleritis,
lagophthalmus, mydriasis, myosis, neuralgia, optic neuritis,
orbital abscess, phlyctenular, opthalmia, ptosis, sclerotitis,
strabismus, uveitis.
   Black, 1915, summarized and listed some 41 articles from the
early dental literature, from 1839 to 1915, which had discussed
the apparent causal relation between diseases of the teeth and
diseases of the eye. Black refers to various eye and ear
ailments, including optic neuritis and even loss of sight, which
were cured by dental treatment. Two of these were cited by Black
as relating to the subject of optic neuritis, McConachie 1903 and
Allport 1904.

IRIDOCYCLITIS de Schweinitz 1915
   de Schweinitz 1915, p. 601, "Nearly 20 years ago W. A. Brailey
and Sydney Stephenson [*System of Diseases of the Eye*, Norris and
Oliver ed., 1898] reached the conclusion that most forms of
iridocyclitis resulted from the action of microorganisms, and it
is safe to repeat, in so far as our present knowledge extends,
that almost every case of inflammation of the uveal tract, that
of uveitis or iridocyclitis, is of septic or toxic origin."
   [p. 602, "... to use Mr. Beumont's apt sentence, 'the
dethronement of iridocyclitis from the position of an independent
disease to the secondary one of a complication', must be kept
constantly in mind."

George E. de Schweinitz served as 75th President of the AMA (1922). [Fishbein 1947]

JACK-BENNY-RULE: ROSENOW AT AGE 39 Edward C. Rosenow 1915
   As impressive as was the body of focal infection work up to this time, it all seems to have merely set the stage for the incredible works and career of E.C. Rosenow, his refinement of the general concepts of oral focal infection in the form of his demonstration of the phenomenon of elective localization of bacteria, and his reported grand strides toward the "perfection" of vaccine therapy.
   Utilizing very specific culture techniques, Dr. Rosenow consistently was able to isolate a type of streptococcus which he referred to as alpha non-hemolytic strepcocci viridans, and which tended to electively locate in organs of laboratory animals which corresponded to diseases of persons from which the organisms were taken.
   In 1915 Dr. Rosenow summarized results of IV injection of laboratory animals, which data was first published by Frank Billings in his Lane Lectures of 1915. Thus it may be seen that this breakthrough achievement was attained during the year Dr. Rosenow had reached age 39, "an age described by none other than Jack Benny as representing the peak of perfection in the human male." [Lewis Flint, *Behavior Patterns of Hydration*, 1964.)

FRANK BILLINGS' FINEST HOUR Billings 1916
   Billings 1916 (Lane Lectures), page v., states "the etiologic relation of focal infection to systemic disease has been a subject of study in the clinical material of Rush Medical College, in affiliation with the U. of Chicago and the Presbyterian Hospital for the past 12 or more years."
   p. 26 cites his own work and that of Rosenow as confirming "the report of Schottmüller [*Münch. Med. Wchnschr.* 1903, L, 845] in the isolation from the blood during life of the patient of a pure culture of streptococcus viridans. Schottmuller isolated a streptococcus from patients with chronic infectious endocarditis, which grew fine colonies on blood agar plates, was non-hemolyzing, but produced a greenish halo around the colonies. In consequence it was named S. viridans and because of its low virulence for animals it was also called streptococcus mitior."
   p. 36, includes elective localization data subsequently published by Rosenow, *JAMA* 1916, p. 1687, which data was the target of Holman's fraud in 1928.

GENESIS OF ELECTIVE LOCALIZATION CONCEPT Billings 1916
   "The acquirement of a selective specific tissue affinity by a strain of streptococci has been noted by Forssner [*Nord. Med. Arkiv.* 1902, xxxv, 1-56]. by culture in kidney and kidney extract, the ordinary streptococcus pyogenes (hemolysans), which had no pathogenic elective affinity for the kidney, was converted into a strain, which injected intravenously into animals constantly produced outspoken anatomical lesions of the kidney.

This Forssner believes is positive proof that the bacteria of a local infection may attain a specific pathogenic and elective tissue affinity."

IRIDOCYCLITIS Irons Brown and Nadler 1916
   Irons Brown and Nadler 1916, reproduced iridocyclitis in 5 of the initial 8 rabbits injected IV with hemolytic streptococci isolated from the inflamed tear sac of a patient with iridocyclitis.
   Cultures of hemolytic streptococci taken from the tear sac subsequently failed to produce iridocyclitis, which the authors attributed to a probable change in the invasive power of hte organism for ocular tissue.

DENTAL SEPSIS AND PHYSICAL DEGENERATION OF AGING Duke 1918
   Duke 1918, p. 7, "One of the main advances of recent years ... has been the disclosure of the fact that small and apparently innocent infections which give rise to little or no local disturbance may likewise be the source of serious generalized disease."
   Duke 1918, p. 17-21, quotes Rush, p. 20
   "Very few men of 50 years or over who show advanced stages of dental sepsis are normal physically. ... Men of advanced age who have worn false teeth for a number of years have better health as a rule than the average of their age who have retained defective teeth."
   p. 39, "The tendency of devitalized teeth to abscess varies in different individuals."
   p. 72 "Streptococcus viridans is found more constantly in the deeper pyorrhea pockets and in alveolar abscesses than other organisms, and usually predominates in number."
   Duke summarized the "most important suggestions" of Rosenow, Billings and co-workers: "First, that the number of diseases caused by streptococci is greater than was formerly supposed; second, that streptococci may acquire affinities for certain tissues, which in many instances is remarkably specific; third, that streptococci may change in their selective affinities, morphology and cultural characteristics and biologic reactions after cultivation in artificial media or after growth in animal tissues.
   Whereas Forssner had earlier shown that a nonspecific streptococcus may acquire an affinity for kidney, (p, 73) Billings and Rosenow concluded "that members of the streptococcus-pneumococcus group may develop affinities for certain tissues, but also while growing in primary foci of infection. ... They found the elective affinity less marked, however, in the strains isolated from the primary foci. The interesting deduction is made by Rosenow ... that a focus in specialized tissue, therefore, would seem less important as a distributor of bacteria than the primary focus."

THE REVOLUTION OF ROSENOW Duke 1918

p. 74, "It has long been known that the tendency of organisms
to localize depends to a certain extent on virulence, and that
the virulence of an organism is changed by environment.
Rosenow's elaboration has been so extensive, however, as to
almost revolutionize former views concerning infection."
    p. 106, Conclusions:
"It is now apparent that many disorders, which in previous
years were considered obscure in origin and incurable, are due
wholly or in part to chronic infection, and that such diseases
can often be cured or retarded in their progress by removal of
the primary source of infection. It is also apparent that the
ocurrence of chronic sepsis is far more frequent than was
formerly suposed. It is so frequent, in fact, that few of mature
age are wholly free from it."
    p. 109: "Oral sepsis ... may have a toxic effect with ensuing
disease in both normal and diseased organs."

RHEUMATIC FEVER AND TONSILLITIS Osler 1918

    In 1918 Osler [Osler, Sir William, *The Principles and Practice
of Medicine*, D. Appleton and Co., New York and London, 1918
(Eighth Edition)], p. 373, stated:
    "The tonsils are culture centres of many septic organisms,
particularly of the streptococcus type. The association of
rheumatic fever and rheumatic affections generally with infected
tonsils is a prevailing view, but it is an old story insisted on
by Lasague and other French writers years ago. A not
innconsiderable number of cases of rheumatic fever begin with
tonsillitis. With organisms isolated from the tonsils
experimental arthritis and endocarditis have been caused. The
removal of the tonsils has been followed by a complete recovery
of sub-acute and chronic forms of arthritis. This is as far as
the evidence goes."

TYPES OF DENTAL INFECTION:
APICAL ABSCESSES Cotton 1919, p. 271

    "... I think we are save in following the dictum of Thoma. He
quotes from Grieves as follows: 'There is to my knowledge no
medicament, nor method, germicidal, oxidizing or electrolytic,
that will revivify the pericemental apex. If it be vital, the
tooth is healthy; if it be diseased, the tooth is next to doomed.
 This is the point in treatment where materia medica stops and
good surgery begins.'"

FILLED TEETH WHERE X-RAYS DON'T GIVE CLEAR PICTURE Cotton 1919

    "... we found after extraction that the roots were eroded,
frequently absorbed, and that the tips of the roots for some
distance were necrotic; and cultures were always positive in
tresting either for the short-chain streptococcus or the
Connellan-King diplococcus ... .with the good results
obtained in ... extracting all such teeth, our position is
impregnable."

SOFT GRANULOMAS, OFTEN ON APPARENTLY VITAL TEETH Cotton 1919
  "These granulomata usually form below the crown of the tooth
and encircle the roots, often running completely around them. ...
 we have repeatedly cultured the apices of these teeth and have
always found them infected. Therefore, even if the granuloma
were removed [by scaling], the accompanying infection would
continue at the apex of the root and the damaging process go on.
  Such a granuloma does not show in the radiogram and can be
easily overlooked. Frequently, there is a faint red line near
the gum margin, or the gum may be somewhat swollen and purple,
but very seldom can pus be squeezed from the gum. The tooth may
have no filling and show no sign that it is diseased, although at
times it has a milky white appearance. It is our opinion that
such a condition is a result of the spread of infection from a
nearby infected tooth, for we have found it only where other
teeth were infected in the same region." Cotton describes a case
from the Spring of 1917 where this had occurred, requiring not
only the extraction of several teeth with apical abscesses, but
also eight molars. "... the result was remarkable. ... His
convalescence was rapid and in the summer he was accepted in the
U.S. Navy as a physically fit indivudual."

UNERUPTED THIRD MOLARS Cotton 1919
  Cotton 1919, p. 274-277, presents five cases over the previous
6 months "where the symptoms were directly due to unerupted
wisdom teeth and where, after extraction of these teeth, the
sympotoms rapidly disappeared. The symptoms varied from mere
headaches and irritability to profound mental disturbances,
lasting for two or three years."

MENTAL ILLNESS AND TEETH Cotton 1919
SYSTEMIC DISEASE AND TEETH Cotton 1919, p. 284
  "That infected teeth alone could cause very serious systemic
diseases was demonstrated by Hastings in 1914 ...." [Hastings TW,
"Complement-fixation tests in chronic infective deforming
arthritis and arthritis deformans", *J. Experimental Med.* XX, p.
52]
  "It can be seen that extracting the teeth, alone, will not
correct a focus in the kidney, liver, or gastro-intestinal tract;
hence there are failures that tend to discredit the whole theory
of focal infection, whereas the cause of our failures may be
found in our lack of attention to these secondary foci."
  In mental disease: "In about 25% of our cases the teeth alone
seem to be the source of infection and, with the removal of this
source, our patients rapidly recover. In speaking of mental
cases we mean the so-called functional group for which no
definite etiology had previously been found.
  "... in another group, about 25%, both the teeth and tonsils
are at fault, and have to be eliminated if we wish to restore the
patients."
  p. 286, "I feel I do not overstate the facts when I say that
insanity can be prevented or cured by a conscientious practice of

the principles discussed in this paper...

p. 287, "We were not the first to show that by eliminating
infected teeth mental diseases could be cured. In 1908 Henry S.
Upson, M.D., of Cleveland Ohio, published his work on the
relation of infected teeth to certain nervous and mental
conditions [Upton, Henry S., *Insomnia and Nerve Strain*,
G.P.Putnam's Sons, N.Y., 1908]. He reported cases of the so-
called functional psychoses as both dementia precox and manic
depressive insanity, which recovered when impacted and unerupted
molars were extracted, and root infections were eliminated. ...
Upson stated that Savage, the English alienist, reported, in
1876, a number of cases of insanity due to infected teeth, which
cases recovered when the infected teeth were extracted; and that
this work was mentioned by Lauder Brunton in an essay on cases of
insanity due to infected teeth. In Thoma's admirable book [KH
Thoma, 1916, Oral Abscesses, Ritter and Co., Boston Mass.] ...
there are a number of cases of insanity which recovered when
infected teeth were extracted ..."

RELATION OF MENTAL TO PHYSICAL DISEASE Cotton 1919
Cotton 1919, p. 288, "We have made the mistake of considering
the mental disease as the principal factor to be studied, but we
have learned that the mental symptoms are merely incidents in the
general infection and toxemia. ... One strain [of S. viridans]
may be more toxic than another and therefore affect the nervous
system. We have only been able to find in one case the organism
in the brain itself, hence we assume that the toxemia is the
causative factor in mental disease. Also we must take into
consideration the constitutional reaction of patients to these
poisons ...

MENTAL ILLNESS AND HEREDITY Cotton 1919
Cotton 1919, p. 289 "Where do we place heredity? ... We do not
underrate heredity nor constitutional factors, but we believe the
former has very little influence either in the etiology or in the
prognosis of mental diseases.

MENTAL ILLNESS & FOCAL INFECTION; CASE STUDIES Cotton 1919
Cotton 1919, p. 301-312, concludes with descriptions of 13 13
additional cases "that illustrate the relation of focal
infectyion to mental condition", in which either removal of
infected teeth, removal of infected teeth and tonsils, or these
in conjunction with autogenous vaccine resulted in dramatic
improvement, usually outright cures.

PULP INVASION: LONG DRAWN-OUT PROCESS Henrici/Hartzell 1919
PULP INFECTED EARLY IN CARIES,PYORRHEA Henrici/Hartzell 1919
Henrici and Hartzell 1919, in a study involving sterile-ly
removed pulps from "clinically vital teeth with grossly normal
roots", comparing teeth with pyorrhea, caries or both, against
"entirely normal" teeth, found infection in zero of 22 normal
teeth, v.s. 42% of 40 teeth with pyorrhea, 43% of 23 teeth with

caries, and 46% of 30 teeth with both pyorrhea and caries.
  "... in approximately one-half the number of vital teeth
invaded by caries or surrounded by pyorrhea, the pulp is already
infected by streptococci, a conclusion so startling that we felt
some hesitancy about placing our work on record at this time.
Nevertheless, we can find no fault in our technique, supported as
it is by a series of twenty-two normal controls with uniformly
negative results.
  "The route of invasion of the pulp from caries is clearly along
the dentinal tubules, and from pyorrhea it must be, as Collins
and Lyne state, 'by esxtension from the gingival tissues.' We
have referred in previous papers to lymphatic channels extending
from the gingival region thru the peridental membrane to the
apical region. ..."
  "From the results of our studies it would sem that the invasion
and destruction of the pulp is frequently a long drawn out
process, microorganisms being present long before actual necrosis
of the tissues takes place. ..."

RHEUMATISM AS CAUSED BY STREPTOCOCCUS Topley 1921
  Topley 1921, p. 344, relates that Springer in 1898 [Aetiol. u.
Klinik des Akut Gelenkrheum, Wien 1898] suggested that "acute
rheumatism is an attenuated pyaemia, due principally to
Streptococci", and that Rosenow had suggested that "Acute
rheumatism is due to streptococci which have peculiar properties
.... the hypothesis that acute rheumatism is caused by a
specific streptococcus, which has undergone variation in a
special direction, receives considerable support from the facts
at present established. The streptococcus which is generally
accepted as the cause of erysipelas, a characteristic and
notifiable disease, is generally acknowledged to be specifically
identical with the S. pyogenes, though here we must also assume
adaptation to special conditions of life."

ERYSIPELAS, PUERPERAL FEVER, SCARLET FEVER Topley 1921
  Topley relates that Newsholme (1895) has drawn attention to the
observed similarity of rheumatism with erysipelas, puerperal
fever and scarlet fever, all associated with streptococci. p.
346

BLOOD, ELECTIVE LOCALIZATION Barnes 1922
HIPPOCRATES AND ABSCESS OF EAR   Barnes 1922, p. 1,
  "Hippocrates mentioned that abscesss of the ear and necrosis of
the jaw may be due to infected teeth. More than 100 years ago
Benjamin Rush advanced the opinion that decayed teeth 'were the
unsuspected cause of general diseases', and reported a case of
rheumatism of the hip-joint cured by the extraction of a decayed
tooth..
  "... Rosenow believes that in regions of low blood supply a
gradation of available oxygen affords optimum conditions for the
growth of bacteria.
  "Dissemination of bacteria from foci of infection occurs by way

of the lymphatics or the blood stream. Experimental evidence
indicates that the latter is the most frequent avenue of
infection and that the invasion is embolic in character!"
  p. 5, Dr. George W. McCaskey of Fort Wayne, regarding
"Rosenow's conclusions in regard to the elective affinity of
bacteria for different organs and structures", "his work has been
so scientific, and his facts so firmly established that I believe
we must either repudiate his facts, or in a general way accept
his conclusion..
  "It was a brilliant conception to find the focal infections
postmortem, collate them with pathology, and proceed to establish
their etiologic relationship by animal experimentation. ..."

RHEUMATISM AND TEETH Mayo 1922
  Mayo 1922, p. 1206, "Hippocrates recorded two cases in which
eradication of infection of the mouth had relieved patients of
rheumatic troubles of the joints."
  "Years ago, I used to like to 'pull' teeth myself. Among other
things, no matter what the disease, I always felt if I could get
the old snags out of the mouth part of the cure would be
accomplished. It cured the patients of many things they did not
know came from infections in the mouth, and it helped me to learn
something of focal infection."

EXPERIMENTS YIELD 2000 RABBITS' FEET PER YEAR Price 1923
  Among the many physicians who were inspired by and were able to
replicate the results of Dr. Rosenow was Weston Price, an
organizer and member of the Research Commission of the American
Dental Association and Fellow of the American College of
Dentists. His 2-volume book, *Dental Infection, Oral and Systemic*
[1923: Cleveland, Penton Pub. Co.], "included clinical resumés of
2000 cases of systemic disease which he was convinced were
incited by dental infections. ... these books contained the
results of 25 years of study and research carried on at his
private laboratory at a cost approximating $250,000. ... The
extent of his studies are impressive since at times he had as
many as 16 persons engaged in investigations and in some years as
many as 500 rabbits alone, amongst other laboratory animals, were
required for inoculation." [H. A. Bartels 1965].
  (see also Price 1939)

SYMPTOMLESS FOCI Price 1923 Chapter LVIII, p. 29
COMFORT AS A SYMPTOM Price 1923 Chapter LVIII, p. 29
  "Local comfort not only is not a certain index of success or
safety, but may constitute both what is probably one of the
greatest paradoxes and one of the costilest diagnostic mistakes
through injury to health, that exists in both dental and medical
practice, because it may mean only the absence of local reaction
... whereas, the absence of this local reaction ... permits
[infection products] to pass throughout the body to irratate and
break down that patient's most susceptible tissue... ."

SMALL QUANTITIES OF INFECTION MAY CAUSE MAJOR REACTIONS

Price 1923, p. 30, "... the evidence at hand strongly suggests that soluble poisons may pass from the infected [root-filled] teeth ... and produce systemic disturbances entirely out of proportion to the quantity of poison involved."

DENTAL INFECTIONS AND PRECANCEROUS SKIN CONDITIONS

Price 1923, p. 35, "The evidence suggests ... dental infections may produce localized ... sensitizations [which] may develop into precancerous conditions."

DENTAL INFECTIONS AND HEART DISEASE

Price 1923, p. 51, discusses the correlation between heart disease and dental infection, as "most strikingly brought out" by Dr. Louis I. Dublin, statistician for the Metropolitan Life Insurance Co. in a paper published in The Nation's Health for August 1922, indicating that the incidence of heart disease as a cause of death increases consistently with age, and that, as shown in Chapter 4 and in Figure 3 of Chapter 9, "100 percent of the individuals suffering from heart involvement have extensive caries. ... the evidence at hand demonstrates that the incidence of death from heart involvements is very greatly reduced ... among the individuals ... who have had their dental infections removed ... ."

SYMPTOMLESS INFECTIONS: ABSENCE OF SYMPTOMS IS A BAD SIGN

Price 1923, p. 52, stresses that symptoms about a tooth root's apex (fistula, area of absorption, history of soreness) are indications of a protective reaction, whereas the absence such symptoms are a bad sign which "argue for the extraction of the tooth ... ." In the case of a patient with heart disease under consideration, Dr. Price argued also for extraction of not only those teeth with putrescent pulps and chronic apical lesions, but also of molar teeth with deep caries involving ... the major portions of crowns of the teeth even thopugh the pulps were vital. ... [due to] the [great] probability of these pulps' dying under any restorations ... . Even a toothless patient with a heart that will work ... is infinitely better than a quantity of gold crowns or any other type of more approved dental restorations [which incapacitate] the patient."

p. 53, "As I dictate this paragraph, my memory goes back to patient after patient whose life has gone out prematurely ... from heart infolvement and other complications ... , and in whose mouth there were teeth which ... had not sufficient evidence of pathology to condemn. As I would now interpret those teeth, what I mistook to be insufficient evidence of pathology, was an inadequate local reaction; and the lack of rarefaction or evidence of condensation of bone were really evidences of that poor defence ... [and] many of those patients ... might have lived for years had I known to put into practice what I am teaching in this book."

THE RELATION OF DENTAL CARIES TO SYSTEMIC DISEASES
  Price, 1923, Chapter IX, p. 154-7, presents statistics
correlating dental caries with rheumatic group lesions,
concluding that they are proportional. Relation of caries to
type of rheumatic group lesions are presented as percentage of
each type with caries in Figure 83 on p. 156, as follows:

Table B1: Relation of caries to type of rheumatic group lesion

Type lesion	Percent with Caries
Digestive Tract	70
Internal Organs	70
Nerves	90
Rheumatism	90
Heart	100
Kidney	100

Note that Dr. Price's works are available through the Price
Pottenger Nutrition Foundation, 2667 Camino del Rio, S., Ste.109,
San Diego, CA 92108-3767; (619)574-PPNF.

ULCERATIVE COLITIS Bargen 1924
  Bargen, JA, *J.A.M.A.* 83 (Aug. 2, 1924, "Experimental studies on
the etiology of chronic ulcerative colitis", provides a brief
summary history of this disease, suggesting its "pedigree" can be
traced back to the "bloody flux" of Sydenheim in 1669.
  Sterile swabs from the base of colon ulcers or easily-bleeding
mucous membranes of patients were cultured in dextrose-brain
broth, as per Rosenow's works, and from 2-8 cc of resulting
diplococcus (predominating or pure) cultures were injected
intravenously in rabbits. Lesions essentially like those in
patients were reproduced in the rabbits and again in several
successive animal passages. The importance of the use of tall
tubes of glucose brain broth, which afforded a gradient of oxygen
tension, was emphasized by the author and echoed by Dr. Rosenow;
it was noted that "failure to detect the causative diplococcus
followed direct [conventional] plating methods".

FRAUD PERPETRATED AGAINST ROSENOW Holman 1928
  Holman 1928 attempted to delineate between the concepts of
focal infection and (Rosenow's) elective localization,
enthusiastically embracing the former including even elements of
Rosenow, but derogatorily rejecting elective localization as "a
theory with little if any experimental basis". Holman's faulty
and even fraudulent case against elective localization, and his
continuing legacy, is summarized and exhibited in "Doctoring the
Numbers (see 2.4, above). Nonetheless, Holman praised Rosenow
etc. for having changed focal infection from a theory to a
principle (which in fact Rosenow did do, primarily through the
proof of elective localization!):

FOCAL INFECTION CHANGED FROM THEORY TO PRINCIPLE Holman 1928
"... what Rosenow and his followers particularly showed and what
all the other investigators of the problem have definitely
demonstrated is that streptococci do localize in various organs
and tissues and can produce lesions at least sufficiently
suggestive of those found in man so that their potential danger
in infected foci cannot be neglected. ... focal infection has
changed ... from a theory to a principle ... of great
importance".
   Bierring 1938 would later properly refer to this Holman
conclusion as "rather significant and somewhat contradictory".

ULCERATIVE COLITIS Bargen 1928
   Bargen 1928 provides details of a series of cases in which deep
intramuscular injections of immune serum were given, in all of
which "there was definite improvement in the general condition.
... At least two of these cases illustrate the futility and
impracticality of ileosigmoidostomy ..."

WROTE BOOK *DENTAL INFECTION AND SYSTEMIC DISEASE* Haden 1928
   Haden 1928, p. 18:
   "Black [*Ophthamol. Rec.*, 1915, 24, 610] mentions articles as
early as 1843 relating dental disease to eye lesions. Garretson
[*Oral Surgery*, Phila. Lippencott and Co., 1890, p. 1364], in
1890, describes various systemic derangements such as spasms,
skin diseases, diarrhea and 'irritation fever', arising from
dental disease. ... Miller [*Dental Cosmos*, 1891, 33, 689] reports
examples of numerous diseases which have arisen from dental
infection. [but] these were all ... due to direct extension of
the infection into surrounding tissues, or into the bloodstream
producing a septicaemia, to the swallowing of pus from around the
teeth, or to reflex irritation from diseases of the dental pulp."
   Haden notes that in England, William Hunter [*Brit. Med. J.*,
1900, ii, 215]] "mentions, in 1900, pleurisy, empyema, nephritis,
pyelitis, perinephritic abscess, cholecystitis, anemia and
endocarditis as not infrequently arising from dental infection
through hematogenous distribution of bacteria. ... Rickman
Godlee [*Lancet* 1903, Vol. 2] expressed the opinion that many of
the chronic diseases of middle life are due to the absorption of
small doses of poison from chronic localized infections. The
conclusions of the English group were drawn entirely from
clinical observations."

ROSENOW'S FUNDAMENTAL CONTRIBUTION Haden 1928, p. 20:
   "Rosenow [*JAMA* 1914 63, 903] made a fundamental contribution to
bacteriology in demonstrating that the bacteria concerned in
chronic foci of infection are very sensitive to oxygen tension,
and that the cultivation of the organisms and the reproduction of
lesions in animals is largely dependent upon the use of proper
laboratory technique. To Rosenow [*JAMA* 1915 65, 1687] is due the
credit for showing that the organisms in chronic foci vary
greatly in their affinity for different tissues of the body."

p. 32, "Several studies have been made of the frequency of dental infection in those suffering from chronic disease. The opinion is quite unanimous that the incidence of chronic foci of infection is very high in such patients. ...

STATISTICAL CORRELATION: SYSTEMIC/TOOTH DISEASES Haden 1928
   p. 33 "The very much higher incidence of dental infection in those with systemic infection than in those showing no systemic disease is emphasized by the findings in 100 patients I reported in making a study of differential leukocyte count. One hundred percent of 47 patients with disease of focal origin had pulpless teeth and 77% had periapical areas of rarefied bone; of 53 patients with no disease of focal origin, only 47% had pulpless teeth and 32% had one or more teeth showing rarefaction of bone at the apex."
   p. 37, "The most important factor perhaps [concerning suitable conditions for the growth of bacteria in chronic foci] is the oxygen tension, as emphasized by Rosenow. ... I have cultures all tissues in deep tubes of glucose brain broth agar and glucose brain broth. [Rosenow, E.C., *J. Dent. Res.* 1919, 1, p. 205]. These mediums afford all gradations of oxygen tension. The brain substance renders the bottom of the tube anaerobic; the top is aerobic, so every degree of oxygen tension between these two points is provided. The hydrogen-ion concentration is approximately 7. The nutritive qualities are especially favorable for the growth of organisms in infections about the teeth. The agar medium shows also the number of bacteria which can be grown in the material inoculated. Only sufficient agar is added to barely solidify. This does not retard growth yet holds the colonies discrete. The broth medium is used for the inoculation of animals, for transplants to blood-agar plates, and for identification of the organisms ... ."

GLUCOSE BRAIN BROTH RECIPE Haden 1928
   "The mediums used are prepared as follows:
   Glucose Brain Broth - Dehydrated bactonutrient broth, 8 gm; sodium chloride, 8 gm; dextrose, chemically pure, 2 gm; Andrade indicator, 10cc; distilled water, 1000 cc. The broth and salt are dissolved by heating. After cooling, the indicator and dextrose are added. The medium is tubed in 6 x 3/4" test-tubes, so that the depth is at least 3-1/2 or 4 inches. Three pieces of calf brain, about 1 cm sq, and 2 or 3 pieces of crushed marble are added to each tube. The tubes are then sterilized for 20 minutes in the autoclave at 20 pounds (9.07 kg.) pressure.
   Glucose Brain Agar - The agar medium is made by adding 7 gm of powdered agar to 1 liter of the glucose brain broth prepared as indicated above. The calf brain and marble are then added and the medium is sterilized."

Table B2: Cultures - 1500 cleanly extracted
          anterior teeth; Haden 1928

	Deep Agar		Broth	
	%	%	%	%
No.colonies:	1+	10+		
			pos	neg
Total No.				
Vital (respond to electric current)	400 14.5	4.8	55.0	45.0
Pulpless, radiograph negative	600 56.7	46.2	83.8	16.2
Pulpless, radiograph positive	500 73.4	62.8	91.0	9.0
Pulpless - all	1100 64.6	53.7	87.1	12.9

PULPLESS TEETH WITH NEGATIVE X-RAYS ARE THE WORST Haden 1928

p. 42, Haden interprets the positive cultures in vital teeth to represent the maximum error in technique, although some may represent actual infection.

p. 44, "The pulpless teeth with negative radiograph constitute the most important group. ... The structural changes which we take as indicating infection [i.e. as in a positive radiograph] are in part evidence only of resistance of infection. ... It seems most probable that pulpless teeth which show no evidence of resistance and yet harbor bacteria are more apt to cause systemic disease, since there is no barrier to the entrance of bacteria and their products into the blood and lymph channels."

p. 47, "The most noteworthy result in the roentgen-ray negative group is [an] incidence of infection ... nearly as high as in the radiographic positive group."

p. 53-4, "the most striking finding here is the very high percentage of positive cultures in the radiographic negative teeth. This is not a surprising result. The organisms commonly are of a low grade of virulence, so might well be present in the periapical tissues for a long time without producing radiographic evidences of bone destruction. Where there is little local resistance to the infection conditions are most favorable for bloodstream dissemination from such a focus. ... Considering the greater chance of dissemination of the bacteria from the radiographic negative tooth, it is apparent that the two groups are of approximately equal importance from the standpoint of systemic disease.

p. 86, Haden found little difference in the incidence of lesions in animals following the injection of material from radiographic negative vs. radiographic positive teeth. In both cases these were consistently and substantially higher than for bacteria from areas of residual infection.

ELECTIVE LOCALIZATION, WHY SOME FAIL TO VERIFY Haden 1928
   p. 86-88, Haden 1928 cites a number of researchers, co-workers
of Rosenow, who "have been successful in demonstrating the
elective localizing property of streptococci. The greater number
of workers elsewhere have, however, been unable to verify his
findings."
   "It seems probable that failures to demonstrate elective
localization are due largely to disregard of certain fundamental
and necessary technical details. It is vitally necessary in
culturing the bacteria previous to inoculation that the
conditions under which the organism was growing in the body be
provided in the culture tube. This requires primarily a gradient
oxygen tension, but also the use of media favorable for the
growth of the organisms. It is very important, likewise, that
the least possible time elapse between the removal of the
infected material from the body and the injection of the
culture."

Table B3: ELECTIVE LOCALIZATION Haden 1928. p. 90

	S		O		N		S/O	S/N
	Specific		Other-Specific		Non-Specific			
	#	%	#	%	#	%		
Kidney	48	85	319	28	1383	27	3.0	3.1
Endocard.	46	57	321	12	1383	16	4.7	3.6
Myocard.	46	37	321	10	1383	9	3.7	4.1
Eye	142	65	225	1	1383	8	65.0	8.1
Stomach & Duodenum	131	61	236	4	1383	16	15.2	3.8

STRIKING EVIDENCE, TRUTH OF ELECTIVE LOCALIZATION Haden 1928
   p. 91 "The results in these 4 groups of cases offer striking
evidence of the truth of the theory of elective localization.
The cultures have been made in a uniform manner. Each rabbit has
been injected intravenously with 5 cc of broth culture, and every
animal has been subjected to a routine autopsy."
   "Various explanations are offered for the tendency to specific
localization. The extent of clumping of the organism, the nature
of the blood supply, the food supply and local tissue resistance,
must all be factors in determining the site of localization. The
most important factor, however, is some peculiar property,
probably of a chemical nature, inherent to the organism. The
localizing tendency of bacteria in certain foci varies from time
to time. Its development is probably dependent upon local
conditions at the site of the focus and also upon properties
peculiar to the tissues and the fluids of the host. Rosenow
[*Dental Cosmos* 1917, 59, 485] has emphasized that 'the focus is
of importance not only as affording the entrance way for
bacteria, but also as a place where varying affinities may be
acquired.'"

MYOCARDIAL DISEASE IS AN EXCELLENT EXAMPLE   Haden 1928-156
   "Many individuals doubtless carry infected teeth throughout
life without showing manifest disease of focal origin, although
marked injury to vital organs may result from the long-continued
absorption of bacterial poisons without being recognized.
Myocardial disease which is responsible for such a high
proportion of deaths after middle life is an excellent example."

EARLY TREATMENT, PULPLESS TEETH, ROOT CANALS   Haden 1928
   "Experimental work emphasizes especially the possible dangers
of focal lesions and the importance of removal before systemic
disease occurs. Failures in obtaining a cure or improvement in
the conditions due to focal infection by removing the focus
should only stress more the importance of the early removal of
dental infection. We should attempt to prevent the development
of systemic disease rather than attempt to cure it after it has
developed.
   "The ideal thing is to remove all dental infection. ...
   "The difficult problem is the pulpless tooth. ... There is no
convincing proof that periapical infection can be cured by root-
canal treatment. Areas of rarified bone at the apices of teeth
resulting from infection may partly or completely fill in
following treatment with different sterilizing agents. This does
not prove that such areas have become bacteria-free, since it is
well known that bone regeneration often takes place in the
presence of active infection. No satisfactory bacteriological
studies have been made after treatment of such areas to prove
they are really sterile."

PULPLESS TEETH WITH NO RADIOGRAPHIC DAMAGE   Haden 1928
   p. 159 "It is especially hard to decide on the best
disposition of pulpless teeth which show no radiographic evidence
of periapical infection. ... The radiographic findings taken as
evidence of infection is in large part evidence of the patient's
resistance to the infection. ... It seems most probable that an
infected tooth which shows no evidence of resistance and yet
harbors bacteria at the apex is more apt to be a focus of
systemic disease, since there is no barrier to the entrance of
bacteria and their products into the blood and lymph channels.
   "The desirable procedure in this group is to remove such teeth
in an attempt to prevent systemic disease from dental infection.
... In the presence of systemic disease of definite focal origin,
all pulpless teeth should be removed subject to the exceptions
previously noted." These exceptions, as discussed earlier on p.
159, refer to patients in whom "the systemic disease of focal
origin may be out of all proportion to the local lesion ...,
especially in older individuals ... [or] in other patients
[where] the structural changes may be beyond repair ..."]
   Haden's concluding paragraph:
   "Careful study of the subject must convince one of the
importance of dental focal infection in the causation of systemic

disease. It is apparent that often serious damage to vital
organs results from focal infection without being recognized
early enough to obtain satisfactory results from removal of the
focus. These facts justify the serious consideration of dental
focal infection as a factor in medicine with especial reference
to its early removal."

PEPTIC ULCER, STREPTOCOCCUS AS CAUSE OF   Nickel 1928
  Nickel 1928, p. 215-6: "Frick [A. Frick, *JAMA* 82:595 (Feb. 23,
1924] stated that according to his clinical experience there
seems to be no doubt that Rosenow's theory of the elective
affinity of a specific streptococcus, of a certain grade of
virulence, for the gastric or duodenal mucosa is correct and that
a specific streptococcus is the common cause of peptic ulcer."
  "Eusterman [Eusterman GB, *Minn. Med.*, 6:698 (1923)] summarized
the clinical evidence for the infectious origin of peptic ulcer
in the light of recent experimental work and expressed the
opinion that in certain types of ulcer it is the only tenable
theory at this stage of medical progress."

METHOD OF SWABBING Nickel 1928
  "If the focus was the tonsil, a culture was obtained by using a
small laryngeal mirror with the mirror so bent as to be almost in
a straight line with the handle. The tongue was depressed with
an illuminated tongue depressor, and the sterilized laryngeal
mirror was then inserted between the tonsil and the anterior
pillar, and pressure applied backward and mesially toward the
base of the tonsil. This procedure caused necrotic and puslike
material to ooze from the depths of the crypts; that material was
then scooped up with the laryngeal mirror and transferred with a
sterile swab from the mirror to a tube containing 2 cc of
gelatin-Locke solution, from which cultures were made in various
mediums." 217

ROSENOW'S GREEN STREPTOCOCCUS Nickel 1928
  "The predominating causative organism in all of these
experiments was found to be a green-producing streptococcus. ...
In primary culture it grew poorly or not at all on a blood-agar
plate, but it grew readily in partial tension mediums, such as
Rosenow's dextrose-brain broth." 224
  "The streptococcus which we have isolated consistently in these
cases is identical with that first described by Rosenow as having
etiologic importance in the production of peptic ulcer in man,
and it provides a means for active immunization with specific
autogenous vaccine." 230
  1928a, p. 232, Nickel presents results for various diseases,
after removal of focus of infection, with and without vaccine
therapy. [Of interest in consideration of Rosenow's later works,
e.g. 1956, which advocated vaccine/antibody therapy but not
removal of foci, are Nickel's comparisons of results with
different combinations of these two variables. Notably superior
results were obtained with both vaccines and foci-removal, while

results for those receiving focus-removal only were far superior to those receiving vaccine only. Thus, for Rosenow's vaccine/antibody combo to be capable of forestalling negative effect of focal infection, without focus removal, this must constitute highly effective medicine.]

Table B4: RESULTS OF VACCINE (Percent Improved) - Nickel 1928
              FOCUS REMOVED VS. NOT REMOVED

Vaccine	61% (216 cases)	26%	(39 cases)
No Vaccine	55% (75 cases)	21%	(28 cases)

Nickel 1928a

  Results, 500 cases: "Of particular interest is the very high average incidence of one or more pulpless teeth in all the groups." P. 252

POST-OP. INFECTION AS HEMATOGENOUS Nickel and Sager, 1928b
  Nickel and Sager, 1928b, investigating the problem of reducing post-operative infection of wounds, demonstrated "that streptococci can localize in tissues with lowered resistance but that they also can have elective affinity for tissues not traumatized. ... These occurrences suggest the possibility that infection may be brought about by other means than faulty [surgical] technic."
  Nickel 1928b, Rosenow in, p. 298, "the results of these experiments indicate clearly that the infection in some instances may be hematogenous in origin. ... The work adds evidence to the importance of the dictum of surgeons that the less tissues are injured, the less is the likelihood of postoperative infection, no matter what the source of contamination may be."

OPTIC NEURITIS White 1928
  "...practically all types of neuritis, no matter whether they are of the ophthalmic, the trifacial, the auditory or the ulnar nerves, arise from some focus of infection." [p. 131] ...

IV DISSEMINATION OF BACTERIA White 1928
  White 1928 cautions that "A primary focus may have produced so many secondary foci that its elimination does not cure the neuritis. The infection is believed at present to usually travel by way or the blood stream". [p. 129]

EMPHASIS ON TEETH White 1928
  p. 132 "Of late the teeth have furnished the foci in so many cases that it is really a great disappointment when a patient comes who has lost all his teeth or with teeth so healthy that there is little hope of finding the trouble there."

NONVITAL TEETH (ROOT-CANALICIZED) White 1928
  "Were I confronted with ... a patient with serious optic nerve disturbance, where after thorough investigation nothing but

devitalized teeth had been found, I should unhesitatingly
advocate their removal. Rice 1926 [*Trans. Amer. Laryng. and
Otol. Soc.*]... aptly states: '... we are eminently justified in
viewing all pulpless teeth with grave suspicion." [p. 133] ...
    p. 134, White quoting Rice: "The conservative dentist will
say, 'This patient is in good health, the pulpless teeth are
symptom-free, and roentgenograms are negative. Why, then,
sacrifice the teeth? On the face of it, the reasoning seems
sound, but on second thought, shall we retain these teeth until a
myocardial disturbance puts in an appearance, or a cholecystitis,
a rheumatoid arthritis, an iritis, a corneal ulcer, renal
calculi, and so on, or shall we practice prophylaxis and remove
the suspicious teeth? ...
    "It is not possible to determine whether a pulpless tooth in
the mouth is or is not sterile. ...
    "It is known, beyond the peradventure of doubt, that dental
foci of infection are among the most active agents that militate
against bodily well being, and graveyards are filled with their
victims."

FIRST PROCEDURE: SUSPICIOUS TEETH OR TONSILS White 1928
    "In all instances, if teeth or tonsils are suspicious enough to
warrant removal, let that be the first procedure." [p. 136] ...
    IRITIS p. 137, cites Irons and Brown (1924) as having found
the "probable source of the infection" in 46 of 50 cases of
iritis, with teeth and/or tonsils to some extent involved in 70%
of the cases.
    p. 136, White!, "... it is practically always possible to
determine the source of the infection. The important thing, in
treating each and every case, is to eliminate the focus, unless
the patient is already much below par."

OPTIC NEURITIS: 26/30 HAD FOCI IN TEETH/TONSILS White 1928
    p. 139, In a series of 30 cases of optic neuritis, White found
foci in teeth and/or tonsils in 26; "... the sphenoids were
opened but twice, and in neither case was it justifiable, as both
would undoubtedly have recovered simply by removal of the focus."

ORAL FOCUS AS POSSIBLE ETIOLIGICAL FACTOR IN M.S. White 1928
    p. 161, in a conversation with (neurologist) Dr. Gilbert
Horrax, discussing a patient diagnosed with MS, Dr. White
"mentioned the infection found in teeth and tonsils and he
unhesitatingly advocated their removal on the theory that this
infection might possibly be a factor in the etiology of the
multiple sclerosis." In response to a direct question, Dr. Horax
said, "I don't believe anyone could say that multiple sclerosis
is caused by focal infection in the teeth or tonsils, but I
should certainly think that this is a possibility which ought to
be eliminated."
    Dr. White reports that in the 8-1/2 months since removal of
foci of infection (teeth and tonsils) "there has been little
change" in previously noted "marked optic atrophy" and that this

had also "somewhat checked the progress of the multiple sclerosis."

FOCUS (USUALLY ORAL) CAUSES OPTIC NEURITIS White 1928

"Some focus in the body is responsible for the optic nerve lesion arising from infection. Invasion is through the blood stream. The accessory sinuses supply but an insignificant number of the foci. Most of the foci are found in teeth and tonsils. The sinuses, from their priority of investigation, have occupied the attention of rhinologists too long to the exclusion of other more frequent seats of infection. Dental infections are easily overlooked. ... Devitalized teeth are a potential source of infection." [p. 163]

"Normal vision was obtained in 63% of the cases undergoing operations, while 20 percent improved. In the remaining 17 percent, which were chronic, further loss of vision was prevented. ... Over 80% of the cases had infected teeth or tonsils or both. this last group included one case with marked optic atrophy with chronic bilateral retrobulbar neuritis diagnosed as MS. Optic atrophy and MS seemed to have been checked over a period of 8 1/2 months; whereas considerable diminution had been seen over the previous 10 months.[p. 165]

ARTHRITIS AND INFECTED TEETH White 1928

Dr. White also relates his personal experience with dental infection. "My knees became swollen and painful. ... as my tonsils and sinuses appeared negative, I had the teeth filmed, and ... the extraction of two of them was advised because of apical infection ... [which extraction] relieved the knees." On a recurrence of the knee infection, dental films were negative; however, Dr. L.M.S. Miner examined both teeth and films, felt two teeth were clinically unhealthy and advised their removal. Prompt relief followed. Two years later this experience recurred.

GALLBLADDER DISEASE Wilkie 1928

Wilkie 1928, p. 481, commenting on Rosenow:

"From the walls of a large number of diseased gall-bladders he was able to cultivate a streptococcus which, on injection into animals, appeared to have a selective affinity for the gall-bladder. ...

"In my own experience I was impressed by the fact that, whilst the bile and gallbladder wall so often proved to be sterile on culture, yet stained sections of the wall revealed the presence of streptococci in the submucous coat. ...

"Illingworth, working in my clinic, was able to show that, using Rosenow's special medium, streptococci could be grown from the wall of the gall bladder in quite a large percentage of cases in which the bile was sterile. He further showed that the organisms of the 'coli' group are relatively infrequent except in active supprative cases.

"... Dr. A. L. Wilkie ... has shown that cholecystitis is

almost invariably an intramural streptococcal infection, and that Rosenow's contention of a selective affinity of this organism for the gall bladder is strikingly true. ... He has brought to light the illuminating and remarkable fact that bile inhibits the growth of this streptococcus. ... This fact accounts for the widespread failure to confirm Rosenow's findings. ... Medical treatment of cholecystitis, to be rational ..., must be aimed at this intramural streptococcus, attacking it through the bloodstream - for example, by vaccine or by some agent which is absorbed by the gall bladder and passes through its wall ... "

   p. 482, Wilkie 1928 refers to W.J. Mayo as one of the first to note curious conditions of the mucous membrane of gall-bladder - small white specks resembling the surface of a strawberry.

   Phases of development of 'multiple mulberry cholesterin stone' begins with streptococcal infection, which may prohibit mucous membrane from absorbing cholesterol from bile; rather lipid accumulates in mucosa, forms lipoid papillomata, which shed off to form nuclei around which cholesterol is deposited.

   "Wilkie has shown in the submucosa and in the cystic gland in every case in every case [of cholesterosis] examined a streptococcus was present."

   p. 483, "Once firmly established infection of the gall bladder is highly resistant to cure by other than surgical means."

   p. 484, the author notes that a large proportion of patients are obese, and suggests that the "wise plan" includes a preliminary course of exercise: "The remarkable improvement in general tone with loss of weight which results makes the operation both easier and safer."

   Wilkie 1928, p. 484, concludes that gall-bladder infection "is usually an intramural streptococcal infection, and is frequently associated with the formation of gall stones.

ULCERATIVE COLITIS Bargen 1929
   Bargen 1929, p. 571, notes a "seemingly significant factor bearing on the causative relation of bacteria to this disease [ulcerative colitis] is the clinical observation that frequently tonsillectomy, removal of infected teeth or acute infections of the upper respiratory tract, cause marked acute temporary exacerbations of the disease. This suggests the presence of the causative bacteria in these foci."

   "Diplostreptococci, in all essentials like those isolated from the rectal lesions, have been isolated from periapical abscesses of teeth or from buried tonsillar abscesses, and cultures of these when injected intravenously have produced in animals lesions like those described. These organisms were agglutinated by the immune rabbit and horse serums. This has been the experience with the use of strains from many patients on several hundred rabbits."

ULCERATIVE COLITIS Cook, 1931
   Cook, 1931, p. 2299
   "Streptococci that were freshly isolated from pulpless,

infected teeth of [15] patients who had ulcerative colitis ...
localized electively, producing lesions in the colon... of 60% of
60 rabbits [4 per patient] that were given intravenous
injections" vs. lower percentages in the stomach or duodenum (6),
kidney (3), gallbladder (0), joints (5) and muscles (8) and none
elsewhere.

COLITIS REPLICATED IN DOGS, VIA TOOTH Cook 1931
Cook, 1931, utilized the methodology of Rosenow and Haden to
culture streptococci from infected teeth of patients who had
chronic ulcerative colitis, injected these into devitalized teeth
of dogs, and thereby produced "a clinical and histopathologic
picture of ulcerative colitis resembling, in every essential
respect, the disease as it occurs spontaneously in man. ... Dogs
used as controls, ... the teeth of which were infected similarly,
but with streptococci from infected teeth of patients suffering
from diseases other than ulcerative colitis, never developed
lesions of the colon."
"Now that ulcerative colitis has been reproduced by methods
which, in every essential respect, simulate the conditions at
hand in patients, the skepticism which still exists as to the
significance of the focus and the inherent specific or elective
localizing power of the diplostreptococcus in the etiology of
this disease should not long survive."
...
"The prevention or elimination of dental foci of infection in
patients who have chronic ulcerative colitis, as in other
diseases in which a focus has been shown to harbor the causative
organism, should prove of great importance as a preventive and
curative measure."

PULPLESS TEETH, SUMMARY OF PREVIOUS WORK Cramer & Reith 1932
Cramer and Reith 1932 summarized previous work on pulpless
teeth. This included Haden 1925, who studied 1307 such teeth
with cultures in deep agar, obtaining growth in 5% of vital, 44%
of roentgenically negative and 63% in roentgenically positive
teeth.

HEART DISEASE Jones and Newsom 1932
Jones and Newsom 1932 claimed to have established "a positive
relationship between experimentally produced focal dental
infection and cardiac hypertrophy..." utilizing "a nonhemolytic
green-producing gram positive type of streptococcus corresponding
in its sugar fermentations to Streptococcus mitus." Their work
built on that of Rosenow and Meisser, who had earlier produced
renal stones in dogs with microorganisms believed to have
selective affinity for renal tissue.

PULPLESS TEETH, SUMMARIES OF 3000 PERSONS Rhoads & Dick 1932
Rhoads and Dick, 1932, p. 1884, undertook to study the
pathologic significance of pulpless roentgenographically negative
teeth. Summarizing studies involving more than 3000 persons, the

authors found "69.2% of pulpless teeth in adults had roentgenographic evidence of periapical bone change. Assuming that root canal filling is undertaken to preserve the teeth and conserve the patient's health, these figures would indicated that the procedure is unsuccessful in the hands of the majority of dentists."

Table B5: PULPLESS TEETH - 3000 PERSONS - Rhoads and Dick, 1932

INVESTIGATOR	number persons	with pulpless teeth	# teeth	# pulpless teeth	% with apical change
Haden	500	455	-	-	most
Tovell			3276	1600	73%
Ulrich				1350	83%
Moorehead	362				
Duke	1000				50-81%
Eusterman	900		2099		
Gould	325				29%
	3000+				

Rhoads and Dick, 1932, cultured green-forming cocci from all of 209 roentgen ray negative pulpless teeth and concluded that "it seems justifiable to regard all pulpless teeth as probable foci of infection, whether they show apical change in the roentgenograms or not. Certainly that position should be taken in the presence of systemic disease of a type usually associated with focal infection."

SUBJECTIVE INSERT: It is difficult to comprehend how all the seemingly irrefutable evidence in support of this connection between teeth and systemic diseases could have been so maligned, and for what reason. It seems clear that the major impetus came from the field of endodontics, determined at all costs to continue the practice of removing and refilling diseased tooth roots.

PEMPHIGUS Welsch 1934
BLOOD Welsch 1934
Welsch 1934, p. 611, "A Streptococcus was isolated from the blood of five of the [7 pemphigus] patients in each of ten trials, whereas cultures from the blood of a sixth patient with

pemphigus were sterile on 4 separate occasions. A characteristic streptococcus was isolated from swabbings of the nasopharynx of these 7 patients in each of the 21 attempts."

BLOOD CULTURE TECHNIC, PEMPHIGUS Welsch 1934
PEMPHIGUS, BLOOD CULTURE TECHNIC Welsch 1934
   Welsch 1934 relates that blood for culture was drawn in amounts of 20 cc as aseptically as possible and put into sterile tubes containing 5 cc of a 2% solution of sodium citrate in a physiologic solution of sodium chloride.
   p. 613, "The organism isolated from these patients with pemphigus is extremely pleomorphic. In the primary culture from the blood it usually appeared as a streptococcus, but in some cultures pleomorphic forms consisting of a mixture of ovoid, coccoid and bacillary forms, and in still other cultures bacillary forms only were obtained. In dextrose-brain broth cultures from the nasopharynx, only the streptococcic forms were found. Early transplants on blood agar plates from the dextrose-brain broth cultures from the nasopharynx and from primary cultures on blood agar plates produced colonies which were indistinguishable form onw another but which on smearing in some instances revealed pure streptococciac forms, in other instances a mixture of coccoid and bacillary forms, and in still others only bacillary forms. Some of the pleomorphic forms revealed a tendency towards clubbing and were diptheroid in appearance. The stable form is the streptoccic form. ... Smears of colonies on blood agar plates, when more than 24 hours old, often revealed coccoid bodies or granules inside the bacillary forms. Immunologically and antigenically, all forms behaved identically.
 The aforementioned changes in morphologic characteristics are common with those observed in other streptococci by Rosenow, Jensen and Morton, Mellon, and Koch and Mellon."
   Welsch 1934, p. 628, discusses how the cataphoretic slowing ability, as discussed previously by Rosenow, indicates that respective streptococci have to varying degrees combined with corresponding "antibodies" thus becoming larger and slower.
   Welsch herein demonstrates specificity of various streptococcal strains as concerns pemphigus, dermatitis herpetiformis, lupus erythematosus, and erythema multiforme, in terms of percent under the average mobility in salt solution.
   p. 629, Dr. L. A. Brunstig, Rochester, Minn.: "It seems to be significant that the organisms have been isolated from the circulating blood on 10 occasions in five of the patients."
   p. 630, comment by Dr. Theodore Cornbleet, Chicago: " ... I think that Dr. Welsch has succeeded in showing that the blood of the patient with pemphigus has specific properties; this is a continuation, of course, of the works of Pehs and Macht."
   p. 612, 2a: provides reference to Kendall, "Mediums for the Isolation and Cultivation of Bacteria in the Filtrable State", Northwestern University Bulletin 8, 1931, Vol. 32.

PULPLESS TEETH - 1800 OBSERVED Swanson and Van Kirk, 1936

Swanson and Van Kirk, 1936, cultured 1800 extracted, pulpless teeth in brain-heart-infusion medium and observed:

"Positive cultures [pure cultures of non-hemolytic diplo-streptococci] resulted for enough x-ray negative [root-filled pulpless] teeth to warrant the statement that absence of x-ray evidence does not guarantee sterility in pulpless teeth. The small difference in incidence of infection [96.4% for root-filled vs. 97.8% for not-root filled] would seem to indicate, conversely, that the sterile pulpless tooth under any circumstances may be an extreme rarity." This referred to the authors having obtained positive cultures in 96.4% of 1220 root-filled teeth and 97.8% of 582 not-root-filled teeth for an overall 96.8% of 1802 pulpless teeth.

ENCEPHALITIS Swanson and Van Kirk 1936
Swanson and Van Kirk 1936, also extracted several pulpless teeth from a 77 year-old encephalitis patient, cultured gram-positive streptococci which were injected intravenously into a rabbit resulting in "definite" disturbance of the central nervous system. This was repeated through 6 animal passages, wherein afinity for the central nervous system was retained.

JAMA QUARTER CENTURY SURVEY ON BILLINGS/ROSENOW Bierring 1938
[Bierring, "Focal Infection: Ouarter Century Survey", the Frank Billings Lecture, presented to the Section in Practice of Medicine, AMA; Walter Bierring served as 87th President of the AMA (1934).]
Bierring 1938 noted in Cecil and Angevine's study, that when small doses (2cc) of a hemolytic strain of streptococci were injected Intravenously, arthritis was produced in 85%.
p. 1623, Bierring salutes Billings's accomplishments, and mentions several diseases discussed by Billings in the context of focal infection.
p. 1623-4, refers to "The brilliant work of Rosenow in demonstrating the transmutability of the streptococcus-pheumococcus group permitted at the the time a better understanding of the changing pathogenicity of these bacteria."
p. 1624, "the unusual results obtained by Rosenow ere evidently due to the use of special culture methods devised by him for excised tissues, blood and other fluids, in which due regard was given to the question of oxygen pressure, particularly in primary cultures. ...

ROSENOW'S WORK CONFIRMED IN DETAIL BY HADEN Bierring 1938
"the work of Rosenow was confirmed in detail by Russell L. Haden. who followed closely certain fundamental details insisted on by Rosenow", in a 1925 study of kidney disease. ...
para, para, para, para,

ULCER,GASTRIC/DUODENAL-PROOF INFECTIOUS THEORY Bierring 1938
"These results were confirmed by a second study of Haden, on the elective localization of bacteria in peptic ulcer."

...
"These results furnished definite confirmatory proof of
Rosenow's theory of elective localization and the infectious
theory of peptic ulcer as well as of the theory that dental
infection is an important factor in the causation of gastric and
duodenal ulcer."

HEART DISEASE Bierring 1938
Bierring 1938 referred to the results of Jones and Newsom's
1932 experimental investigations as "distinctly suggestive of
selective tissue affinity and elective localization" as concerns
the relationship between dental infection and cardiac disease.

HOLMAN CONCLUSION SIGNIFICANT, CONTRADICTORY Bierring 1938
Bierring 1938 refers to Holman's 1928 final comment as "rather
significant and somewhat contradictory: 'What Rosenow and all
the other investigators of the problem have definitely
demonstrated is that streptococci do localize in various organs
and tissues [of laboratory animals] and can produce lesions at
least sufficiently suggestive of those found in man so that their
potential danger in infected foci cannot be neglected."
Bierring refers to Holman's 1928 article as having "recognized
that a certain general bacterial adaptation to environment is
accepted by everyone" while it nonetheless asserted "that the
factors on the side of the host are more variable and therefore
far more important."

ROSENOW MEDICAL GUIDE OF FUTURE; CLINICAL SUM. Bierring 1938
Bierring 1938, p. 1626, "Any impartial view of the mass of
experimental and clinical studies that have been recorded must
recognize that this evidence is supportive of the fundamental
conception of an infectious process, in that many pathogenic
bacteria possess a predilection for certain tissues. ... [e.g.],
the pneumococcus is prone to localize in the lungs", etc.
However, "organisms of the streptococcus may invade almost any
tissue of the human body. ...
"The results of experiments which have been cited emphasize the
importance of foci of infection as places in which bacteria may
grow and acquire elective pathogenic properties which determine
their mode of action and distribution after their entrance into
the blood stream.
"Within the inner circles of the bacteriologist and the
immunologist, specific tissue affinity and elective tissue
localization are still subjects of controversy, yet the tenets of
both sciences offer definite confirmation regarding this
fundamental concept of focal infections, and perchance it is safe
to assume that the 'Rosenow heresy' may yet become the medical
guide of the future."
Bierring 1938, p. 1626, According to Biering "any impartial
reviewer must admit" that numerous critical clinical observations
over the previous 25 years lend "the fullest support to the
dictum spoken by Billings in 1932, 20 years after his original

contribution: 'Focal infection as an etiologic factor of general disease is now an established pathological principle."

ARTHRITIS, INITIATING AND CONTRIBUTING CAUSES Bierring 1938
   Bierring cites studies implicating focal infection in diseases of the nervous system, ocular disease, dermatology (cutaneous disorders may also act as a foci), subacute bacterial endocarditis, anemias, chronic arthritis and the relation of this to diminished blood supply due to bacterial emboli or their toxins; and discusses many initiating and contributing causes of chronic arthritis including age, heredity, nutrition, infection and trauma.

RHEUMATOID ARTHRITIS Cecil and Angevine 1938
   Cecil and Angevine 1938, p. 579, regarding 200 cases of typical rheumatoid arthritis, "every case in the series showed or had shown at some time previously, several characteristic fusiform fingers, which, in our opinion, are a typical manifestation of this syndrome. The sedimentation rate was accelerated in 93% of these patients."
   The authors note that "clearly these were cases of well established arthritis ... so well established so as to perhaps not be affected by removal of primary (originating) foci."
   The authors said they were unable to confirm the role of focal infection in rheumatoid arthritis, based on a study of 200 cases.
  However, they stated "Undoubtedly there are cases of infectious arthritis which result from focal infection."

TEN YEARS WORK, 200 CASES, CONFIRMS ROSENOW Goldberg, 1938
   Goldberg, 1938, based on 10 years' research into dental infections and their relations to systemic disease, concluded:
p. 275 "In cases of dental infection with systemic manifestations it is advisable to remove all dental foci, after which the patient is given a rest for at least four weeks. In many cases there is complete recovery from the systemic disturbance following the removal of infected teeth, while in others there is not. If the patient on his return does not show marked signs of improvement in his systemic condition, the use of an autogenous vaccine is indicated. Vaccines are administered by the physician. In no instance has the use of autogenous vaccine been followed by deleterious results"
   Reporting on 200 cases, 62 were given autogenous vaccines, of which only 8 showed no results, 54 good results. Of 426 total teeth cultured, 333 of 361 (92%) nonvital teeth and 43 of 65 (66%) of vital teeth yield positive cultures. Of the total 426 cultures, 335 (79%) yielded nonhemolytic streptococci, or 87% of those (335 of 378) yielding growth of any type.

RHEUMATISM, FOCAL INFECTION AND   Jarløv and Brinch 1938
   Jarløv and Brinch 1938, per *JAMA* 111, p. 290, assert that a causal connection between focal infection and diseases of the joints is highly probable." [see ROSENOW, "Testimonials"]

RHEUMATISM   Quinoz 1938
  Quinoz, 1938, per *JAMA* 111, p. 2250, studied 50 cases of
rheumatism, caused by tooth infections in 30, tonsils in 17 and
both in 3.

DIET, HARMFUL IMPACT OF MODERN DIET ON PRIMITIVES Price 1939
Weston Price 1939 In *Nutrition and Physical Degeneration*, 1939,
1970, Dr. Price discussed discussed the deleterious impact of
modern diets on primitive peoples, and the benefits of vitamins.
  (see also Price 1923)

ASTHMA   Cooke 1940
  Cooke 1940, p. 139, regarding 241 cases of asthma from his
clinic, with a post op period of from 6 months to 10 years, "In
117 cases in which all indicated surgery had been done, definite
and satisfactory improvement was reported in 88%; whereas in 124
cases in which, for one reason or another, the necessary surgery
was not completed only 37% had definite improvement."

TEETH, DEFINITE RELATIONSHIP TO GENERAL DISEASE   Miller 1940
  p. 478-9 "The work of Billings, Rosenow and others who
developed the theories of focal infection, has had a profound
influence, not only upon the development of oral surgery, but
upon dentistry and its importance to general health service.
Since 1910, when the theory that infection of the mouth was
responsible for many systemic diseases was advanced, it has
definitely been established that diseases of the teeth and of
their supporting tissues have an important relationship to
general health."

FROM TEPIDITY TO WHOLE-HEARTED ACCEPTANCE   Slocumb 1941
  Slocumb etal 1941, "... from the clinical standpoint alone, as
... concerns the three clinical entities of heart disease,
chronic infectious arthritis and glomerulonephritis ... we
progress from tepidity toward relative enthusiasm to whole
hearted acceptance of the concept of focal infection."

GLOMERULONEPHRITIS, ACUTE   Slocumb etal, 1941
  Slocumb etal, 1941, relate (unpublished data) R.M. Woods and
M.W. Binger's experience with 21 cases of acute
glomerulonephritis wherein noticeable improvement was noted
following removal of a focus of infection (14 tonsillectomy and 7
mastoidectomy); moreover 84% of a total 61 cases studied had
developed during acute inflammations of the upper part of the
respiratory tract.

GLOMERULONEPHRITIS, CHRONIC   Slocumb etal, 1941
  "It is widely accepted that chronic glomerulonephritis ... is
caused ... by repeated or continued toxic assaults on the kidneys
which originate in acute or chronic foci of infection. ... Of the
patients suffering from chronic nephritis who come to us with

intermittent exacerbations of the acute phase, more than 80% have evidences of chronic infections about roots of teeth, in the tonsils or in the sinuses."

ARTHRITIS Slocumb etal 1941
   Slocumb etal 1941 respond to Reiman and Havens, who ignored early emphasis in reporting on "striking benefits" of application of the focal infection theory, and focused on a portion which failed to improve.
   - points out inconsistancy of allowing acute foci of infection and not chronic in that it is "difficult clinically to distinguish sharply the stage in which chronicity begins ... "
   - assess the effects of removal of foci in heart disease, infectious arthritis and glomerunephritis.

HEART DISEASE Slocumb etal 1941
   "On the basis of our clinical experience we feel ... that in heart disease focal infection can be considered to be a factor only in an occasional case of coronary thrombosis or acute pericarditis, and in the small group of cases in which emphysema and pulmonary hypertension result from chronic bronchitis secondary to infection in tonsils or sinuses."

CHRONIC INFECTIOUS ARTHRITIS Slocumb etal 1941
   The authors agreed with Hensch 1938. [Hensch, PS, *Is Rheumatoid (Atrophic) Arthritis a Disease of Microbic Origin?*, London, Oxford U. Press, 1938]. Hensch had summarized some 21 arguments for the microbic theory, and opposition to them, p. 35-62, and had stated "that the evidence for infection, though very impressive, is incomplete." Nonetheless he concluded "as a practicing physician I have committed myself to the microbic theory."

SURGERY AS AUTOHEMOTHERAPY; 3-7 DAY RULE Slocumb etal 1941
   Slocumb etal 1941, relate an experience that might be due to an inadvertant form of autohemotherapy. p. 2163, "We encounter many patients who report diminution in symptoms of chronic infectious arthritis after any type of surgical intervention or even general anesthesia has been carried out, but the improvement persists for from 3 to 7 days and then is gradually lost." [This period is consistent with Florence Sabin's finding that antibody is produced for 3-4 days in the reticuloendothelial system.]

AUTOTHERAPY Welsch 1946
   Welsch 1946, p. 11, Table 2, indicates 10 of 129 dead mice were eaten by mates before cultures could be made for streptococci.

BLOOD CULTURE - VALUE OF ROSENOW'S BROTH Welsch 1946
   p. 10, in 22 of 22 pemphigus patients, the characteristic streptococcus was isolated from nasopharynx swabbings, and in 16 of 22, from the blood. Welsch notes "Cultivating the blood in anaerobic ampules of Rosenow's dextrose-brain broth has been the

most satisfactory method of isolating the streptococcus from this
material [Rosenow 1934, *J. Infect. Dis.*, 91-122]

PEMPHIGUS CAUSED BY ROSENOW'S STREPTOCOCCUS Welsch 1946
   Welsch 1946, p. 39, demonstrated a specific relationship
between pemphigus and Rosenow's characteristic streptococcus in a
number of ways:
(1) precipitin reactions between
   (a) both nasopharyngeal washings and blister fluid of patients
who had pemphigus and
   (b) serums of animals immunized with the specific streptococcus
(2) precipitin reactions between
   (a) serums from patients who had pemphigus and
   (b) both alkaline-saline extracts and specific polyscaccharide
substance of the streptococcus
(3) cataphoretic mobility-reducing action tests; and
(4) other intradermal tests with dead organisms and immune horse
serum.
   Welsch 1946 also noted that a similar streptococcus was
isolated from patients with dermatitis herpetiformis, disseminate
lupus erythematosus and erythema multiforme exudativum resp.
   Welsch 1946, p. 40, concluded "If the material presented here
is to be accepted as factual, pemphigus must be considered a
streptococcal disease in which the streptococcus is present on
the mucous membranes and in foci from which repeated showers of
organisms enter the bloodstream."

RHEUMATIC FEVER AND TONSILLITIS British Med. Journal 1954
   In 1954 an editorial in the British Medical Journal noted that
epidemics of rheumatic fever were observed to follow epidemics of
streptococcal infection; and that a reduction in streptococcal
carrier and infection rates in rheumatic fever victims, through
prophylaxis with sulphonamide or penicillin, had been associated
with a reduction in the incidence of recurrences. Moreover,
other studies indicated that children from lower rental areas
were found to have lower tonsillectomy rates and higher
streptococcal-carrier and rheumatic fever rates than children
from higher rental areas, leading some to the conclusion that
tonsillectomy protects against rheumatic fever by reducing the
streptococcal carrier and infection rates.

ARTHRITIS Castiglioni 1958
EPILEPSY Castiglioni 1958
   Castiglioni, Arturo, *A History of Medicine*, NY, Alfred A Knopf,
1941, 1958, p. 622, Benjamin Rush (1745-1813) "was probably the
first to record that general disease (arthritis, epilepsy) could
be relieved by the extraction of decayed teeth."
   p. 837, refers to Austin Flint (1812-1886), "His *Principles and
Practice of Medicine* was long a leading textbook on the subject."

CIRCULATION/SPREAD OF PATHOGENS FROM FOCI Störtebecker 1967
MYASTHENIA GRAVIS Störtebecker 1967

EPILEPSY FROM TEETH THRU VEINS Störtebecker 1967
   Störtebecker 1967 discussed how "the cranial and vertebral
venous systems provide a pathway for the dissemination of
bacterial products from dental and urogenital foci of infection
to all parts of the central nervous system [which communications
might be] potentially significant in the pathogenesis of
disseminated sclerosis, epilepsy, myasthenia gravis and other
neurological disorders ...   There is a vertebral venous system
that follows the spine externally and internally, and a cranial
venous system that is situated extracranially and intracranially.
 The two systems communicate directly with each other at the base
of the skull throught the foramen magnum. The flow in this joint
system is unimpeded as there are no valves directing the
circulation."
   Störtebecker also related how Batson in 1940-1943 demonstrated
that a contrast medium could be injected into the dorsal vein of
the penis and traced through the entire intraspinal vertebral
venous system to the skull and sometimes the venous system of the
face, similarly demonstrating a flow from the pelvic veins to the
vertebral venous system in monkeys. "Batson considered this mode
of flow as very probable in certain malignant metastases, such as
carcinoma of the prostrate gland."
   Störtebecker also offered that "Sicher's comments on the
anatomy of the veins in the head and their role as pathways for
the spread of toxic-infections substances are highly
significant". Sicher had related "The danger of a retrograde
spread of infection is [grave] because the veins of the face have
few if any valves, which in other veins prevent a backflow of
blood ...
   p. 306, "We know that a superior labial furuncle can cause
meningitis. ... the spread must take place along the venous
system." A venous route for brain abscess infection from foci
in ear, sinuses and jaw (including wisdom teeth) is also
discussed.

OPTIC NEURITIS Störtebecker, 1967
MULTIPLE SCLEROSIS Störtebecker, 1967
   p. 307,Störtebecker, 1967 discusses the possible role of dental
infection in some forms of disseminated sclerosis and cranial
lesions; "In cranial lesions, such as eye muscle paresis and
optic neuritis, it is advisable to seek infectious foci within
the cranial venous system.

EPILEPSY Störtebecker 1967
MENTAL ILLNESS Störtebecker 1967
   p. 310, "The dissemination of bacterial products must also play
a role in epilepsy ...   I have observed in epileptic patients an
encouraging regression of clinical and electroencephalographic
signs and symptoms following the elimination of dental infectious
foci. ..." Störtbecker relates Bering's positive reactions in
intracutaneous tests with antibodies against alpha streptococci
in 78% of epilepsy patients v.s. 7% of controls. [Bering, EA,

Jr., *J. Neurol. Neurosurg. & Psychiat.* 14:205, 1951,
"Confirmation of the Rosenow antibody-antigen skin reaction in
idiopathic epilepsy."]   "... An established lesion in the
central nervous system cannot be cured by removing the infectious
foci.... All we can do in these cases is to arrest progression
of the disease .... Our primary aim should be prophylactic - to
prevent the outbreak of the disease. Neurological disorders and
mental illness exact an enoumous social and economic toll. The
inclusion of a thorough dental exam with every medical checkup is
therefore imperative in an effective program of prevention and
eradication of infectious foci."

AUTOIMMUNITY AND INFECTIOUS FOCI Störtebecker 1967
  "... Autoimmune mechanisms must also be considered in
connection with infectious foci. "
  It is noted that as early as 1915 Dr. Rosenow had specifically
discussed "local infection due to intravascular dissemination of
bacteria; the association of diptheroid bacilli with various
disease conditions" [15R1]. The intravascular dissemination of
bacteria in these various disease conditions provides a logical
explanation as to why autohemotherapy has been reported
successful in many of these same conditions; the causative
organism is in the blood, which circumstance enables the blood to
act as an autogenous vaccine when reinjected extravascularly.

MENTAL DISEASE USUALLY ASSOC. WITH PHYSICAL Pauling 1968
  p. 265 "The proper functioning of the mind is known to require
the presence in the brain of molecules of many different
substances. For example, mental disease, usually associated with
physical disease, results from a low concentration in the brain
of any one dof the following vitamins: thiamine (B1), nicotinic
acid or nicotinamide (B3), pyridoxine (B6), cyanocobalamin (B12),
biotin (H), ascorbic acid (C) and folic acid. ... [see also
MENTAL ILLNESS file]

ENDOCARDITIS Jones, etal, 1970
  Jones, etal, 1970, discuss the need for control of bacteriemia
associated with the extraction of teeth, particularly bacterial
endocarditis, relative to patients (a) with prosthetic
cardiovacscular appliances, and (b) with no evidence of pre-
existing heart disease; note that "cases of bacterial
endocarditis have occurred even in patients 'protected' by
antibiotics."

STOMATITIS Morse 1977
ECZEMA Morse 1977
ACNE ROSACEA Morse 1977
BRONCHITIS, CHRONIC Morse 1977
DYSHIDROSIS Morse 1977
  Morse 1977, p. 441, refers to Welsch, who was able to produce
subacute bacterial endodarditis in dogs by placing streptococci
in their teeth.

p. 441, Henoq and associates [*Rev. Stomatol. Chir. Maxillofac.* 73:21-30, 1972] obtained positive skin reactions with microbes cultured from infected root canals in "all" tested patients with stomatitis, eczema, acne rosacea, chronic bronchitis, and dyshidrosis. "The authors discussed the possibility of treating certain allergies by removal of dental foci and the use of desensitization."

p. 442, reports results of Dietz [*Oral Surg.* 57:877-883 (1952)] which implicated pathologic pulps as a source of antigens in skin, as disclosed by skin reactions.

FOCAL INFECTION CONCEPT RELATED TO AUTOIMMUNITY Morse 1977
p. 443-4, Morse 1977 discusses "newer concepts of focal infection": "One concept states that microbes disseminate into the bloodstream from an original site (e.g. root apex). They then arrive at a secondary site and interact with the host's antigens (e.g. joint proteins) so that the host's tissues are altered. The host's immunologic cells then react to the changed proteins ('autoantigens') and mount an immunologic attack against these proteins. This occurs even after the original inciting microbes have been destroyed. This reaction is a microbially incited autoimmunity. Another possibility is that microbial products result in an allergic reaction." [How about an old fashioned infection, plain and simple?]

CONTEMPORARY SUPPORT FOR FOCAL INFECTION Morse 1977
HIVES Morse 1977
p. 444 "Klotz [in Frazier CA, 1973] discussed the finding of clinical allergists that 'foci' of infection, particularly in the teeth, tonsils and sinuses, can be the principal etiologic factors of recurrent or resistant urticaria (hives). Removal of the original foci often resulted in clinical cures. DiStefano [1971] also analyzed cases of allergic skin manifestations that were apparently caused by teeth with infected pulps.

EYE CONDITIONS Morse 1977
"Sarmanz and Bartha did an analysis of 1010 eye diseases with respect to the frequency of dental 'foci'. They found that eye conditions involving the uvea were often related to dental foci. In a recent paper, Sela and Sharav [*Isr. J. Dent. Med.* 24: 31-35, 1975] analyzed cases of uveitis that apparently were related to dental foci."

BLOOD, MICROORGANISMS IN Morse 1980
Morse 1980, p. 324,
"Bacteremia, anachoresis, cavernous sinus thrombosis and focal diseases are all dependent on the presence of microorganisms in the bloodstream."

DANGER OF MULTIPLE EXTRACTIONS Morse 1980
p. 325, "According to Bender and co-workers ... Bacteremias following extraction varied from 51.5% (single extractions) to

93.4% (multiple extractions, heavy trauma)."

DENTAL INFECTION AS CAUSE OF SYSTEMIC DISEASE *Lancet* 1980
   Editorial, *The Lancet*, May 31, 1980, 1175: "The only systemic
disease with which dental sepsis has commonly been associated is
bacterial endocarditis, but there are indications that dental
infections may be causally related to as much wider spectrum of
disorders." Pyrexia of undetermined origin, brain abscess and
subdural abscess are specifically discussed, with possible
implication of Streptococcus milleri on one occasion; it is
reported that treatment of pyorrhoea in some cases and
symptomless dental infection in others yielded beneficial
results. The editor concludes: "The ætiological role of chronic
dental infection in systemic disease has probably been
underestimated in the past. The organisms involved are
fastidious... "
   [This is precisely how Dr. Rosenow repeatedly described the
disease-causing oral bacteria with which he worked -
"fastidious"].

LEUKEMIAS, BACTERIAL ENDOCARDITIS Arens, 1981
   Arens, 1981, Chapter 2, p. 16-23, lists as conditions in which
bacteriemia from oral foci may be dangerous, p. 23 leukemias, and
bacterial endocarditis.

PATHOGENIC BETA-HEMOLYTIC STREPTOCOCCUS Brook 1981
   Brook 1981, p. 377, "Removal of the tonsils and adenoids is
associated in many instances with a reduction of pathogenic
organisms such as Group A beta-hemolytic Streptococci and S.
aureus."

CALL FOR REAPPRAISAL FOCAL INFECTION Thoden van Velzen 1984
   Thoden van Velzen and co-workers 1984 cite the "rather recent
increase of knowledge in several pertinent fields: which enables
a reappraisal of the focal infection concept.
   - cite "the divergent properties of the different microbial
species on the one hand, and those of individual hosts on the
other [as] a possible explanation of the inconstancy of focal
infection phenomena."

LOCUS MINORIS RESISTAENTIAE Thoden van Velzen 1984
CIRRHOSIS OF LIVER - ALCOHOL, FOCUS Thoden van Velzen 1984
PULPITIS DUE TO TRAUMA, & FOCUS Thoden van Velzen 1984
   - when "disseminated bacteria [in the bloodstream] meet with
favorable conditions, they tend to localize at that spot and,
after a certain time lag, start multiplying." This might be a
"locus minoris resistaentiae" resulting from "local inflammation
or degenerative processes such as liver cirrhosis due to alcohol
intoxication or pulpitis due to trauma..."
   - cites improvements in anaerobic culturing techniques of the
previous 15 years, and "it has become clear during recent years
that anaerobes are responsible for a significant number of

clinical infections. Most of the anaerobic bacteria implicated
are normal inhabitants of the body surfaces, prominent among
which are plaque components."

DISEASES, SEVERAL, & FOCAL INFECTION Thoden van Velzen 1984
ANGINA   Thoden van Velzen 1984
RHEUMATIC FEVER   Thoden van Velzen 1984
THROMBOSIS   Thoden van Velzen 1984
ERYTHEMA NODOSUM   Thoden van Velzen 1984
BELL'S PALSY   Thoden van Velzen 1984
MENINGITIS   Thoden van Velzen 1984
FACIAL NEURALGIA   Thoden van Velzen 1984
PNEUMONIA   Thoden van Velzen 1984
ARTHRITIS   Thoden van Velzen 1984
MYOCARDITIS   Thoden van Velzen 1984
IMPLANT PROSTHESIS   Thoden van Velzen 1984

Thoden van Velzen 1984:
 - Within the context of focal infection, discusses (1)
endocarditis, myocarditis, brain vessel infections and abscesses,
lung infections, liver cirrhosis, pulpitis, (2) angina, rheumatic
fever, diffuse glomerunophritis, pneumonia, thrombosis, several
dermatological diseases, uveitis and iridocyclitis and other
diseases of the uveal tract, arthritis, hepatitis, erythema
nodosum, meningitis; (3) myelin sheath injury, facial neuralgia,
Bell's palsy (a demyelinating disease), fever of unknown origin

Thoden van Velzen 1984:
 - cites primary objections to theory
1) oral infection is ... "often not accompanied by secondary
metastatic disease", and
2) "in many cases ... removal of all potential foci is not
followed by healing of the 'secondary' affliction.

Thoden van Velzen 1984:
 - cites "three pathogenic pathways leading to focal infection:
1. metastatic infection due to transcient bacteriemia, including
myocarditis, endocarditis, brain abscesses, metastatic lung
infections, liver cirrhosis, pulpitis, transplants and implant
prostheses
2. metastatic inflammation " immunological injury
3. metastatic injury   " microbial toxins

MENINGITIS AND TEETH Thoden van Velzen etal, 1984
   Thoden van Velzen etal, 1984, "recently it has been suggested
that in some cases meningitis might be the result of immune
complex mediated injury secondary to dental foci. [Hedström SA,
Nord CE and Ursing B, *Scand. J. of Infect. Dis.* 12 (1980), 117-
121] Four patients are described who recovered rapidly following
the administration of anti-inflammatory drugs and appropriate
dental treatment. "Although it has to be conceded that proof of
a causal relationship of dental foci of infection and metastatic

immunological injury is far from complete, the available evidence seems to support such a hypothesis."

MENINGITIS FROM DISTANT OR ADJACENT INFECTION Francke 1987
   Francke 1987, p. 175, on meningitis, notes some signs "suggest distant or adjacent sources of infection and, therefore, resident flora are likely causes."

SCLEROSIS, PROGRESSIVE SYSTEMIC & ORAL INFECTION Janssens 1987
   Janssens X etal 1987 discuss oral disease (teeth) manifestations of progressive systemic sclerosis, without asserting teeth may serve as infective focus.

ARTHRITIS Lens 1988
MENINGITIS Lens 1988
ENDOCARDITIS Lens 1988
   Lens 1988, p. 1, refers to arthritis, meningitis, endocarditis and uveitis as diseases mentioned in connection with the hypothesis that dental infections may function as a source of inflammatory processes elsewhere in the body.
   Lens 1988 presented experimental evidence of dissemination of antigenic material from the gingiva to other sites in the body, evidence in support of the concept of focal infection.
   Specifically the authors experimentally induced an inflammation in the knee of mice and then injected antigen in the gingiva. This resulted in a sustained increase of the antigen in the blood and 24 hours later an exacerbation of the knee inflammations.
   Arthritis references, per Lens 1988:
Reich, H. von, 1974, *Dtsch. Zahnaertzl.* Z 29, 1043-4
Shimizu, K, Toyota Y, Koh, T, etal, 1977, *Bull. Jossai Dent Univ.* 6, 421-4.

SCLEROSIS, SYSTEMIC & ORAL INFECTION Wood & Lee 1988
   Wood R and Lee P 1988 discuss oral disease (teeth) manifestations of progressive systemic sclerosis, without asserting teeth may serve as infective focus.

OPTIC NEURITIS Bocca M etal 1989
   Bocca M etal 1989:   Abstract: Bocca etal examine the presence of dental diseases in patients with optic neuritis or uveitis, in comparison to a control group. Possible interactions between opthalmic and dental pathologies are analyzed to highlight possible clinical signs which may be useful for identification. {MEDLINE/kw: optic neuritis focal infection}

OPTIC NEURITIS Ilewicz L etal 1990
   Ilewicz L etal 1990: Abstract: Ilewicz etal sought to demonstrate relations between foci in the oral cavity and certain inflammatory diseases of the eye (intraocular and retrobulbar optic neuritis, iritis, retinitis and keratitis. Positive results were obtained in 31 of 43 patients with electrocutaneous test, the test for pulp viability with faradic current).

OPTIC NEURITIS   Chaabouni M etal 1991
  Chaabouni M etal 1991: Abstract: Chaabouni etal discuss 4
patients with acute dental infection and unilateral inflammation
of the optic nerve. "The first symptom was in all cases a sudden
fall of visual acuity. The visual field is always altered.
Papilloedema is observed in three eyes. The treatment is of the
dental infection at first, secondly, corticosteroids are
associated. An improvement is noticed in 3 cases. ..."

OPTIC NEURITIS   Philippe J etal 1991: Abstract: Philippe,
etal., discuss case of 23-year-old woman with decreased vision
and central scotoma, disclosed by fundus examination as
unilateral acute edematous optic neuritis. A nasolabial cyst of
probable dental origin was diagnosed and excised with systemic
antibiotics. "The prognosis was excellent with recovery of a
normal visual acuity and normal fundus appearance. There was no
evidence of any recurrent episode. The nasolabial cyst was the
cause likely of the neuritis. Nevertheless, multiple sclerosis
must be considered. Only long-term absence of neurological signs
could prove that the maxillary lesion was directly responsible
for the optic disorder."

ORAL FOCI AND FEBRILE EPISODES IN LYMPHOMA WITH CHEMOTHERAPY
  Laine PO etal, *European J. of Cancer, Part B. Oral Oncology*,
1992 Oct., 28B: 103-7, implicated oral foci as the source of
infection causing febrile episodes in lymphoma patients receiving
cytostatic drugs, for non-Hodgkins lymphoma or Hodgkin's disease.
  We may note that Dr. Rosenow's early work encompassed
Hodgkin's, with the implication that the oral foci may not only
be causing the febrile episodes but perhaps also the lymphoma
itself.

MYOCARDIAL/CEREBRAL INFARCTION Asikainen and Alaluusua 1993
  Asikainen and Alaluusua 1993 states "Oral bacteria may spread
into the blood stream through ulcerated epithelium in diseased
periodontal pockets and cause transient bacteraemias ..." and
discusses "the new association between dental infections and
myocardial/cerebral infarction [which] have offered new
challenges for cooperation between dental and medical
researchers."

BACTERIOSPERMIA AND SUBFERTILITY IN MALES
  Bieniek KW and Riedel HH *Andrologia*, 1993 May-Jun, 25(3)159-62,
diagnosed bacteriospermia in more than 70% of subfertile
patients, and noted that a high incidence of potential dental
foci was found in all patients. In a test group of 18 patients,
the oral foci were removed; six months later, about 2/3 of
spermiograms proved sterile. In the control group, findings of
spermiograms remained poor. MEDLINE ABSTRACT: "This study
indicates that a direct causal relationship exists between
bacterial colonies (dental foci) and therapy-resistant

bacteriospermia which probably leads to subfertility.

CORONARY HEART DISEASE De Stefano etal 1993
  De Stefano etal 1993 concluded that "Dental disease is associated with an increased risk of coronary heart disease, particularly in young men. Whether this is a causal association is unclear."

PULMONARY COMPLICATIONS Ballou etal 1994
S. MILLERI AND ORAL FOCI Ballou etal 1994
Balloul H, etal., *Archives de Pediatrie*, 1994 Mar, 1(3):264-7. (French). "Septicemia due to Streptococcus milleri with pulmonary complications". The authors discuss the role of S. milleri in septicemia that is often complicated by abscesses. "Two foci of dental infection were found and treated by tooth extraction." Patient was also given some combinations of six medications, and case brought to a successful conclusion. Abstract does not indicate just what aspect of regimen is thought to have been decisive; reasons for apparent resistance to treatment are discussed.
  This article supports a connection between S. milleri and S. rosenow, i.e., that the former may be a form of the latter.

HEART DISEASE Debelian GJ 1994
MYOCARDIAL INFARCTION Debelian GJ 1994
CEREBRAL INFARCTION Debelian GJ 1994
ENDOCARDITIS Debelian GJ 1994
BRAIN ABSCESSES Debelian GJ 1994
IMPLANT INFECTIONS Debelian GJ 1994
  Debelian GJ etal, "Systemic diseases caused by oral microorganisms.", *Endodontics and Dental Traumatology*, 1994 Apr., 10(2):57-65; MEDLINE ABSTRACT: "Human endodontic and periodontal infections are associated with complex microfloras ... . These infections are predominantly anaerobic, with gram-negative rods being the most common isolates. The anatomic closeness of this microflora to the bloodstream can facilitate bacteremia and systemic spread of bacterial by-products and immunocomplexes. A variety of clinical procedures such as tooth extraction, periodontal and endodontic treatment, may cause translocation of microorganisms from the oral cavity to the bloodstream. ... in patients with ineffective heart valves or vascular diseases, bacteremia can be a potential danger, leading most commonly to infective endocarditis and myocardial or cerebral infarction. Other forms of systemic diseases such as brain abscesses, hematologcal infections and implant infections have also been related to oral microorganisms."

MENTAL ILLNESS IN ELEPHANT Holden 1994
  Science magazine [Holden C., 265, 1529 (9 Sept. 1994)] noted that after a rampaging circus elephant was killed in Honolulu in August, an autopsy was conducted "to see if there was a biological cause for her aberrant behavior. They found no sign

of disease, but she had previously suffered a tusk abscess."

SINUS ABNORMALITIES, ORAL FOCI AS CAUSE OF Abrams 1996
  Abrams, JJ and RM Glassberg, <u>Amer. J. Roentgen.</u> 1996 May, 166
(5): 1219-23, conclude: "We have demonstrated a twofold increase
in maxillary sinus disease in patients with periodontal disease
and have shown a causal relationship." The authors highlighted
the implications particularly for those planning implant surgery.

LEUKEMIA IN CHILDREN, ORO-DENTAL "MANIFESTATIONS" Nikoui 1996
  Nikoui M and Lalonde B, J. Canadian Dental Ass., 1996 May,
62(5):443-6, 449-50, review oral conditions related to leukemia,
with the presumption that the former are caused by the latter.
The authors note that leukemia accounts for about 30 percent of
childhood cancer cases in Canada, and that leukemia and
associated therapies are are more likely to be associated with
oral problems ("complications") than all other types of cancer.
(per MEDLINE abstract)

PLEASE NOTE THAT THIS CHRONOLOGY DOES NOT ATTEMPT OR PRETEND TO
BE COMPREHENSIVE. SEE "MEDLINE" FOR "FOCAL INFECTION" SINCE
1966, AND INDEX MEDICUS FOR EARLIER CITATIONS.

APPENDIX B2: FOCAL INFECTION BIBLIOGRAPHY

Alexander 1869: Amaurosis from neuralgia of dental nerves. Alexander in Amer. Jnl. Med. Sciences. --Dental cosmos, 1869, p. 161

Allport, Frank, [Dental Review 18 (April 15, 1904), #4, Chicago, Ill., U.S.A., "The Relation of Odontology to Opthamology and Otology.", 305-315]

Allport 1904: The relation of odontology to ophthalmology and otology. Allport, Frank, Dental Review, 1904, p. 305

Anderson, WAD, Pathology, 1971, p. 289.

Arens, DE, WR Adams and RA DeCastro, Endodontic Surgery, Harper and Row, Philadelphia, 1981, Chapter 2, "Medical Considerations and Contraindications".

Austin, Louie T., D.D.S., and Thomas J. Cook, D.D.S., Rochester, Minn., "Bacteriologic Study of Normal Vital Teeth", J.A.D.A. 16: 894-6 (May) 1929

Austin, Louie T., D.D.S., Rochester, Minn., "Relationship of Dental Sepsis to Systemic Disease", J.A.D.A., 27, May 1940, 684-688.

Ball LC and Parker MT, J. Hyg. (Camb.) 1979; 82, 63-78

Bargen, JA, J.A.M.A. 83 (Aug. 2, 1924), "Experimental studies on the etiology of chronic ulcerative colitis"

Bargen, JA, Archives of Internal Medicine 1928, 50-60, "Specific serum treatment in chronic ulcerative colitis"

Bargen, JA, Archives of Internal Medicine, 1929, 559-572, "Chronic Ulcerative Colitis"

Barnes, AR and AS Giordano, J. of the Indiana State Med. Assoc. XV (Ja. 15, 1922), 1-7, "Bacteria Recovered Postmortem with Special Reference to Selective Localization and Focal Infection."

Bartels, H. A., "Historical Portraits in Dental Culture - Weston Price (1870-1948)", NYJD 35(3), March 1965, 97-8

Batson, O.V., "Function of the vetebral veins and their role in the spread of metastases. Ann. Surg. 112:138, 1940; "Role of the Vertebral veins in metastatic processes." Ann. Intern. Med. 16:38, 1942; "Vertebral vein system as a mechanism for spread of metastases."

Amer. J. Roentgen. 48:715, 1943; per Störtebecker 1967

Beaumont 1913: Beaumont, British Med. Jnl., Sept. 26, 1913, p. 525

Bierring, Walter L., "Focal Infection: Quarter Century Survey", JAMA 111 (Oct. 29, 1938), 1623-1627.
  "The work of Rosenow was confirmed in detail by Russell L. Haden [1925], who followed closely certain fundamental technical details insisted on by Rosenow." (Bierring 1938)

Billings, Frank, Arch. Int. Med. 4 (Nov. 1909), 409, "Chronic Infectious Endocarditis".

Billings, Frank, Arch. Int. Med. April 1912, 484-498, "Chronic Focal Infections and their Etiologic Relations to Arthritis and Nephritis".

Billings, Frank: "Chronic focal infection as a causative factor in chronic arthritis", JAMA LXI (Sept. 13, 1913), 819-826.

Billings, F., FOCAL INFECTION, The Lane Medical Lectures (Sept. 20-24, 1915), D. Appleton and Co., NY & London, 1916, p. 36.

Billings, Frank, [JAMA 1922;78:1097-1105]

Black, Arthur D., Ophth. Rev. XXIV Dec., 1915, 610-622.

Black, G.V., 1915, 1936: Special dental Pathology, Black, G.V., p. 370

Blanc 1871: Chronic ophthalmia cured by taking out of a tooth. Abstract. Blanc in Revue de Therapeut.Medico-Chirurg., Aug., 1871. --Dental Cosmos, 1871, p. 634

Blayney, J.R., Dental Cosmos LXXIV, 635-653 (July 1932).
Bocca, M, etal, Minerva Stomatologica, 1989 Oct, 38(10):1117-20, "The correlation between dental pathology and opthalmic pathology". {MEDLINE/kw: optic neuritis focal infection}

Brailey, W. A. and Sydney Stephenson [System of Diseases of the Eye, Norris and Oliver ed., 1898], per de Schweinitz, G.E., Ophthal. Rec. XXIV, Dec. 1915, 603-610.

Breslau 1913: Connection between ocular diseases and inflammatory conditions of the teeth. Seydel, F., Breslau. From Deutsche Monatsschrift fur Zahnheilkunde. -- Dental Cosmos, 1913, p. 106

British Medical Journal, May 8, 1954, p. 1081-2, Editorial: "Social Incidence of Rheumatic Fever".

Brook, Itzhak, The Laryngoscope 92 (1981) 377-382, "Aerobic and anaerobic bacteriology of Adenoids in Children: A comparison between patients with chronic adenotonsillitis and adenoid hypertrophy."

Brook I, and PA Foote, Jr., Laryngoscope 96 (Dec. 1986), 1385-8, "Comparison of the Microbiology of Recurrent Tonsillitis Between Children and Adults."

Castiglioni, Arturo, A History of Medicine, NY, Alfred A Knopf, 1941, 1958, p. 622, Benjamin Rush (1745-1813)

Cecil RL and DM Angevine, Annals of Int. Med. 12 (Nov. 1938), 577-584, "Clinical and Experimental Observations of Focal Infection, with an analysis of 200 cases of Rheumatoid Arthritis", p. 579,

Chaabouni M, etal., Revue de Stomatologie et de Chirurgie Maxillo-Faciale, 1991, 92(4):259-61, "Optic neuropathy of dental origin. Apropos of 4 cases". {MEDLINE/kw: optic neuritis focal infection}

Cohen, Stephen and Richard C. Burns,

Pathways of the Pulp, C.V. Mosby, St. Louis, 1987, p. 378; 1980.

Cook, Thomas, J.A.D.A. 18 (1931), 2290-2301, "Focal infection of the teeth and elective localization in the experimental production of ulcerative colitis".

Cooke, Robert A., Proc. Dental Centennial Celebration, 1940: Maryland State Dental Assoc. and A. D. A. , 134-140, "The Role of Allergy in Medico-Dental Problems".

Cotton, H.A., "The Relation of Oral Infection to Mental Diseases", J.Dental Res. 1:269 (1919).

Cramer HC amd AF Reith, JADA 19 (June 1932) 976-982, "Quantitative Bacteriologic Study of Pulpless Teeth Correlated with Dental Roentgenograms".

Davis, D.J., in discussion following Mayo CH, Dental Rev. XXVII (1913), 281-297, p. 323.

Davis, C.G., Inflammation of eye cured by extraction of a tooth. Dental Cosmos, 1876, p. 110

De Stefano, F., et al., BMJ 306 (1993), 688-691, "Dental disease and risk of coronary heart disease and mortality"

De Dio, Robert M, et

al., Arch. Otolaryngol. Head, Neck surg. 114 (July 1988), 763-5, "Microbiology of the Tonsils and Adenoids in a Pediatric Population"

de Schweinitz, G.E., Ophthal. Rec. XXIV (Dec. 1915), 603-610, "Concerning Focal Infections in their Relation to Certain Disorders of the Uveal Tract."

Delestre 1869: Amaurosis from dental irritation. M. Delestre in Med. Times and Gazette. --Dental Cosmos, 1869, p. 161

Dental News Letter 1847: Painful affection of the eye cured by the extraction of a tooth. Dental News Letter, 1847-48,46.

DeWitt 1868: Amaurosis of the right eye relieved by the removal of the filling from a carious tooth of the corresponding side and its final cure by the extraction of the tooth. F. M. DeWitt in Am. Jnl. Med. Sciences. -- Dental Cosmos, 1868, p. 272

Dietz, Oral Surg. 57:877-883 (1952) per Morse, D. R., Oral Surg. 43, 436-451, 1977; and per Grossman 1960.

Dimmer 1913: Metastatic ophthalmia following tooth extraction. Dimmer in

Wiener Vierteljahrs-- Fachblatt. --Dental Cosmos, 1913, p. 959

Duke, William W., Oral Sepsis In Its Relationship to Systemic Disease, C.V.Mosby, St. Louis, Mo. USA, 1918, pp. 17-20.]

Dutrow 1915: Report of a case of reflex ocular disturbance due to impacted third molar. Dutrow, H.V., Ophthalmic Record, May, 1915, p. 253

Editorial: "Focal Infection", JAMA 150 (Oct. 4, 1952), 490-1.

Eusterman [Eusterman GB, Minn. Med., 6:698 (1923)] summarized per Nickel AC and AR Hufford, Arch. Int. Med.41 (1928), 210-230, p. 215

Fishbein, Morris, The American Medical Association 1847-1947, A History of the A.M.A., W.B. Saunders Co., Phila. & London 1947, p. 224

Flint, Austin, A Treatise on the Principles and Practice of Medicine, 3rd Ed., Henry C. Lea, Phila., 1868, p. 688

Forssner [Nord. Med. Arkiv. 1902, xxxv, 1-56] per Billings 1916 (Lane Lectures)

Francke, O.C.. Bull. Hist. Dent., 21, 73-79 (1974), p. 73-4]

Freeman, J., "Toxic Idiopathies", The

Lancet, July 31, 1920, p. 229-235.

Freeman, John, "Skin reactions in asthma", protein idiopathies. The Practitioner 116:73-8, January 1926

Frick A, JAMA 82:595 (Feb. 23, 1924) per Nickel, AC and AR Hufford, Arch. Int. Med.41 (1928), 210-230, p. 215

Friedman PJ, "Correcting the literature following fraudulent publication", JAMA 263, No. 10 (March 9,1990), 1416-1419

Frühauf, Amaurosis cured by the extraction of fangs. Excerpt. Deutsche Vierteljahrschrift für Zahnheilkunde. -- Dental Cosmos, 1873, p. 662

Garfield, E. and A. Welljams-Dorof: "The Impact of Fraudulent Research on the Scientific Literature", JAMA 263 (March 9, 1990), 1424-1426.

Gilmer 1915: chronic oral infections. T.L. Gilmer, Archives Internal Med., 1912, p. 499.

Goldberg, Harry A, Am. J. Orthodontics 24 (March 1938), 272-80, "Ten Years' Research of Dental Infections and Their Relations to Systemic Disease".

Goulden 1911: Some inflammatory eye

conditions due to oral sepsis. Goulden, C., from Proceedings Royal Society of Medicine, London, Feb., 1911. -- Dental Cosmos, 1911, p. 216

Greger B, G Döller, WD Schareck, GH Müller, J Mellert, UT Hopt, and H Bockhorn, Transplantation Proceedings xix (October 1987) 4057-4060, "Incidence and Clinical Course of CMV- (and Herpes Simplex-) infections under Triple Drug Therapy"

Guthof, Otto, Zentralblatt fur Bakteriologie, Parasitenkunde, Infectionskrankheiten und Hygient, Abt. IU, Origl 166 (1956), 553-564, "Ueber pathogene 'vergrünende (Viridescent) Streptokokken'".

Haden, Russell, L., Dental Infection and Systemic Disease, Lea and Febiger, Philadelphia, Pa., U.S.A. 1928, p.159

Hancock 1859: Two cases of amaurosis depending on dental irritation. Case of ptosis and diverging strabismus from decayed teeth. Henry Hancock in London Lancet. --Dental Cosmos, 1859-60, p. 50

Harris, Malcolm, Royal Soc. of Health Journal 86 (1966), 79-81, "Dental Infection and the Eyes".

Hastings, TW, J. Exper. Med. XX (1914) p. 52-71, "Complement Fixation Tests in Chronic Infective Deforming Arthritis and Arthritis Deformans"

Hatton, Edward H., "Focal Infection", in Black, G.V., G.V. Black's work on Operative Dentistry, and Special Dental Pathology combined, Vol. 4 (1936), p. 414-416.

Henoq and associates [Rev. Stomatol. Chir. Maxillofac. 73:21-30, 1972] per Morse, D. R., Oral Surg. 43, 436-451, 1977.

Henrici, Arthur T. and Thomas B. and Hartzell, "The Bacteriology of Vital Pulps", J. Dent. Research 1:419-422 (Dec.) 1919

Hensch 1938. [Hensch, PS, Is Rheumatoid (Atrophic) Arthritis a Disease of Microbic Origin?, London, Oxford U. Press, 1938]. per Slocumb et al 1941,

Herrick, James B., in discussion following Mayo CH, Dental Rev. XXVII (1913), 281-297, p. 323.

Herschfeld, JJ, Bull. Hist. Dent. 33:35-45 (1985); reprint of Hunter 1911.

Hippocrates, Teachings of, Adams edition, pp. 127, 300, 360.

Hirsch, Edwin F., Frank Billings, The Architect of Medical Education, An Apostle of Excellence in Medical Practice; A Leader in Chicago Medicine, University of Chicago, 1966.

Hogg 1857: Amaurosis from decayed teeth. Excerpt. Tabez Hogg in London Lancet. -- Dental News Letter, 1857-58, p. 160

Holden C., Science 265, 1529 (9 Sept. 1994)

Holman, W.L., "The Localization in Animals of Bacteria Isolated from Foci of Infection", JAMA 88 (Feb. 5, 1927), 424-5.

Holman, W.L., "Focal Infection and 'Elective Localization', A Critical Review", Archives Path & Lab. Med. 5 (1928), 68-136; see table, p. 133.

Hughes RA, British Journal of Rheumatology 33 (1994), 370-7, "Focal Infection Revisited".

Hunter, William, Odont. Soc. Trans., Jan. 1899, per BMJ, 28 July 1900, 215-6.

Hunter, William, Dental Register 65 (1911), 579-611, "The Role of Sepsis and Antisepsis in Medicine and the Importance of Oral Sepsis as its Chief Cause".

Hunter, William,

Lancet 1:79 (Jan. 14) 1911.

Hutchinson 1875: On the kind of teeth usually associated with cataract. Jonathan Hutchinson in British Journal of Dental Science. -- Dental Cosmos, 1875, p. 326

Hutchinson, S.J., Lagophthalmus due to dental irritation. Med. and Surg. Reporter., Excerpt. Dental Cosmos 1886, p. 123

Ibershoff 1915: Carious teeth as a factor in ocular diseases. Ibershoff, A.E., Jnl. Ophthal. and Oto-Laryng.m May, 1915, p. 141 and July 1915, p. 209

Ilewicz L, Ciechocinska J, Chrusciel H, Czasopismo Stomatologiczne, 1990 Sep, 43(9):513-6, "Relationship between grade I and II inflammatory foci and certain inflammatory opthalmic diseases". {MEDLINE kw: optic neuritis focal infection}

Irons EE, EVL Brown and WH Nadler, J. Infectious Disease 18 (1916), 315-334, "The Localization of Streptococci in the Eye, A Study of Experimental Iridocyclitis in Rabbits."

JAMA 150 (Oct. 4, 1952), Editorial:

"Focal Infection", 490-1.

JAMA 263, No. 10 (March 9,1990) addresses the question of fraudulent or otherwise invalid scientific research.

Janssens, X, et al., Clinical Rheumatology, 1987 Dec 6(4):532-8, "Disease manifestations of progressive systemic sclerosis (scleroderma): sensitivity and specificity" {MEDLINE/kw: sclerosis teeth}

Jarlov E., Brinch O, Focal infection and arthritis, Danish Section, Association Internationale Pour les Recherches sur la Paradentose, Copenhagen: Lassen and Stiedl, 1938; per Hughes, R.A., Brit. J. Rheum. 1994:33:370-7; see FOCAL UPDATE]; abstr.- JAMA 111 (July 11, 1938), 290, "Focal Infections - Considerations on Causes and Nature of Diseases of Joints".

Jones, N.W. and S.J. Newsom, Archives of Pathology 13 (1932), 392-414, "Experimentally produced focal (dental) infection in relation to cardiac structure"

Jones, et al., 1970, p. 454-459, [bacterial endocarditis; bacteriemia in]

Kempton, H.T., Loss of

sight from decayed teeth. London Dental Review. --Dental Cosmos, 1862-63, p. 548

Koecker 1842: Case of deafness and lost sight cured by proper dental treatment. Amer. Jnl. Dental Science, 1842-3, p. 243

A case of amaurosis consecutive to the extraction of a tooth. From La Stomatologia, Milan, July, 1906. -- Dental Cosmos, 1907, p. 875

Lardier, P., Amaurosis from a carious tooth. Excerpt, in L'Union Medical. --Dental Cosmos, 1875, p. 389

Lens JW, W Beertsen, Journal of Periodontal Research Jan. 1988; 23 (1):1-6, "Injection of an antigen into the gingiva and its effect on an experimentally induced inflammation in the knee joint of a mouse."

Lewis, Dean D., in discussion following Mayo CH, Dental Rev. XXVII (1913), 281-297, p. 323.

MacWhinnie 1913: Teeth and their relation to the eye. MacWhinnie, A.M., New York Medical Jnl., Oct. 18, 1913, p. 755

Marshall, J.S., Amaurosis from diseased dental pulp. Dental Cosmos, 1883, p. 425

Marx, Jean, Science 247, p. 1540 [genetics alone insufficient]

Mayo, Charles H., "Local Foci of Infection Causing General Systemic Disturbances", The Medical Herald 32 (1913) 370-373. [1913b]

Mayo, CH, "Focal Infection of Dental Origin", Dental Cosmos 64 (1922), 1206-1208.

Mayo, Charles H., "The Relation of Local Foci of Infection to General Systemic Conditions, Constitutional Diseases Secondary to Local Infections", Dental Rev. XXVII (1913), 281-297; discussion 309-327. [1913a]

McConachie 1903 [McConachie, A.D., Dental Cosmos, 1903, p. 941, "Reflex Neuroses of Dental Origins as Manifest in Eye, Ear, Nose and Throat Diseases."], p. 942

McConachie 1903: Reflex neuroses of dental origin as manifest in eye, ear, nose and throat diseases. McConachie, A.D., Dental Cosmos, 1903, p. 941

Medical Times. Aug. 1968. 854 [History]

Merritt 1911: Severe pain in eye caused by congested tooth pulp. Merritt, A.H., Dental Cosmos, 1911, p. 1445

Mervis, J., Nature 359 (29 Oct., 1992), p. 787.

Metchnikoff [Ann. d. l'inst. Pasteur, xii, 1898] per Mayo CH, Dental Rev. XXVII (1913), 281-297.

Miller, Howard C., in Proceedings, Dental Centenary Celebration, 1940, Maryland State Dental Association and A.D.A., 475-481, "Oral Surgery and Its Relation to Dentistry and Medicine", p. 478-9

Moorehead, Frederick B., in Discussion, Mayo CH, Dental Rev. XXVII (1913), 281-297.

Morse, D. R., Oral Surg. 43 (March 1977), 436-451, "Immunologic Aspects of pulpal-periapical diseases."

Morse, D. R., in Cohen, S. and R. C. Burns, Pathways of the Pulp, C.V. Mosby, St. Louis, 1980, p. 324; 1987, p. 378.

Newman HN, "Focal Infection Revisited", Periodontal Abstracts 41 (1993), 73-7

Newman HN and Williams, 1992, per Newman HN, "Focal Infection Revisited", Periodontal Abstracts 41 (1993), 73-7.

Nickel AC and AR Hufford, Arch. Int. Med.41 (1928), 210-230, "Elective Localization of Streptococci Isolated

from Cases of Peptic Ulcer", p. 215 [1928a]

Nickel AC and WW Sager, Mayo Clinic, Staff Meetings, Proceedings, Oct. 16, 1928, 297-299, "The Infection of Artificially Produced Sterile Abscesses by the Intravenous Injection of Bacteria."[1928b]

Osler, The Principles and Practice of Medicine, D. Appleton and Co., New York and London, 1909 (Seventh Edition) p. 440

Osler, Sir William, The Principles and Practice of Medicine, D. Appleton and Co., New York and London, 1918 (Eighth Edition)

Parker MT and LC Ball, J.Med. Microbio. 1976; 9:275-302, "Streptococci and Aerococci associated with systemic infection in man".

Peck, Edw. S., Pathological relations between diseases of the teeth and of the eye, arising from rheumatism and gout. Dental Cosmos, 1905, p. 103

Pfeiffer MP & Snodgrass GL, "The continued use of retracted invalid scientific literature", JAMA 263, No. 10 (March 9,1990), 1420-5

Philippe, J, et al., J Francais D Opthalmologie, 1991,

14(1):32-5, "Maxillary cyst of dental origin with uncommon ocular complication" {MEDLINE kw: optic neuritis, dental}

Pierce, Charles H., The Journal-Lancet, Aug. 1, 1915, 414-419, "The Practical Value Of Autogenous Vaccine Therapy, With Cases"

Power 1884: On the relations between dental lesions and diseases of the eye. Abstract from paper by Henry Power. London Medical Press. -- Dental Cosmos, 1884, p. 308 (accomodation,

Poynton and Paine, Lancet Oct. 28, 1911, pp. 1189-1191, per Mayo CH, Dental Rev. XXVII (1913), 281-297.

Price, Weston, Nutrition and Physical Degeneration, 1939, 1970 [available through Price-Pottinger Foundation, San Diego, CA.]

Price, Weston, Dental Infection, Oral and Systemic, 1923: Cleveland, Penton Pub. Co. [available through Price-Pottinger Foundation, San Diego, CA.]

Quinoz, D, (abstr.), JAMA 111 (Dec. 10, 1938) 2250, "Rheumatism from Focal Infection"

Rhoads, P.S. and G.F. Dick, JADA 19 (November 1932), 1844-1893, "Roentgenographically

negative pulpless teeth as foci of infection: Results of quantitative cultures"

Rosenow, E.C., J. Infect. Dis. i (1904), 280-312, per Mayo CH, Dental Rev. XXVII (1913), 281-297.

Rosenow, E.C., in discussion following Mayo CH, Dental Rev. XXVII (1913), 281-297, p. 321

Rowntree, Leonard G., Amid Masters of TWENTIETH CENTURY MEDICINE, Charles C. Thomas, Springfield Ill. 1958]

Rush, Benjamin, Medical Inquiries and Observations, I (1818), p. 199; reprinted in Duke, William W., Oral Sepsis In Its Relationship to Systemic Disease, C.V.Mosby, St. Louis, Mo. USA, 1918, pp. 17-20.

Salter, S.J.A., Amaurosis consequent on acute abscess of antrum produced by a carious tooth. London Lancet. --Dental Cosmos, 1862-3d, p. 548

Schottmüller [Münch. Med. Wchnschr. 1903, L, 845] per Billings 1916 (Lane Medical Lectures).

Sela and Sharav [Isr. J. Dent. Med. 24: 31-35, 1975] per Morse, D. R., Oral Surg. 43, 436-451, 1977.

Sirletti, Amaurosis following dental disease. Excerpt in Arch. Clin. Ital. dei Med. Condotti. -- Dental Cosmos, 1878, p. 685

Slocumb, Charles H., Melvin W. Binger, Arlie R. Barnes and Henry L. Williams: "Focal Infection", JAMA 117 (Dec. 20, 1941), 2161-2164.

Springer in 1898 [Aetiol. u. Klinik des Akut Gelenkrheum, Wien 1898] per Topley WWC and HB Weir, J. Path. and Bacteriology 24 (1921), p. 344

St. Bartholomew's 1881: Sympathetic Ptosis from decayed teeth. Excerpt from St. Bartholomew's Hospital Reports in Lancet. --Dental Cosmos, 1881, p. 497

Stevens, E.W., Diseases of the eye in relation to the teeth. Dental Cosmos, 1901, p. 108

Störtebecker, T.P., "Dental significance of pathways for dissemination from infectious foci", J. Canad. Dent. Ass. 33: 301-311 (1967)

THE LANCET, Editorial, May 31 1980, p. 1175 [focal infection]

The Lancet 1985, p. 1403-4 [On S. Milleri]

Thoden van Velzen, S.K., L. Abraham-Inpijn and W.R. Moorer, J. Clin.

Periodont. 11 (1984) 209-220."Plaque and systemic disease: a reappraisal of the focal infection concept"

Topley WWC and HB Weir, J. Path. and Bacteriology 24 (1921) 333-346, "The Lesions Produced in Rabbits by the Inoculation of Streptococci Isolated from Rheumatic and Other Lesions in the Human Subject".

Tribbles, S.G., Two cases of ocular diseases associated with pyorrhea alveolaris, Brit. Med. J., April, 1914, p.755

Tunnecliff, Ruth and Carolyn Hammond: Presence of bacteria in pulps of intact teeth. J. Am. Dent. & Dental Cosmos 24:1663-1666 (Oct.) 1937

Utz, U., et al., Nature 364, 243-246 (1993): Discusses "skewing of the TCR repertoire [which] could contribute to the pathogenesis of MS and other T-cell-mediated diseases. ... other T-cell-mediated autoimmune diseases such as diabetes, thyroiditis or rheumathoid arthritis."

Van Buren, Abigail (Dear Abby), Los Angeles Times, Oct. 2, 1994, E2: "Bad Teeth Are Not Just an Imperfection"

Van Kirk LE and WF Swanson, J. Dental Research 15 (Sept. 1936) 315-6, "Experimental Encephalitis in Rabbits: Intravenous injection of streptococci from pulpless teeth in human encephalitis".

Waksman, B. H., Nature 337, 599 (1989): discusses possible relationship between a retrovirus related to HTLV-I and MS, suggesting possible applicability of drugs "being developed for the distantly related AIDS virus"; discusses possibility that "immunological reaction to tissue antigen triggered by viral infection in early life in genetically predisposed individuals" may explain "the pathogenesis of the characteristic inflammatory destructive lesions of MS, rheumatoid arthritis, insulin-dependent diabetes, chronic thyroiditis and other similar diseases".

Watson 1851: Amaurosis from dental irritation. Dental News Letter, 1851-52, p. 296

Welsch, Ashton L., "Specificity of Streptococci Isolated from Patients with Skin Diseases: Studies on Pemphigus, Dermatitis Herpetiformis, Lupus Erythematosus and Erythema Multiforme",

J. Investigative Dermatology 7: 7-42 (1946).

Welsch, Ashton L., Archives of Dermatology and Syphilogy 30 (Nov. 1934) 611-629, "Specificity of a Streptococcus Isolated from Patients with Pemphigus."

White, Leon E. (1928): "The location of the focus in optic nerve disturbances from infection", Ann. Otol. Rhinol. Laryngol. 27 (1928), 128-164. [28Q3]

Wilkie DPD, Brit. Med. J. 1 (1928), 481-4, "Some Aspects of Gall-Bladder Disease"

Wood R, Lee P, Oral Surg, Oral Med, Oral Path, 1988 Feb 65(2):172-8, "Analysis of the oral manifestation of systemic sclerosis (scleroderma)" {MEDLINE/kw: sclerosis teeth}

Wood's Amer. Ency. ... 1915: Dental amblyopia. Wood's Amer. Encyc. of Ophthalmology, Vol. V, p. 3817

Woods, Hiram, Ocular phenomena accompanying three cases of gastro-intestinal disorder, Ophthalmic Record, 1915, p. 547

Wright, C.E., Sclerotitis relieved by extracting a carious tooth. Western Jnl. of Medicine. --

Dental Cosmos, 1870,
p. 496

Wright, C.E.,
Sclerotitis relieved
by extracting a
carious tooth.
Excerpt.Medical
Record. --Dental
Cosmos, 1870, p. 103

Wright, G.H.,
Influence of maxillary
changes on the eye,
Dental Cosmos, 1912,
p. 266

Yang et al., Am J.
Neph. 1994, 14(1):72-5
[transplant
complications]

APPENDIX C: MICROBIAL VARIATION: DISSOCIATION & TRANSMUTATION
  Of Butterflies, Slime-Molds Microbes -- Going Through A Phase

WHAT IS LIFE? - THE ROSENOW TANGENT

Examples of organisms which exist in different embodiments are
common in nature. Thus we have the butterfly and caterpillar,
the house-fly and its worm-like larvae, the protozoan and
sporatozoan forms of the creature that causes malaria, the
multicellular mobile colony and unicellular spore of the slime
mold (e.g., see Hapgood, Fred, Science Digest, April 1982, p.
32).

It may at first seem somewhat off the wall, but transitions
between viral and bacteriological forms seem reminiscent of slime
molds; these may exist in individual independent one-celled
organisms, and also as a conglomerate, relatively complex animal
organism with distinct structure, specialized components, and
locomotive movement. The most evident difference is size, but
there would also appear to be some differences in transitions
between sub-celled and cellular "organisms" and between single-
celled and multi-celled ones. The apparent similarity is none-
the-less striking. What seems particularly relevant is Dr.
Rosenow's assertion that the polio-related streptococcus with
which he dealt could be grown in large or small forms depending
on the culture media. This would indicate that all the
components necessary for complete replication of the larger form
exists in the smaller one, and raises two interesting
possibilities:

(1) that the "virus", at least in some cases, is the actual
lowest form of life, and not the bacterial cell;

(2) that other viruses may also have conglomerate forms
analogous to Rosenow's polio creatures, which conglomerate forms
may now be thought of as secondary invaders.

ON THE REPRODUCTION OF VIRUSES - THE LONG WAY

O.K., if the filter-passing phase of an organism is synonymous
with a virus, if the larger phase is synonymous with a bacteria
or streptococcus or perhaps even staphylococcus (to each his or
her own); and if in the latter cases replication can be observed,
then replication on the viral level would not even be necessary;
or vice-versa, and continually-generated supplies of one or the
other could flow into the medium favorable to the other and be
transformed. Thus there would be no need for viral-infected
cells to act as "virus factories" as is so often pictured - busy
little factories enslaved by some whip-cracking hateful fiendish
little scraps of molecules - evil acids. Maybe that is the way
it is. Maybe both phases replicate.

Note how Tulasne's 1949 diagram of dissociation (discussed
below) could be interpreted as comprising a viral factory.

MEDLINE ON L-FORMS, VARIATION, DISSOCIATION 1977-1994

A scan of citations derived in MEDLINE with keyword "L-form" discloses that L-forms are being implicated in the current literature in a number of conditions, e.g., secretory otitis media, idiopathic hematuria, tuberculosis, lymphadenitis, staphylococcic sepsis, burn wound infection, in bone marrow, and in diseases in fish and pigeons.[MEDLINE: kw L-forms bacteria]

For the period 1990-1994, MEDLINE lists 71 items on the "subject" of "l-forms"; 2001 items with "l-forms" as a "keyword" and 202 items with "l-forms of bacteria" as "keyword". These include reference to the possible role of oral foci as a reservoir for systemic disease; e.g., Avdonina LI, et al.., 1992 noted that "The regularities of the pathologic process development in periodontal tissues of subjects without tuberculosis were found to fully conform to the current concept of a latent tuberculous infection. The periodontal foci of infection may be regarded as reservoirs of persistent mycobacteria, whose main form, L variant, was detected in 71.68 % of cases."

APPENDIX C1:   DISSOCIATION CHRONOLOGY

EVERYTHING OLD IS NEW AGAIN

This chronology incorporates key early works on the subject of
dissociation, plus selected items (1977-1994) accessed through
MEDLINE on the subjects of "L-forms", bacterial variation, and
microbial dissociation.

DISSOCIATION: NO BIG THING! Hadley 1927
For a comprehensive discussion of the immense body of work on
(horizontal and vertical) transmutations prior to 1927, including
investigators prior to the last turn of centuries, see Hadley,
Phillip: Microbic dissociation; the instability of bacterial species
with special reference to active dissociation and transmissible
autolysis. J. Infect. Dis. 40:1-312, 1927.

Hadley, p. 5, discussed in detail "an ever-increasing mass of
evidence pointing to the instability of bacterial species [which]
... may have a more significant bearing on problems of virulence,
infection and immunity than many have supposed."
In reaction to the advocacy of extreme variability by Nägeli in
1877, Hadley contrasts Cohn's "equal vehemence on the conservatism
of bacterial types", which position was joined by Robert Koch and
his disciples who "succeeded in forcing upon the bacteriological
world a saner - perchance too sane - view definitely opposed to that
of Nägeli and his colleagues. ... . the Cohn views gradually became
established as a sort of dogma...". [p.8]
Hadley laments that "The dogma of the absolute constancy of
specific bacterial types was strongly entrenched." [p. 9]
"What is 'the normal' bacterial type? .. is there such a thing
...? I believe that a careful consideration of the data assembled in
the preceding pages tends to establish the view that 'normal
culture' or 'normal type' in the absolute meaning of these terms and
as commonly employed, is something of a myth. ... Shall we regard as
'normal' the disease form, the convalescent form or the old
laboratory form? Also what shall we say regarding the intermediates
and the filtrable forms? ... bacteriologists for the most part have
been chiefly interested in their culture tube collections. It is
these organisms - often tame, domesticated things - that have been
set up as 'types' and as standards of normality. It would seem to
me much more accurate ... to regard a culture as normal relative to
a given condition of environment... ."[286]
Hadley cites "evidence that microbic dissociation, as an adaptive
reaction, stands in close relation to a type of reproduction about
which we as yet know little." [p. 288]
"... it is becoming increasingly clear that we shall never know
what a bacterial species really is until we acquaint ourselves with
the outermost limits of its variability ... ."
"The truth we shall eventually come to .. is that the free-living
microorganism is potentially a kaleidoscopic thing, in which the
power of responding successfully to a changing environment by
alterations in the body state, both morphologic and biochemical -
and even by self-destruction, if need be, in order to generate
another and more stable type - stands as its one most important

attribute. ... [288-9]

"...most cultures, when first secured from their natural habitat
and placed upon the usual cultural mediums, possess great potential
variability. Each apparent species is surrounded by its small group
of satellites to each of which we unwisely attempt to assign a
classificatory niche." Hadley suggests we concentrate not on
methods of classification but rather "on the one thing that is most
essential - the problem of the nature and origin of variations. ...
there is no class of organisms more favorable than bacteria for
studying the possible influence of environment in determining the
trend of hereditary variation." [p.290]

"...it may eventually be demonstrated, not that a foreign
filtrable virus gives rise to dissociation and to autolysis in the
d'Herelle sense; but on the contrary, that the fundamental
physiologic reaction, of which both microbic dissociation and
transmissible autolysis are only different modes of expression,
gives rise to the filtrable virus." [p.296]

NOW YOU SEE IT ... VIRUS OR BACTERIA? Kendall 1931

The essential distinction between what we commonly perceive of as
viral and bacterial forms may simply be phasal. As Kendall stated
in 1931 in Science magazine, "It is postulated that a majority, if
not all, known bacteria can and do exist in a filterable and in a
non-filterable state." [p. 139]

"The belief that bacteria may have a filterable state is a very
old one." Kendall goes on to list types: B. typhosus, coccus from
influenzal cases, Rosenow's poliomyelitis streptococcus, Dochez's
scarlet fever streptococcus, B. paratyphosus alpha, Noguchi's
leptospira icteroides, Staphylococcus aureus, B. typhosus and coccus
from the "flu" cases, have thus been ... made filtrable, filtered
and recovered."

"... both staphylococcus 'phage' filtrates, and Bedreska
'staphylococcus antivirus" have yielded perfectly typical cultures
of Staphylococcus aureus upon cultivation in the proper manner."
[p.134]

"... bacteria within the intestinal canal are in an environment
that should encourage their continued existence in the non-
filterable state. Rather the contrary condition would appear to
prevail in the respiratory tract." [p.137]

"the problem of immunity, in light of these observations, takes on
a new aspect. On the one hand, the beneficial effects reported
during the use of phage and Bedreska Antivirus for therapeutic
purposes would seem to be related, not to enzymes or toxins, but
rather to the presence of viable, filterable stages of bacteria,
although, of course, enzymatic and toxic effects are not disproven
by any means." [p.138]

[In suggesting that the beneficial action of a suspected antitoxin
may actually be that of an antibacterial vaccine (filterable stage
of the bacteria), Kendall allows for the removal of the only
exception that Wright had possibly allowed for the action of serum
therapy to be other than that of vaccine therapy!]

In this article, Kendall described his so-named "K-medium": small
intestine (of man, swine, dog or rabbit) "thoroughly extracted with
alcohol to remove water and alcohol soluble extractives, followed by

extraction with benzol to remove excess of lipoidal substances.
This residue, dried, can be kept indefinitely. The addition of
Tyrode solution, or even normal saline to this powdered extract
substance, makes a rather turbid medium which can be autoclaved
without apparent harm." [The reader is kindly referred to Kendall
1931 for further instruction.]

   Kendall attested to the sterility of his media: "Mediums used for
cultivation were autoclaved at fifteen pounds steam-pressure for
twenty minutes. Therefore they were initially sterile."

   And he asserted the reversibility of the process: "... the
filterable state is readily induced by inoculation of the cocci in
the special medium. the converse process, transformation of the
filterable to the not-filterable state, is a relatively slow
procedure. It can be done, however, by inoculation of K medium
growth upon intestine-proteose-peptone-agar, possibly better upon
blood agar and usually, except for vary fastidious microbes, as will
appear later, upon plain agar." [p.133]

   VIRUS AS PHASE McKinney 1937

   McKinney 1937 [McKinney HH, J. Heredity 28 (1937), 51-57, "Virus
Mutation and the Gene Concept"] p. 56
   "In view of the evidence that active virus is not a constituent of
normal susceptible tobacco plants, that the virus regenerates true
to a measurable type, that it mutates, that the mutants and
submutants also regenerate true to their respective types and
manifest more or less orderly relationships to each other, it is
difficult to believe that the primary virus and its many strains
represent closely related enzymes of the ordinary sorts. ...
   "It is possible that virus generation involves some unique system
of precursors. However, the evidence now available tends to favor
the view that the virus and its mutants embrace the essential
elements of lineage or inheritance. This view is based on the
evidence that the virus, its mutants and sub-mutants, regenerate
true to measurable types and because the mutants and sub-mutants
tend to retain certain characters of the strains from which derived.
  It would seem that these combined features and not Mendelian
segregation must serve as the basic test for inheritance, otherwise
we would be forced to take the absurd position that inheritance does
not exist in the bacteria and other asexual organisms.
   "It is possible that the virus represents a filterable form of
some larger organism, or it may represent a degenerated organism
which has retrogressed by a series of mutations to a stage where a
few genes or perhaps a single gene remains to perpetrate as a virus.
  However, it does not seem necessary to assume that the virus
represents a stage in a degeneration process, since it may represent
a stage in a progressively complex evolutionary development from
molecules, and it may possess a simple metabolism. In any case, the
primary virus and its mutants doubtless reflect a series of closely
related compounds which function essentially as genes. The several
characters of a given virus may reflect properties of a single
compound and changes in any of these characters - mutations - may
reflect changes in this compound."

PLEURO-PNEUMONIA/POLIO: GLOBOID, SMALL; VIRUS? Britannica 1944

<u>Encyclopedia Britannica</u>, Vol. 9, 1944, p. 239, "Filter-passing viruses": Filtrable viruses "appear to be of various natures, and the only property common to them is minuteness. ... Those occasioning bovine pleuro-pneumonia and human poliomyelitis are globoid in shape and just on the margin of visibility with the best microscopes. ... In some cases, small bodies of definite size, shape and staining characteristics are always to be seen in the cells at the seat of the lesion. Whether these represent the microbe or granules in the cell contents** (check word) produced under the influence of the virus is a matter of opinion."

NATURE OF DISSOCIATION TO FILTRABLE FORMS Tulasne 1949

PLEURO-PNEUMONIA-LIKE FORMS PRODUCT OF REVERSIBLE DISSOCIATION
  Tulasne R [<u>Nature</u> 164 (Nov. 19, 1949), "Existence of L-Forms in Common Bacteria and their Possible Importance"] discusses the dissociation of Proteus vulgaris in the presence of high concentration of penicillin into "pleuropneumonia-like", "dwarf, submicroscopical, 'filtrable' forms", "easily identified ... as colonies of the type L" and shown by ultramicroscopical and histochemical study to comprise "desoxyribonucleic granulations ... having the aspect and the dimensions of a normal Proteus 'nucleus' (about 0.2-0.3u). ... In the case of a transfer to a medium without penicillin, quite normal Proteus cells soon appear, each of which seems to originate from one of the pleuropneumonia-like bodies." ...

Figure C1: Reversible dissociation of Proteus (R.Tulasne, NATURE 164, 19 Nov. 1949).

· Hence a bacterium as common as *Proteus* gives, under the action of penicillin, dwarf, submicroscopical, 'filtrable' forms with possible reversion from the dwarf to the normal form (see diagram).

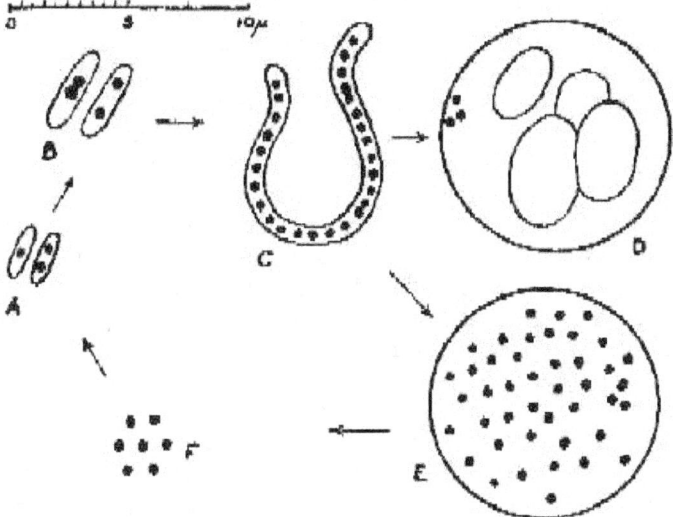

A, Normal *Proteus* cells, resting phase ; *B*, normal *Proteus* cells, lag phase ; *C*, swarming filament ; *D*, large body in lysis ; *E*, large body with desoxyribonucleical granulations ; *F*, pleuropneumonia-like body (desoxyribonucleical granulations)

Observations concerning such transformations ... are not exceptional"; probably in the near future they will become very common." Tulasne goes on to cite reports of such transformations in cultures of Streptobacillus moniliformis; Bacteroides sp., spontaneously or under penicillin action, with possible reversion to "normal" form; some Gram-negative and Gram positive sporulated bacteria; typhoid bacilli; Pasteurella pestis and Salmonella enterididis. "... Thus it seems to be clear that the appearance of such submicroscopical forms is a general phenomenon ... .

"We are of opinion that these submicroscopical forms of bacteria may be considered as normal resistance forms which the micro-organisms adopt against various noxious agents. They are selected by those agents but not produced by them. They are formed by bacteria which are nearly reduced to nuclei.

"The existence of such submicroscopical, filtrable forms of bacteria may have great importance for the pathology of infection. It is probable that they can be selected under various influences or appear spontaneously 'in vivo', and it is quite possible that their pathological potentialities are different from those of corresponding visible forms. Indeed it may be that the whole problem of the 'filtrable forms' of bacteria (especially those of Mycobacterium tuberculosis and of Treponema pallidum) should be entirely re-investigated. This may well lead to the solution of some outstanding general problems of pathology and epidemiology".

In 1951 Dr. Rosenow investigated the ineffectiveness of penicillin in an epidemic of influenza. [51R4] We are referred to the works of Tulasne who demonstrated that the action of penicillin in the case of Proteus was not destructive but rather dissociative and reversible.

HISTORY OF L-FORMS, 1935-1951 Dienes & Weinberger 1951

Louis Dienes and Howard J. Weinberger, Bacteriological Reviews 15 (1951), "The L Forms of Bacteria", 245-288
p. 245 "In 1935 Klieneberger isolated from cultures of Streptobacillus moniliformis a strange organism which she designated as L1. This organism differed in many respects from bacteria and resembled the organisms of bovine pleuropneumonia. ... " The authors relate that all investigators including Klieneberger have now concluded that L1 "was a growth form of the bacillus. ... Apparently the bacteria undergo a strange transformation in response to various influences, and they survive and multiply as tiny soft forms often unrecognizable with the usual bacteriological methods. The study of these forms is in a preliminary stage and their significance in the life and activity of bacteria is not known. ...
p. 250, notes that Heilman and others were able to regain the bacilli after making transfers from single L1 colonies, demonstrating clearly that the bacilli grow from L forms. Heilman also studied growth requirements, finding that "The bacillus grew on certain media in the absence of native animal proteins. The L1 grew only if such proteins were present." [Might this logically have potential implications for "in vivo" growth? ... also below]
[It is noted that Heilman co-authored 5 articles with Rosenow between 1934-1939, two on myasthenia gravis; and that this was

essential formative work preceding his herein identification with L-forms; the clear implication is that Rosenow's work was involved with L-forms - but too early.]

The authors note "Strains isolated from pathological processes are usually highly pleomorphic [with a greater tendency to produce L1 colonies], while strains isolated from the pharynx of rats are often only slightly pleomorphic and produce few L1 colonies.

PENICILLIN "The bacillus is very sensitive to penicillin; the growth of some strains is inhibited by the presence of 0.02 unit per ml of the medium. L1 grows even in the presence of 10,000 units of penicillin per ml., and strains of L1 occurring spontaneously in a culture are just as resistant as those developing in the presence of penicillin."

p. 251, in the case of <u>Bacteroides</u>, the authors note "Both the bacillary and the L forms of <u>Bacteroides</u> grow only under anaerobic conditions and the L forms only in the presence of animal serum."

p. 262, is noted "After the discovery of the L1, the next L type culture observed was obtained by Dienes from a bacillus cultivated from a human dog-bite wound."

p. 265, "... it is of interest that the initial stages of [L-form] development were observed in several genera and families. Thus, this ability to transform into such forms may well be a general property of bacteria."

p. 269, "It is apparent that the small forms are reproductive [and] that they multiply by division like bacteria. ... Dienes impression is that the small forms are often elongated and distinctly bacillary. They may grow into short curved filaments and sometimes have the appearance of tiny bipolar stained bacilli.

"The small forms gradually swell into the large forms and in most cultures the majority of the organisms are in various stages of this process. ... All transitional forms present from the smallest to the largest in cultures and organisms of varying size may be seen in short chains."

[Note similarity to Rosenow 1916 (16R4, 1203), "In all the liquid mediums during the early days of growth, chains are often found in which there are single members of all sizes and shapes - large diplococci, large coccus forms, small diplococci and small coccus forms."]

p. 272, "The change of structure [to L-forms] and slowing down of the metabolism may secure the survival of the bacteria in conditions in which the usual bacterial form cannot survive."

272-3, "Although the rigid bacterial membrane is lacking in the pleuropneumonia-like organisms and L forms, a definite cell boundary is clearly seen in stained preparations and with electron microscope, both in the small organisms and the large bodies. The boundary between the individual organisms inside the large bodies, regardless of whether they develop into bacilli or into L forms, only becomes visible when the smaller forms have segmented from each other. The L forms once separated do not coalesce with each other to form larger ones. The large body is derived from a single small organism which probably undergoes multiplication remaining inside of a common envelope.

p. 276, "Pleuropneumonia-like organisms cultivated from urinary infections often are indistinguishable morphologically from L type cultures. ..."

[L forms] belong to the smallest living forms capable of independent life."
  p. 283, "... it is difficult to believe that the similarities between the L type cultures and the pleuropneumonia organisms extending to so many points are accidental. These characteristics represent a simplification of the bacterial structure, and when bacteria are transformed into L forms, they assume these properties.
  It is very likely that the origin of a similar complex group of properties is the same in the pleuropneumonia group. This group probably descended at some time from the bacteria and became stabilized to live in this form. If this supposition is correct ... the pleuropneumonia group ... represents a growth form which various bacteria can take up. ...
  "The speculations just discussed suggest further speculations concerning the development of the viruses. Two aspects of the problem should be distinguished. One is the phylogenetic development of the viruses developed from other microorganisms by gradual loss of properties as a consequence of parasitism. The discovery of the L forms and their properties gives support to this idea. The other aspect of the question is whether viruses develop from bacteria at the present time. The observations made thus far with the L forms offer no evidence for this supposition. We have no information on the role of L forms in the pathogenic action of bacteria. Well-controlled, positive observations on this point would be of great interest. Until they are made, speculations have little value.
  "It is outside the scope of this review to discuss the possible relationship of the L forms to the so-called filtrable forms of bacteria, to bacterial gonidia and to various pleomorphic forms described in the literature. Klieneberger suggested in a recent paper [Klieneberger-Nobel, E., 1951, "Filterable forms of bacteria.", Bact. Rev. 15, 77-103] that some of these are probably analogous to the L forms. She feels especially justified to identify the filtrable G forms of Hadley [Hadley P, Delves E and Klimek, J, 1931, "The filterable forms of bacteria: I. A filterable stage in the life history of the Shiga dysentery bacillus. J Infect Dis., 48, 1-159] with the L forms, and she regards the discovery of the latter as confirmation of the older observations. The reviewers do not agree with Klieneberger's conclusions. ... Unless a technic is devised by which the filtrable forms can be produced regularly so that their properties may be studied, their very existence remains questionable."

PLEURO-PNEUMONIA AGENT AS SMALLEST BACTERIA De Robertis 1970

De Robertis EDP, Nowinski WW, and Saez FA, CELL BIOLOGY, Fifth Edition, W.P. Saunders, Philadelphia 1970, p. 9: "Among agents that have the smallest living mass, the best suited for study are microbes of the so-called pleuro-pneumonia group (PPLO) ... . These agents range in diameter from 0.25u (the limit of resolution of the optical microscope) to 0.1 u; thus their size corresponds to that of some of the large viruses."

DISSOCIATION - TOO COMMON TO BE MUTATION DeLong 1977
DISSOCIATION AS FORM OF REPRODUCTION DeLong 1977

De Long, R. [J. theor. Biol. (1977) 64, 761-764, "On Bacterial Dissociation"]: "One of the most common phenomena found among bacteria is dissociation... .

"Bacterial dissociation is characterized by many changes occurring in a population simultaneously. These changes are readily reversible. The changes occur in the absence of any known mutagens. Dissociated bacteria have been designated as smooth (S) and rough (R) forms depending on their colonial morphology. Some of the simultaneous, associated changes occurring along with colonial morphology are as follows: (1) cellular morphology, (2) antigenicity, (3) synthesis, (4) virulence and (5) cellular division. The percentage of bacteria in a population manifesting such changes is large. Populations of bacteria shift from S to R and R to S quite readily along with the associated changes and at high percentages (50% to 100% is not uncommon)."

De Long argues that the frequency of dissociation is far too great to be explained by the hypothesis of mutation, and that "the back mutational rate's frequency makes the mutational hypothesis seem almost ludicrous". DeLong calculates that the probability of both direct and reverse mutation occurring would be less than 1 x 10 (-16), and thus that dissociation relates to a "more encompassing mechanism". The author suggests dissociation may relate to bacterial reproduction, and points out that "Such characteristics as virulence, antigens, syntheses and diagnoses are dependent on whether the bacteria are of the S form or the R form."

De Long's assertion that the frequency of dissociation requires classification other than as a type of mutation finds support in Schrödinger's What is Life?, where it is maintained that mutations must be rare.

BACTERIAL L-FORMS - "IRRESISTABLE ... BEAUTIFUL" Madoff 1986

Madoff, Sarabelle, ed., The Bacterial L-Forms, Marcel Dekker, Inc., N.Y. and Basel, 1986
Lewis Thomas, in the Forward, declares: "L-forms are charming creatures ... absolutely irresistible. They are ... beautiful, nothing less. ... There is a shared hunch that they may turn out to be significant pathogens in certain chronic human diseases, perhaps including genitourinary disorders, even rheumatoid arthritis (my own hunch)."
p. 2, Madoff cites the mid-1930s work of Klieneberger and Dienes as having "ushered in a new era in the world of microbiology" after the former isolated pleuropneumonia-like organisms from a culture of streptobacillus moniliformis. Dienes demonstrated their reversion to the bacillary form [termed "revertant bacteria"] and also "established that bacteria could continue to multiply in the absence of their rigid cell wall". Madoff provides a listing of some 24 bacterial genera from which L-forms have been derived, illustrating that this quality is quite general: Agrobacterium, Bacillus, Bacteriodes, Bartonella, Bordetella, Brucella, Clostidium, Corynebacterium, Erysipelothrix, Escherichia, Flavobacterium, Haemophilus, Listeria, Neisseria, Proteus, Pseudomonas, Salmonella, Sarcina, Serratia, Shigella, Staphylococcus, Streptobacillus, Streptococcus, Vibrio.

Madoff offers that "L-forms probably represent a polygot mixture of considerable variability." As for the induction of L-forms, "The penicillins are the most effective inducing agents. Other antibiotics that interfere with cell-wall synthesis ... have also been used." It is noted that some species "require increased osmotic protection for L-form growth." Among other agents, the combination of sucrose and sodium chloride has been reported to be successful. [This is noted in possible relation to Dr. Rosenow's work with dextrose in culture media, and sodium chloride in storage menstruum.

As for size, the author notes "Although 'elementary bodies' as small as 200-300 nm are seen, the size of the smallest units capable of cell division remains uncertain. Mechanisms of cell replication, as in mycoplasma, appear to vary from binary or asymmetric division to budding or segmentation of the small dense bodies from large spherical forms. ... In summary, L-form processes indicate that if there are orderly mechanisms in the life cycle of L-forms they are not entirely clear. It is not yet known how the genome segregates in the formation of the new and viable L-form elements."

ROLE OF TEMPERATE PHAGE IN BACTERIAL DISSOCIATION Mil'ko 1986

Mil'ko & Egorov [ibid, 1986(4):6-19, "Role of temperate phage in bacterial dissociation"]; Medline abstract: "... dissociants may appear in bacteria population from spontaneous mutations and transfer of genetic material (conjugation, transformation, transduction). ... The role of temperate phage has been shown in splitting of bacteria into variants in the genera Mycobacterium, Corynebacterium, some Bacillus, Clostridium, Staphylococcus, some enterobacteria, Yersinia, Vibrio Pseudomonas, Rhizobium, Nostoc..."

LARGE QUANTITIES OF VIRUSES IN NATURAL WATER Bergh et al. 1989

1989 Bergh et al. 1989, per Sherr 1989, found 3 to 7 orders of magnitude more femtoplankton (viruses of <0.2 um in size) in natural waters than expected. Bergh et al. referred to these as bacteriophages. As per other items in this section, it might be suggested that these may be viral analogs to larger identifiable bacterial types, rather than "bacteriophages".

MOLLICUTES VARY WITH ENVIRONMENT CHANGE Rosengarten 1990

Rosengarten R and Wise KS [Science, 1990 Jan 19, 247(4940):315-8, "Phenotypic switching in mycoplasmas: phase variation of diverse surface lipoproteins"]
Medline abstract: "The ability of some microorganisms to rapidly alter the expression and structure of surface components reflects an important strategy for adaptation to changing environments, including those encountered by infectious agents within respective host organisms. Mycoplasma hyorhinis, a wall-less prokaryotic pathogen of the class Mollicutes) is shown to undergo high-frequency phase transitions in colony morphology, opacity, and expression of cell-surface-protein-antigens which spontaneously vary in size ...".
 This is seen as "part of a complex system that controls interactions of these organisms with their hosts."

VARIABILITY IS INHERENT, COMMON, REVERSIBLE Pavlova 1990

   Pavolva IB, et al. [Zhurnal Mikrobiologii, Epidemiologii i
Immunobiologii, 1990 Dec.(12):12-5], present an electron microscopy
study of bacterial development, asserting that "heteromorphous
growth of cells is inherent in the normal cycle of development of
bacteria in the population and that this process is reversible. It
has certain regularities, common for different bacteria, in the
variability of the natural L-transformation of bacteria."

ENVIRONMENT/DISSOCIATION VARIANTS AND SURVIVAL Mil'ko 1992

   Mil'ko ES & Egorov NS [Biologicheskie Nauki, 1992(5):89-96, "The
effect of physicochemical environmental factors on the growth of
gram-positive bacterial dissociants"]; Medline abstract:
   "The growth of R- [rough], S-[smooth] and M (g)- dissociants of
Streptococcus lactis, Bacillus coagulans, Rhodococcus
rubropertinctus under the action of some physico-chemical factors:
temperature, pH, ultraviolet (UV) rays, high concentration of NaCl
and storage have been compared. R-variants gain selective advantage
under the influence of UV-irradiation, high temperature and storage;
S-variants-- at decreasing of active pH of medium; M (g)-variants --
at decreasing of growth temperature, high values of pH, increased
NaCl concentration. The dissociation has been concluded to enlarge
the limits of the species survival."

MOLLICUTES ARE TRUE EUBACTERIA Bove 1993
   Bove JM [Clin. Infect. Dis., 1993 Aug, 17 Suppl 1:S10-31,
"Molecular features of mollicutes"] states "It is now firmly
established that the mollicutes are true eubacteria. They have
evolved regressively (i.e. by genome reduction) from gram-positive
bacterial ancestors ... specifically, from certain clostridia. Many
of their properties, such as small genome size, small number of rRNA
operons and tRNA genes, lack of a cell wall, fastidious growth, and
limited metabolic activities, are seen as the result of this
evolution. Other properties, such as the anerobiosis of their
earliest evolving members ... have been inherited from their
eubacterial ancestors. However the mollicutes are not simply wall-
less gram-positive bacteria. They have properties of their own. ...
[including] peculiar systems for pathogenicity, cell adhesion,
antigenic variation ..."

DISSOCIATION AND THE ROLE OF ENDOTOXIN Hurley 1993
   Hurley JC [Lancet, 1993 May 1, 341(8853):1133-5, "Reappraisal of
the role of endotoxin in the sepsis syndrome", discusses evidence
that release of endotoxin from gram negative bacteria "is not
directly responsible for complications of sepsis syndrome", but
"rather ... is a marker for transition of gram-negative organisms to
cell-wall-deficient forms (L-forms) that may persist undetected
despite antibiotic therapy directed against the parental form. This
transition has two consequences in compromised patients: L-forms
cause organ failure and the serve as a sanctuary from which cell-
wall-intact revertants may arise."

CELL WALL DEFICIENT FORMS - STEALTH PATHOGENS Mattman 1993
   L. H. Mattman, Cell Wall Deficient Forms - Stealth Pathogens, CRC
Press, Boca Raton Fla. 1993
   Mattman's "dual thrust" is "to describe the unrecognized
omnipresent role of wall-deficient-organisms..." and "to note that
the majority of unexplained negative cultures concern infection with
these variants." The author notes that shapes "are almost endlessly
variegated: and that "Binary fission ceases; budding is one of the
common forms of reproduction. ...These variants are critically
important in septicemia, menengitis, urinary tract infection, heart
valve infection, arthrides, blinding ocular inflammation, and a host
of other maladies."
   p. 123 The author relates that "L-Forms circulating in the blood
were demonstrated in several general classes of thromboembolic
disease", with specific mention of post-operative pulmonary emboli,
thrombophlebitis and blood clots. It is noted that "Altemeier
noticed that Enovid (Norethnodrel and Mestranol) is a growth factor
for certain wall-deficient bacteria. Thus an explanation exists for
thrombi which have been reported in relatively young women taken
birth control pills."
   p. 166 The author notes that presumed causative agents for
arthritis were cultured as early as 1893 and "observed in direct
stains and cultures in 1896"; that streptococci produce rodent
arthritis, and "that both L-Forms and parent Group A streptococci
produce rodent arthritis when injected intraarticularly into
rabbits."
   p. 209, notes that in the 1920s Kendall [JAMA 99,(1932) 67-69,
"Filtrable forms of bacteria and their significance"] had "found
that filtrable units of the Staphylococcus, Streptococcus and
Salmonella typhi could be coaxed back to their parent forms. ...
Although William H. Welch regarded Kendall's work as a distinct
advance, great skepticism was expressed by most microbiologists.
Unfortunately, this was just prior to the demonstration by
Klieneberger and by Dienes that filtrable organisms could be grown
on solid medium and their sequential reversion steps followed."
   The work of P. Hadley and co-workers, with filtrable units of
Shigella shiga, and works of F.R. Heilman of Mayo is also noted.
Heilman had co-authored five articles between 1934 and 1939 with
E.C. Rosenow, and the cited Hadley work refers to a 1917 Rosenow
article [Rosenow and Towne, J.M. Res. 36, 175]

SIZE, VIRULENCE CHANGES FROM NASOPHARYNX TO BLOOD Weiser 1993
   Weiser JN, et al. [J. Infect. Dis., 1993 Sep, 168(3);672-80,
"Relationship between colony morphology and the life cycle of
Haemophilus influenzae: the contribution of lipopolysaccharide phase
variation to pathogenesis"] discusses variants with
lipopolysacchaide (LPS) of differing molecular weights, appearance
either transparent (heavier LPS) or opaque (lighter LPS),
colonization abilities and virulence.
   "Colonies of Haemophilus influenzae are heterogenous in appearance
because of phase variation in opacity. ... The more transparent
variants expressing a higher-molecular-weight LPS were serum
sensitive and could efficiently colonize the infant rat nasopharynx
after intranasal inoculation. In contrast, the fully opaque variant
expressing a smaller-molecular-weight LPS was serum resistant,

unable to colonize the nasopharynx, and more virulent when
intraperitoneally administered. Organisms disseminating into the
blood-stream from the nasopharynx changed phenotype from transparent
to opaque. ..."

PHASE VARIATION, INTERACTION WITH PNEUMOCOCCUS Weiser 1994
  Weiser JN, et al. [Infection and Immunity, 1994 Jun, 62(6):2582-9,
"Phase variation in pneumococcal opacity: relationship between
colonial morphology and nasopharyngeal colonization."] relates that
electron microscopy "suggests that autolysis occurs earlier in the
growth of the transparent variant". The authors note an apparent
"selective advantage" for this variant in its "efficient and stable
colonization" of the nasopharynx; and conclude "that phase variation
which is marked by differences in colonial morphology may provide
insight into the interaction of the pneumococcus with its host.

APPENDIX C2: MUTATION CHRONOLOGY

   THE THING IS WITH US: TRANSMUTATION IMPLICATION

   In that Hadley, Rosenow and others including Landsteiner have
demonstrated or discussed transformations from one bacterial or
viral species to another, e.g. from pneumococcus to streptococcus,
etc.; and further in that the work of Kendall, Hadley, Rosenow and
others has demonstrated that each species may possess various phases
from filtrable to bacterial, etc.; one may readily speculate that
many of the various forms and sizes of pathogenic organisms resident
in man may be mutations of a single organism (bacteria,
streptococci, pneumococci, viruses, etc.) - a continually mutating,
pervasive, ever-present shadow of the living being. THE THING IS
WITH US.

   1894 - SMITH ON MODIFICATIONS IN MIXED CULTURES [Smith, Theobald,
Assn. American Physicians, Transactions ix (1894) 85-89,
"Modifications, Temporary and Permanent, of the Physiological
Characters of Bacteria in Mixed Cultures."]

VARIABILITY AS FACTOR IN EPIDEMICS, INFECTIOUS DISEASES
   "The variability of pathogenic bacteria is a most suggestive
subject when brought together with the phenomena presented by the
transmission of infectious diseases and the rise and decline of
epidemics. ..."

VARIABILITY, TRANSMUTABILITY AND HISTORY OF MICROBIOLOGY
   "To trace the development of ideas concerning the variability and
transmutability of bacteria would be equivalent to writing a fairly
complete history of microbiology. I must therefore content myself
with the bare mention of the more recent methods used to produce
varieties before entering upon the more restricted theme of this
paper. These methods consist in the passage of bacteria through a
series of animals (Coze and Feltz, DaVaine, Pasteur and his pupils),
exposure to heat (Pasteur), to compressed air and oxygen (Chauveau),
to chemicals of various kinds (Chamberland and Roux, Troje), to
sunlight (Laurent), and the fluids of the living animal
(Gramatschikoff). In 1891 I quite accidentally discovered that
certain pathogenic bacteria which had resisted tenaciously the
modifying influence of several of the methods just cited were
markedly changed in impure or mixed cultures." [p. 85]

MIXED CULTURES AND VIRULENCE
   "... cultures of Hog cholera which had become attenuated,
presumably due to their existence in mixed culture with Proteus
vulgaris, did after time enjoy a recuperation of virulence.
Originally cultivated in March-April, 1891, they were found
attenuated by Dec. 1891 and used as vaccines for immunization until
October 1892 when recuperation of virulence had taken place."[p.93]
   Smith refers to the 1885 works of Gustav Hauser on 3 species of
the bacteria genus Proteus, who noted a swarming on 5% gelatin which
produced "multitudinous forms of growth" [p. 94]: "Hauser's work
naturally raised a number of questions, since the great range of
forms found in the culture, including cocci, bacilli, spirilla, and

sprulina, seemed to call forth once more the much debated, but now apparently dead, issue of variability of the morphological characters of bacteria." Hauser had noted (after 60 transfers to fresh media over a years period) a striking change from one form which had not liquified gelatin to a form which did, and the simultaneous disappearance of the non-liquidifying form.[p. 95]

"It is more than probable that we have to do here with a bacillus undergoing variation more promptly and transmitting such variations more readily than any other form hitherto carefully studied."[p.99]

Smith deduced from the above-referred attenuation and subsequent resurgence of virulence of hog-cholera bacilli that "bacteria may be influenced and modified when not actively multiplying."[p.101] He also reasoned that if Hog-cholera bacillus was changed when grown with Proteus, might not the nature of Proteus be changed to resemble hog cholera?[102]

IMMUNIZING, BACTERICIDE POTENCY OF BLOOD SERUM
"We have been impressed with the remarkable immunizing potency of the blood serum under certain conditions, and we have been surprised by its equally remarkable bactericide powers. Slowly we are coming to learn that the more subtle influence is exerted by biological, rather than by physical and chemical forces, and that in the action of like or related energies upon one another, the solution of many difficult problems in biology and medicine will be found."[p. 103]

A MISSED THEORY MAY BE MORE FRUITFUL THAN CRUDE EMPIRICISM
"I cannot refrain from agreeing with P. Ehrlich, however, when he states that progress in knowledge or insight can take place only from a theoretical point of view, and that even a missed theory may be more fruitful than crude empiricism which records the facts without even a crude attempt at interpretation."[p. 104]

MODIFICATION OF BACTERIA IN SOIL AND IN ANIMAL BODY
Smith discusses the intermingling and modification of bacteria both in the soil and in the human or animal body.

SELF-LIMITING NATURE OF DISEASE; SEASONALITY; MIXED CULTURES
Smith notes "If it is possible that bacteria may be modified when not actively multiplying, and if bacteria may acquire invasive properties in the soil ... it is not difficult to understand how epidemics and epizootics may appear and, after prevailing for a time, again disappear. The pathogenic powers temporarily acquired in the soil would be lost after a time in the human or animal body, and the resulting disease would thus be self-limited. ... If we assume the modification of bacteria by bacteria in the soil, the much-debated hypothesis of Pettenkoffer concerning the influence of season and locality on disease would perhaps appear to bacteriologists in a much more acceptable aspect."

This may "account for the occasional springing up of infectious diseases whose etiology is involved in obscurity, such as diarrhoeal and dysenteric diseases, or those whose appearance is governed by unknown factors, such as Asiatic cholera."

MIXED CULTURES AND PATHOLOGICAL INVESTIGATIONS
"In conclusion, I wish to call attention briefly to the possible

application of mixed cultures in the investigation of purely
pathological problems. ... Experiments in the hands of one may fail,
while in the hands of another they may succeed because a less
virulent race of bacteria has been used. ...

"To reduce or perhaps increase the virulence of bacteria in mixed
cultures will undoubtedly meet with many obstacles in practice ...
In any case prolonged cultivation may be necessary to induce
modification, and for this an extra supply of patience will be
useful in these days of hurried work and still more precipitate
publication."[p. 105]

1943 - LURIA'S "PECULIAR PHENOMENON" SUPPORTS HADLEY/ROSENOW

[Luria, SE, Delbrück M and Anderson TF, "Electron microscope
studies of bacterial viruses." J. Bact. 46:57-77, 1943.]

p. 57 "Ruska (1041) published micrographs of suspensions of
bacterial viruses, in which 'sperm-shaped' particles can be seen.
Ruska suggested that these particles should be interpreted either as
the virus itself or as bacterial constituents."

p. 58-9, authors discuss two viral strains "which are active on
the same host (Escherichia coli strain B)" and which "received
particular attention". Of these, one is noted to "present a very
peculiar aspect", that of being "quite variable. Four frequent
configurations can be described schematically as x-shaped, z-shaped,
inverted z-shaped, and diplococcus-shaped.

p. 62 "The use of two different and unrelated viruses acting on
the same host eliminates the possibility that the particles might be
natural protoplasmic components of the bacterium."

p. 65 "Finally, a point may be mentioned which seems to us
perhaps of the greatest consequence. We have seen that the new
virus is liberated from within the cell. On the other hand, the
pictures of bacteria infected with virus y and taken at fifteen
minutes showed that the adsorbed virus particles, or at least most
of them, do not penetrate into the interior of the cell but remain
on the outer surface of the cell wall. This observation creates a
difficulty in interpreting virus growth. ... The pictures here
reproduced, if interpreted on the assumption that one virus particle
enters the cell, would indicate that the entry of one virus particle
bars the entry of other virus particles by making the bacterial
cell-wall impermeable to them. The highly peculiar phenomenon of
mutual exclusion between virus particles attacking a cell would thus
be explained by a mechanism alternative to that proposed in a
previous discussion (Delbruck and Luria 1942). An interpretation of
this kind, for the correctness of which the experiments offer as yet
hardly more than a hint, would suggest an analogy with the
fecundation of monospermic eggs, and would lend support to those
theories of the systematic position of virus which consider it as
related to the host rather than as a parasite (cf. Hadley, 1928).
[Hadley, P., "The Twort-d'Herelle Phenomenon. A Critical Review and
Presentation of a New Conception (Homogamic Theory) of Bacteriophage
Action." J. Infectious Diseases 42, 263-434.]

It is noted that the Luria article ends here - leaving open the
question of whether the Hadley (and Rosenow) position may be the
correct one.

   1944 - AVERY ET AL. VERIFY MUTANT PNEUMOCOCCI   [Avery, OT, McLeod CM and McCarty M, "Studies on the chemical nature of the substance inducing transformation of pneumococcal types.", J. Exp. Med. 79:137-158, 1944]

   Avery et al. 1944 note "Among microörganisms the most striking example of inheritable and specific alterations in cell structure and function that can be experimentally induced and are reproducible under well defined and adequately controlled conditions is the transformation of specific types of Pneumococcus."
   The authors attribute the first description of this phenomenon to Griffith 1928 [Griffith H., J. Hyg., Cambridge, Eng., 1928, 27, 113.] No reference is made to the prior works of Rosenow on transmutations, nor is the methodology identical to that of Rosenow.
   The significance of inclusion of reference is the acceptance of the fact of mutability, which fact supports Rosenow's claim that such is possible and was accomplished more than a decade prior to Griffith's work, by Rosenow. (see above)

1945 LANDSTEINER ON THE BOUNDARY BETWEEN LIVING AND LIFELESS

   The renowned Karl Landsteiner in 1945 discussed transformations of bacterial types, including conversion of one type of pneumococcus into another in vivo by Griffith in 1928, and in vitro by Dawson and Sias in 1931; and "an apparently analogous transformation of a virus, namely the change of rabbit fibroma virus into that of myxamatosis has been described by Berry and Dedrick ..."
   "The biological significance of Griffith's phenomenon lies in the initiation by certain substances of inheritable changes in unicellular organisms so that there is reproduced indefinitely in subsequent generations the agent which induces the change, along with the type-specific polysaccharide, not previously present. This calls to mind the effects of plant viruses, bacteriophages and filtrable tumor agents. All these active principles are - under the control of living cells - endowed like genes with the capacity for causing the reproduction of their own kind, and have raised the fundamental issues regarding the boundary between living and lifeless matter." [p. 235-6]

1946 HERSHEY - MUTATIONS ARE A GENERAL BIOLOGICAL PHENOMENON

   [Hershey, AD, "Spontaneous Mutations in Bacterial Viruses", Cold Spring Habor Symp. Quant. Biol. 11:67-76]

   It is noted that Luria and Hershey are credited contemporarily with having discovered the mutability of viral forms, this in 1945. Thus through Hadley is established the link between contemporary perspectives on mutation and the early works of Hadley and Rosenow.

   p. 75, Hershey claims: "If it may be assumed that there is anything in common in the transformations of pneumococcal types [and various viral transformations including those] described in this paper, it now appears for the first time that a biological phenomenon of general importance is involved. ... In view of the generality of this phenomenon, it will be surprising not to find that some counterpart to it already exists among the more familiar genetic mechanisms."

1968 VARIATION: MORPHOLOGY/CULTURE/PHYSIOLOGY/COLONY/VIRULENCE
   Bryan AH, Bryan CA and Bryan CG, <u>Bacteriology</u>, 6th edition, Barnes and Noble, New York 1968, p. 22-24: "The amazing phenomena whereby bacteria may undergo changes in morphological, cultural, and physiological characteristics, in colony formation, and in virulence, etc., come under the heading of variation. ... Mutations or transmissible variations are apt to become permanent. They seem to arise suddenly and spontaneously. ... Temporary changes often occur in morphology or physiology, usually due to environmental conditions. ...
   "G colonies ... are minute colonies of very small cells varying greatly in morphology. They may revert to the larger colony forms. It has been suggested that these represent growth from minute filterable gonidia (intracellular granules). ... "

1991 TRANSFORMATION OF S.VIRIDANS INTO PNEUMOCOCCUS
   Chalkey L et al., "Relatedness between Streptococcus pneumoniae and viridans streptococci: transfer of penicillin resistance determinants and immunological similarities of penicillin-binding proteins.", <u>Fems Microbiology Letters</u>, 1991 Dec. 15, 69(1):35-42. This study "strongly suggested the presence of genes homologous to the pneumococcal PBP 1a and 2b genes in viridans streptococci, and documents that penicillin resistance determinants can be transformed from viridans streptococci into the pneumococcus."

1993 "VIABLE ANTIGENS IN CONSTANT TRANSMUTATION"
   Kaufmann SH, "Immunity to intracellular bacteria", <u>Annual Review of Immunology</u> 1993, 11:129-63, "Research on the immune response against intracellular bacteria not only helps us to better understand how the immune system deals with 'viable antigens' in constant trans-mutation, it also forms the basis for the rational design of control measures for major health problems."

1994 - CONFIRMATION OF ALTERED SPECIFICITY IN USUAL CULTURES
   Cvitkovitch DG and Hamilton IR, <u>Oral Microbiol. Immunol.</u>9:209-217, 1994 "Biochemical change exhibited by oral streptococci resulting from laboratory subculturing", has recently confirmed the difficulty/impossibility of preserving bacterial specificity with usual culture technique. In a study of 4 types of oral streptococci freshly isolated from dental plaque - Streptococcus mutans, S. Gordonii, S. mitis, and S. sanguis - the authors demonstrate how "continued laboratory subculturing of oral streptococci results in the selection of strains that possess different properties than those growing <u>in vivo</u> in dental plaque."

APPENDIX D: REPRINTS OF ARTICLES BY E.C. ROSENOW & B. RAPPAPORT

D1: Rosenow's landmark 1915 article, data from which was also featured in Frank Billings's 1915 Lane Lecture Series entitled "Focal Infection" and 1916 book of the same name:

> Rosenow, E.C., "Elective Localization of Streptococci", *The Journal of the American Medical Association*, Vol. LXV (65), No. 20, November 13, 1915, 1687-1691. Copyright 1915, American Medical Association. Reprinted with permission.

D2: Rappaport's report on the results of Rosenow's therapeutic vaccines following the onset of poliomyelitis, pus 100% success with prophylaxis in the studied population, incorporating case studies which must be termed "miraculous":

> Rappaport, Benjamin, "Further Observations on Acute Poliomyelitis Treated with Thermal Antibody", *Quarterly Bulletin, Northwestern University Medical School* 28, 1954, p. 57-60. Permission to reprint granted by Northwestern University Medical School.

D3: Rosenow's next-to-last published article, focusing on MS, with particular emphasis on proof of etiology and vaccine preparation details:

> Rosenow, E.C., "Studies on the Etiology and Specific Treatment of Multiple Sclerosis", *Ohio Medical Journal*, 53(7), July 1957, p. 783-5. Reprinted by permission of the *Ohio State Medical Journal*.

D4: E.C. Rosenow's last published article, comprising a concise summary of results of various diagnostic and clinical studies, including reference to a wide range of diseases including carcinoma:

> Rosenow, E.C., "Studies on Specific Prevention and Treatment of Diverse Diseases Shown Due to Specific Types of Nonhemolytic Streptococci", *American Practitioner and Digest of Treatment* (Philadelphia), 9(5), May 1958, pp. 755-761. [58R1] Reprinted by permission of *Clinical Pediatrics* (successor publication).

D5: *DENTAL CENTENARY CELEBRATION* -1940, reprinted by permission of *The Maryland State Dental Association*:

> Rosenow, E.C., Focal infection and elective localization in relation to systemic disease; review and results of further studies, Proceedings, Dental Centenary Celebration, Maryland State Dental Association, 1940, pp. 261-282, 1940.

APPENDIX D1:   *The Journal of the American Medical Association*, Vol. LXV, No. 20, November 13, 1915, 1687-1691.

ELECTIVE LOCALIZATION OF STREPTOCOCCI*

EDWARD C. ROSENOW, M.D.
ROCHESTER MINN.

The general systemic distribution of micro-organisms in certain diseases with a localized focus is well established, but the factors which determine the localization of bacteria after they gain entrance into the circulation are obscure.

In this paper I wish to record a summary of the results obtained from the intravenous injection, under a standard technic, of streptococci isolated from appendicitis, ulcer of the stomach and duodenum, cholecystitis, rheumatic fever, erythema nodosum, herpes zoster, epidemic parotitis, myositis and endocarditis, and to discuss the bearing of these results on localization of streptococci.

TECHNIC

The streptococci were usually grown from sixteen to twenty-four hours at 37 C. in tall columns of ascites (10 per cent) dextrose (0.2 per cent) broth)2.6+ to 0.8+) to which sterile tissue (guinea-pig kidney or heart muscle) was often added; the sterility of the ascites fluid and broth containing the tissue was always proved beforehand. After incubation smears were made, the cultures were centrifuged in the containers in which they were cultivated,[1] the supernatant fluid was decanted and the sediment suspended in sodium chloride solution so that 1 cc of the suspension contained the growth from 15 cc of broth. The doses for rabbits (ear vein) were usually from 0.5 to 3 cc and for dogs (leg vein) from 1 to 5 cc of this suspension. The injections were made quite rapidly through a rather fine needle (22 gage), usually within an hour after the suspension was made. Blood agar plate cultures were made at the time the suspensions were injected to study the character of the organisms, to test their viability and to save them from [for?] further study. This is an important precaution because negative results have at times proved to be due to early death of the recently isolated organisms in the broth cultures. In the accompanying table, "when isolated" indicates the first or second and, occasionally the third or fourth cultures, or the first culture after one animal passage. "Later" indicates that the strains were cultivated for a week or longer. "After animal passage" indicates usually from the second to the sixth animal passage.

The strains tested from appendicitis, ulcer of the stomach, cholecystitis, rheumatic fever, erythema nodosum, myositis and endocarditis include strains isolated from the characteristic lesions as well as from the apparent atrium of infection. Those from herpes zoster were from the tonsils and spinal fluid, and those from epidemic parotitis were obtained by catheterizing Steno's duct and from the tonsils. The strains from miscellaneous sources were usually from tonsils approaching the normal condition; and the laboratory strains were streptococci or pneumococci cultivated on artificial mediums for a long time and had lost all apparent virulence. The figures in the lowest line of the table represent the average percentage incidence of lesions in individual organs following injection of various strains of streptococci except those from the specific disease. Thus the first figure indicates that 5 per cent of the animals, injected with the various strains except those from appendicitis, showed lesions in the appendix.

Care was exercised to obtain growths from the depths of the supposed primary focus with as little contamination from the surface as possible, the cultures being made from the material expressed from the tonsils or from emulsion of extirpated tonsils after thorough washing in sodium chloride solution. The material from the depths of pyorrheal pockets was obtained by means of a pipet.

For the study of pathogenicity of the cultures, dogs and rabbits were chiefly used, being killed with chloroform at the desired time, usually in from twenty-four to forty-eight hours. Postmortem examinations were always made as soon after death as possible. A thorough inspection in a bright light with the unaided eye or with the aid of a hand lens was made for focal lesions. The exact character of the lesions and the presence of the streptococci in each of the various diseases have been determined by microscopic study of sections. Cloudy swelling is not included in the results given in the table. Hemorrhage, localized necrosis, exudation and infiltration were the usual lesions. Thus, in case of the joints, hemorrhage about the joint or turbidity of fluid, as determined with a pipet, or both, were considered as evidence of arthritis. Hemorrhages in the pericardium and turbidity of pericardial fluid, due to leukocytes, were considered as evidence of pericarditis. The postmortem study of animals often symptomless is essential to obtain accurate knowledge of the pathogenicity of a culture, and must supplant the older method of merely finding out whether a culture produces death or not, a method still too much in vogue. The table includes data only from those animals in which the postmortem was comprehensive, and does not include some of the earlier experiments, especially on endocarditis. [p.1688:] Increase in mortality rate, earlier death and greater degree and distribution of lesions following standard dosage were considered as proof of high virulence. Changes in the spleen and liver were so rare following injection of the strains as isolated, except those from cholecystitis, that they are not included in the table. Acute splenitis and such changes in the liver as focal necrosis, parenchymatous and bile duct hemorrhages and acute degeneration with marked acidity occurred, however, after the strains had acquired greater virulence from animal passage. In the earlier experiments not sufficient attention was paid to the occurrence of lesions in the thyroid, thymus, suprarenals and lymphatic glands. Later a closer search for lesions in these structures was made, especially after it was found that lesions in the thyroid followed intravenous injection of bacteria isolated from goiter. It must be said, too, that strains of streptococci from rheumatic fever, myositis and cholecystitis produce hemorrhages in the thyroid quite commonly, while those from other sources rarely produce them.

RESULTS

A study of the table shows that streptococci from the various
diseases often have a most striking affinity or tropism for the
organs or tissues from which they are isolated. Thus, fourteen
strains from appendicitis produced lesions in the appendix in 68 per
cent of the sixty-eight rabbits injected, which is in marked
contrast to an average of only 5 per cent (given in lowest line of
table) of lesions in the appendix in the animals injected with the
strains as isolated from sources other than appendicitis. Eighteen
strains from ulcer of the stomach or duodenum produced hemorrhages
in 60 per cent and ulcer of the stomach or duodenum in 60 per cent,
a combined total of 74 per cent of the 103 animals injected, in
contrast to an average of 20 per cent hemorrhages and 9 per cent
ulcer following injection of other strains. Twelve strains from
cholecystitis produced lesions in the gallbladder in 80 per cent of
the forty-one animals injected, in contrast to an average incidence
of lesions here of only 11 per cent with the other strains. Twenty-
four strains from rheumatic fever produced arthritis in 66 per cent,
endocarditis in 46 per cent, pericarditis in 27 per cent, and
myocarditis in 44 per cent of the seventy-one animals injected, in
contrast to an average of arthritis in 27 per cent, endocardial
lesions in 14 per cent of the animals injected with strains [p.
1689:] from sources other than rheumatic fever. Six strains from
erythema nodosum produced lesions of the skin in 90 per cent of
twenty animals injected, in contrast to an average of 2 per cent in
the animals injected with the strains from sources other than
erythema nodosum and herpes zoster. Eleven strains from herpes
zoster produced herpetiform lesions of the skin, lips, tongue or
conjunctivae in 77 per cent of the sixty-one animals injected, in
contrast to the average of only 1 per cent of what seemed to be
herpes of the skin with the other strains. Nine strains of
streptococcal organism from epidemic parotitis produced lesions in
one or both parotid glands in 73 per cent of the nineteen animals
injected intravenously, in contrast to no instance of lesions here
with the other strains. Three strains from cases of true myositis
produced myositis in 75 per cent and myocarditis (chiefly of the
right ventricle) in 35 per cent of the forty animals injected, in
contrast to an average of myositis of 12 per cent, and myocarditis
of 10 per cent following injection of strains from sources other
than myositis or rheumatic fever; and eight strains of *Streptococcus
viridans* from chronic septic endocarditis produced lesions in the
endocardium in 84 per cent of the forty-four animals injected, in
contrast to an average of 15 per cent with the strains other than
those from endocarditis. The results following injection of the
miscellaneous strains (usually the first culture from tonsils) and
the laboratory strains serve as a basis of comparison with those
following injection of the strains from the various diseases, and
correspond roughly with the total average incidence of lesions in
the various organs as given in the lowest line of the table.
  While the incidence of lesions in the organs following injection
of the strains isolated from such organs is high, as shown by these
figures, the appearances at the necropsy are even more significant.
  In many instances in which the animals survive the injection for

some time, no other focal lesions could be found except those in the organ in question; and when the animal died early, these lesions were the marked feature and the associated ones were relatively insignificant. Frequently the injection of a very small dose was sufficient to prove the elective localization. This elective property was shown not only by the cultures from tissues and foci but also by the bacteria contained in the foci, directly injected in other animals.

In many cases of both acute and chronic diseases the apparent atrium of infection was found to harbor streptococci having elective affinity; in the former usually only at the time of the attack, in the latter in some instances for months. The elective affinity, however, was less marked in the strains isolated from the supposed focus than in the strains isolated from the lesions in the various organs. The rather wide range of lesions, as indicated in the table, following the injection of the strains from herpes zoster and parotitis is due to the fact that often primary mixed cultures from tonsils and pyorrheal pockets were injected.

Attempts to find a method which would preserve the original tropic property, while only partially successful, have shown that it may be preserved for some weeks in the deeper colonies of the original shake cultures and for as long as seven months by keeping the suspensions containing sterile tissue in the ice chest, thus maintaining the bacteria in a condition of latent life.

The localization of the strains from appendicitis, ulcer of the stomach and cholecystitis as isolated, after cultivation and after animal passage, is of particular interest and will be discussed in a separate paper. It should be stated here, however, that these strains resemble one another very closely indeed in cultural and other respects. Those from appendicitis are the least virulent, those from ulcer occupy a middle position and those from cholecystitis are the most virulent. The virulence seems to be one of the factors that determines their place of survival after intravenous injection. Now if the localization is dependent to a certain extent on virulence, than the occurrence of ulcer and cholecystitis should become greater as the strains from the appendix are passed through animals, and appendicitis should occur oftener after the strains from ulcer and cholecystitis lose virulence from cultivation on artificial mediums. This is found actually to be the case (see figures in table). In this connection other facts should be mentioned. None of the strains from appendicitis produced pancreatitis. The strains from appendicitis produced pancreatitis. The strains from ulcer and cholecystitis as isolated (mostly those from acute cases) produced pancreatitis in 3 per cent and 5 per cent, respectively, of the animals injected. After animal passage, pancreatitis occurred in 15 and 19 per cent, respectively, while after cultivation on artificial mediums pancreatitis in no case was obtained.

Lesions in the intestines, exclusive of the duodenum, were more common with the strains from cholecystitis and rheumatism than with those from appendicitis, and all the strains produced intestinal lesions (chiefly of the mucous membrane and lymphoid structures) quite commonly after they had been passed through animals, whereas, after cultivation for a time, no noteworthy lesions were found in the intestinal tract.

The streptococci studied by me from parotitis resemble the organism described by Herb[2] and, like hers, produced the characteristic picture of mumps in dogs when injected into Steno's duct. Intravenous injection of these organisms produced marked edema and hemorrhage in and surrounding the parotid. The affinity was so great that the streptococci were found in pure culture in the enlarged parotid in three of five full-time puppies removed from the uterus of a dog which was chloroformed during a marked parotitis following injection into Steno's duct. Antigens prepared from a number of these strains were found to bind specifically complement in serum from parotitis (Howell).

Lesions in the skeletal muscles occurred in 75 per cent of the animals injected. The number of lesions in the muscles and myocardium in the animals injected with strains from myositis was often in proportion to the quantity injected, and occurred mostly in the tendinous portion and in the right ventricle.

Lesions in the kidney were especially common after injections of streptococci from rheumatic fever (39 per cent) and from endocarditis (20 per cent). These occurred chiefly in the medullary portion (Rosenow[3]) in the former and in the glomeruli in the latter.

Lesions in the lung, consisting usually of hemorrhages and edema, were rare following injection of the strains when isolated and after they were cultivated on artificial mediums but, just as was found previously (Rosenow[3]) they occurred oftener after the virulence was increased by animal passage.

That the streptococci are the underlying cause of the diseases from the lesions of which they were isolated [p. 1690:] is indicated further by the fact that they have elective affinity for the corresponding structures in animals. Moreover, the fact that the same streptococcus may be made to localize in different organs is in consonance with the knowledge that streptococci may cause diseases with different symptomatology. The possibility, however, that they are secondary invaders to some ultramicroscopic, filterable organism has to be considered. Filtrates of the streptococcal cultures from various diseases were injected intravenously. In some instances the filtrates produced lesions in the organs from which the strains were isolated; the lesions, however, were not due to living organisms because the broth which was inoculated and incubated with the tissues failed to produce any lesions. The results, while inconclusive, may be said to indicate that streptococci produce substances which cause injure specifically in the tissues from which the strains are isolated.

GENERAL DISCUSSION

The results obtained are in harmony with the facts that (1) "septic sore throat" is due to streptococci having peculiar properties;[4] (2) certain epidemics of throat infection, due to streptococci, are more frequently complicated by sinusitis than others; (3) distinct differences in the character of the lesion in the lung and mortality rate in pneumonia, as shown by Cole,[5] are due to pneumococci so nearly alike as to require sensitive biologic tests to differentiate them; (4) hemolytic streptococci frequently have a marked affinity for joints, and (5) Friedländer bacilli in arthritis show elective affinity for joints in animals when other strains do not (Dick[6]). The "organotropic" condition of streptococci is analogous to the affinity of the tetanus toxin for the motor ganglion cells, of the diptheria bacillus for the faucial tonsils, of the meningococcus for the meninges, of the pneumococcus for the lung, of the typhoid bacillus for lymphatic tissues, of the virus of rabies for the central nervous system, of the organism of anterior poliomyelitis for the anterior horns of the spinal cord, of the malarial parasite for the red blood corpuscle, and of the *Trichina spiralis* for muscles. The results, moreover, are in accord with the well-known fact that chemicals when injected intravenously also localize unequally in various organs.[7] The changes in the distribution of lesions as the streptococci are altered by cultivation on artificial mediums or by animal passage are similar to the changes in localization of various chemicals or dyes depending on chemical constitution, as observed by Ehrlich.[8] In my experiments advantage was taken of the opportunity afforded to study the nature of selective action from the standpoint of living bacterial.

Flexner[9] has shown that the functioning organ may be especially favorable to the growth of certain bacteria although the organ extracts may inhibit their growth; hence the growth of bacteria in various organs may be related to function and blood supply. Streptococci of low virulence but highly sensitive to oxygen are found to produce lesions in tissues whose blood supply and there oxygen and food requirements are low (heart valves, tendinous portion of muscles and the structures about joints). Streptococci of greater virulence are found to produce lesions in tissues whose blood supply and therefore oxygen and food requirements are high (kidney, lung, etc.); hence localization and production of injury seem to be closely related to the amount of available oxygen in a given tissue. The fact that lesions occurred far more frequently in the right ventricle (containing venous blood) than in the left ventricle (containing oxygenated blood) is in accord with this hypothesis. Might not the predisposing action of trauma (locus minoris resistentiae), of exposure to cold and of a drunken bout, to infection be best explained on the basis of lack of oxygen?

The changes observed, as hemorrhage, cloudy swelling and necrosis, from a purely chemical[10] as well as from a colloid-chemical[11] point of view, are identical with the changes of tissue asphyxia. I have found that pneumococci when grown and autolyzed under anaerobic conditions produce a much larger quantity of toxic material than when grown or autolyzed under aerobic conditions. Moreover, pneumococcus extracts proved to be toxic to warm-blooded animals (guinea-pigs), have the same inhibitory effect on the development of fertilized eggs of arbacia as does lack of oxygen. Since bacteria and their products are powerful reducing agents,[12] one of the chief effects of the bacteria and their products very likely is interference with the normal cell respiration, and possibly the greater the virulence the more powerful this interference.

Although the circulation is an important factor in determining localization, the tissues themselves play an even more important rôle. The question whether the lesions in the organ for which a particular strain appears to have elective affinity are due to the lodgment of a larger number of bacteria here than in the other organs, or whether the bacteria lodged in equal numbers in the various organs but survive only in the one showing lesions, is now under study. The evidence already obtained, however, points strongly to the former mechanism. It appears that the cells of the tissues for which a given strain shows elective affinity take the bacteria out of the circulation as if by a magnet -- adsorption.

This remarkable tropic condition tends to disappear quite promptly both on cultivating the streptococci on artificial mediums and on passing them successively through animals, and this may occur without demonstrable changes in morphology, grouping or character [p.1691:] of chain formation. I have previously shown[13] that the ability of *Streptococcus viridans* and staphylococci to produce lesions in the endocardium is due partly to physical clumping. Evans[14] has shown that the action of vital stains of the benzidin group is related to the size of colloidal particles. A careful study of smears of the suspensions injected in these experiments revealed no constant relation between localization and clumping or size of the bacteria.

Individual variations in resistance to infection were found in the injected animals. The effects of these conditions in the host as determining factors in localization are important; they are probably expressions of differences in metabolism, oxidation rates, etc., which influence the soil for bacteria. The tendency of virulent bacteria, temporarily or permanently, to render this soil less favorable for their growth is well established. There is some evidence, on the other hand, which goes to show that certain bacteria of very low virulence (commonly found in chronic foci of infection) tend actually to make this soil more favorable. But in the light of my results, it must be considered that differences in the host may afford the peculiar type of reaction, or that the individual harbors a particular form of focus of infection which is favorable for bacteria to acquire elective properties. The following facts support the latter view: (1) the common occurrence of certain noncontagious diseases, such as herpes zoster, ulcer of the stomach, etc., during definite age periods; (2) the fact that foci of infection afford opportunity for bacteria to grow under varying grades of oxygen pressure and in mixed culture, both of which have been shown to cause changes in virulence and other properties of bacteria,[15]
including the streptococcus group;[16] (3) the occurrence of systemic infections such as rheumatic fever, appendicitis, ulcer of the stomach, etc., usually after the acute symptoms in follicular tonsillitis (hemolytic streptococci), have subsided, and (4) the finding in the focus and involved tissues at the time of the systemic infection, streptococci having elective affinity for these structures in animals.

Since different bacteria may acquire simultaneously affinity for the same tissue, diseases which resemble each other more or less closely, such as the different forms of arthritis, may be due to bacteria of different species each having elective affinity for the particular structures involved.

The figures in the lowest line of the table represent the results of numerous experiments (833) with streptococci (220) from a wide range of sources, and may therefore be regarded as an index of the liability of the various organs to infection. Thus, joint lesions occurred more often (27 per cent) than lesions in other organs, corresponding to the frequent occurrence of spontaneous arthritis in man and animals. The occurrence of lesions in the stomach (20 per cent), valves of the heart (14 per cent), myocardium (12 per cent) and skeletal muscles (12 per cent) correspond in a general way to the occurrence of infection in these organs in may. The very infrequent involvement of the skin, tongue and the parotid in animals is in keeping with the rarity of embolic infections in these structures. The character of the lesions and their occurrence simultaneously in the joints, heart, muscles and kidney, and the development of chorea (7 per cent mostly in young rabbits) following injection of the streptococci from rheumatic fever, parallels quite closely the phenomena of rheumatic infection as observed in man. The strains from erythema nodosum resemble those from rheumatic fever, producing a relatively high incidence of arthritis, pericarditis and myositis, a fact which supports the view held by clinical observers,[17] that the causative agents of rheumatic fever and erythema nodosum must be similar.

The tendency to localize electively within a limited range, "monotropism," is most highly developed in the relatively nonvirulent strains isolated from chronic lesions. In the more virulent strains from acute lesions and after animal passage, this tendency is less highly developed, the lesions occurring over a wider range, "polytropism." The fact that the elective property is more highly developed in streptococci isolated from the organ involved, than in those isolated from the probable focus of infection, is in accord with the results obtained by Forssner,[18] who showed that when streptococci are grown in kidney and kidney extracts they acquire a special predilection for the kidney when injected intravenously. Since the bacteria which have been grown in a given tissue acquire greater affinity for this tissue, the likelihood of these bacteria to involve other structures is relatively slight; hence the secondary focus, a cholecystitis, for example, would appear to be less important as a distributor of bacteria than the primary focus; if, however, the secondary focus happens to be in a joint, of which there are many, it may play an important rôle in causing extension to uninvolved joints and in preventing recovery.

The bearing that these results have on the specific treatment of these diseases is evident. The injection of a streptococcus vaccine or antistreptococcus serum without regard to the tropic condition of the infecting strain or the one used in their preparation is, in the light of these results, far from an exact method of treatment. However, the occasional, seemingly good result observed by some may be due to the use of a serum or vaccine made from strains in the same tropic condition as the one infecting the individual so treated.

The results detailed in this and in previous papers seem to bring the necessary experimental proof that chronic foci of infection play a most important rôle in causing systemic disease, a fact which has been observed and frequently commented on by different observers, but has been recognized in its full clinical significance especially by Billings.[19] A focus, such as a pocket in the tonsil which cannot heal for mechanical reasons and which is constantly filled with pus and necrotic material, teeming with bacteria, must be regarded in the light of these findings as a culture tube with a permeable wall affording abundant opportunity for the entrance of bacteria and their products.

* From the Memorial Institute of Infectious Diseases, Chicago, and the Mayo Foundation, Rochester, Minn.

1.   The common 8-ounce nursing bottle is used both as a culture flask and centrifugal tube, and serves the purpose admirably.

2.   Herb, Isabella C.: Experimental Parotitis, *Arch. Int. Med.*, September, 1909, p. 201.

3.   Rosenow, E.C.: Experimental Infectious Endocarditis, *Jour. Infect. Dis.*, 1912, xi, 210; Immunological Observations in Staphylococcus and Pneumococcus Endocarditis, ibid., 1909, vi, 245; Transmutations Within the Streptococcus-Pneumococcus Group, ibid., 1914, xiv, 1.

4.   Davis, D.J., and Rosenow, E.C.: An Epidemic of Sore Throat Due to a Peculiar Streptococcus, *THE JOURNAL A. M. A.*, March 16, 1912, p. 773.   North, Charles E.; White, Benjamin; and Avery, Oswald T.: A Septic Sore Throat Epidemic in Cortland and Homer, N. Y., *Jour. Infect. Dis.*, 1913, xiv, 124.   Rosenow, Edward C., and Moon, V.H.: On an Epidemic of Sore Throat and the Virulence of Streptococci Isolated from the Milk, *Jour. Infect. Dis.*, 1915, xvii, 69.

5.   Cole, Rufus M.: Pneumococcus Infection and Lobar Pneumonia, *New York Med. Jour.*, 1914, xcix, 23.

6.   Dick, George F.: Multiple Arthritis Due to a Friedländer Bacillus, *Jour. Infect. Dis.*, Chicago, 1914, xiv, 176.

7.   Brown, W. H., and Pearch, Louise: On the Pathological Action of Arsenicals upon the Adrenals, *Proc. Nat. Acad. Sc.*, 1915, i, 462. Corper, H.J.: Action of Sodium Sulphocyanate in Tuberculosis, *Jour. Infect. Dis.*, xvi, 38.

8.   Ehrlich: *Studies in Immunity*, Transl. by Charles Boduan,, New York, John Wiley & Sons, 1910.

9.   Flexner, Simon: The Bacillus (Leptothrix?) Pyogenes Filiformia and Its Pathogenic Action, Jour. Exper. Med., 1896, i, 211.

10.   Hoppe-Seyler, F.: Bemerkungen zur vorstehenden, IV Mittheilung von Herrn T. Araki, über die Wirkungen des Sauerstoffmangels, Ztschr. f. physiol. Chem., 1894, xix, 476. Araki, T.: Ueber die Bilding von Milchsäure und Glycose im Organismus bei Sauerstoffmangel, Ztschr. f. physiol. Chem., 1891, xv, 335 and 546.   Fletcher, W.M. and Hopkins, Goland: Lactic Acid in Amphibian Muscle, Jour. Physiol., 1906-7, xxxv, 247.   Woodyat, R.T.: The action of Glycol Aldehyd and Glycerin Aldehyd in Diabetes Mellitis and the Nature of Antiketogenesis, *THE JOURNAL A. M. A.*, Dec. 17, 1910, p. 2109.   Graham, Evarts A.: Late Poisoning with Chloroform and Other Alkyl Halides in Relationship to the Halogen Acids Formed by Their Chemical Dissociation, *Jour. Exper. Med.*, 1915, xxii, 48.

11.   Fischer, Martin H.: *Edema and Nephritis*, New York, John Wiley & Sons, 1915.

12.   Smith, T.: Reduktionserscheinungen bei Bakterien und Bexiohungen zur Bakterienzeile, nebst Bemerkungen über Reduktionserscheinungen in steriler Bouillon, *Centralb. f. Bakteriol. u. Parasitenk.*, Part 1, 1896, xix, 181.

13.   Rosenow, E.C.: Experimental Infectious Endocarditis, *Jour. Infect. Dis.*, 1912, xi, 210; Immunological Observations in

Staphylococcus and Pneumococcus Endocarditis, ibid., 1909, vi, 245.

14. Evans, H.M., and Schulemann, W.: The Action of Vital Stains Belonging to the Benzidine Group, *Science*, 1914, N. S., xxxix, 443.

15. Smith, T.: Modification, Temporary and Permanent, of the Physiological Characters of Bacteria in Mixed Cultures, *Tr. Assn. Am. Phsicians*, Philadelphia, 1894, ix, 85.

16. Rosenow, E.C.: Transmutations Within the Streptococcus Pneumococcus Group, *Jour. Infect. Dis.*1914, xiv, 1.

17. Osler, William: On the Visceral Manifestations of the Erythema Group of Skin Diseases, *Am. Jour. Med. Sc.*, 1904, cxxvii, 1.

18. Forssner, G.: Renale Lokalisation nach intravenöse Infektionen mit einer dem Nierengewebe experimentell angepassten Streptokokkenkultur, *Nord. Med. Ark.*, 1902, 3. f., ii afd. 2, No. 18, p. 1; abstr., *Inn. Med.*, 1902, lv, 45.

19. Billings, Frank: Chronic Focal Infections and Their Etiologic Relations to Arthritis and Nephritis, *Arch. Int.Med.*, April, 1912, p. 484; Chronic Focal Infection as a Causative Factor in Chronic Arthritis, *THE JOURNAL A. M. A.*, Sept. 13, 1913, p. 819; Focal Infection: Its Broader Application in the Etiology of General Disease, ibid., Sept. 12, 1911, p. 899.

ELECTIVE LOCALIZATION OF STREPTOCOCCI

Source of Streptococci		Strains (320)	Animals Injected	Appendix	Stomach Hemor.	Stomach Ulcer	Duodenum	Gallbladder	Pancreas	Intestines	Joints	Endocardium	Pericardium	Myocardium	Muscles	Kidney	Lung	Skin	Tongue	Eye	Parotid
Appendicitis	When isolated	14	68	68	6	1	1	0	9	59	21	0	9	12	0	0	0	0	0	3	0
	Later	8	26	15	19	15	4	0	0	22	19	0	12	23	0	0	0	0	0	0	0
	After animal passage	7	22	45	45	50	45	0	20	36	20	0	20	25	10	0	0	0	0	0	0
Ulcer of stomach in man	When isolated	18	123	2	50	60	20	3	7	16	12	4	5	0	5	0	0	0	0	0	0
	Later	8	22	5	5	0	5	0	0	18	14	0	0	0	0	0	0	0	0	0	0
	After animal passage	7	29	0	23	33	30	15	15	21	5	0	3	3	8	15	0	0	0	0	0
Cholecystitis	When isolated	12	41	0	29	15	80	5	17	17	10	0	2	7	6	5	2	0	0	0	0
	Later	5	14	14	28	14	7	0	0	21	14	0	0	0	7	0	0	0	0	0	0
	After animal passage	4	16	0	21	12	56	19	13	15	19	0	13	0	13	6	0	0	0	0	0
Rheumatic fever	When isolated	24	71	8	23	18	3	3	13	68	46	27	44	27	39	4	0	0	0	10	0
	Later	8	16	0	14	21	0	0	0	21	21	0	28	0	31	0	0	0	0	0	0
	After animal passage	5	19	21	37	21	5	21	0	37	53	32	37	16	42	21	0	0	0	11	0
Erythema nodosum	When isolated	6	20	0	10	0	0	0	5	20	20	10	0	35	10	5	80	0	0	5	0
	Later	3	9	0	22	0	11	0	0	11	11	0	0	0	0	0	22	0	0	0	0
	After animal passage	6	14	0	21	0	50	0	7	50	14	7	14	50	7	43	43	0	0	6	0
Herpes zoster	When isolated	11	61	10	29	8	16	2	8	11	5	11	5	11	5	21	70	13	15	0	0
	Later	6	15	0	13	7	7	13	7	60	7	0	20	40	7	20	7	0	13	0	0
	After animal passage	4	7	0	28	10	0	0	0	43	0	14	0	28	0	43	28	14	0	0	0
Mumps	When isolated	8	19	15	21	5	21	42	10	42	15	0	37	3	5	15	15	0	0	0	73
	Later	6	8	12	0	0	0	12	12	24	24	0	12	12	0	12	12	0	0	0	24
Myositis	When isolated	3	40	2	4	10	2	7	7	20	10	0	35	75	2	0	7	0	0	8	0
Endocarditis	When isolated	8	44	0	7	0	5	0	15	15	84	4	20	0	20	20	2	0	0	0	0
Miscellaneous	When isolated	34	41	3	17	0	4	0	4	17	20	0	15	7	7	7	0	0	0	0	0
"Lab." strains	Before and after animal passage	5	100	2	18	5	2	2	2	42	43	0	15	12	10	17	2	0	0	8	0
Average percentage of animals injected with non specific strains showing lesions in individual organs				5	20	9	11	6	8	27	14	2	10	12	9	11	2	1		3	0

APPENDIX D2:   *Quart. Bull., N.U. Medical School 28, 1954, 57-60*

FURTHER OBSERVATIONS ON ACUTE POLIOMYELITIS
TREATED WITH THERMAL ANTIBODY[1]

BENJAMIN RAPPAPORT, M.D.

FORTY-SIX consecutive cases of acute poliomyelitis have been treated with thermal poliomyelitis streptococcal antibody. Twenty of these cases occurred in 1946 and were published in 1948 (1).

The thermal antibody used in these studies was supplied by Dr. E. C. Rosenow of Longview Hospital, Cincinnati, Ohio. It was prepared from a mixture of strains of the specific type of streptococcus isolated from nasopharynx or spinal fluid during life or from spinal cord of persons that succumbed to epidemic poliomyelitis one or more years previously. The freshly isolated streptococci were stored meanwhile at 10 C. in very dense suspension (1000 organisms per cc.) of glycerol, two parts, and saturated NaCl solution, 1 part. The antibody as used was prepared by diluting the dense glycerin NaCl solution suspension of the streptococcus is isotonic NaCl solution to 10 billion streptococci per cc. and heating in the autoclave at 17 lbs. pressure for 3 hours after adding 1.5 per cent H_2O_2 and then bringing the pH to 6.5 or 7.0 (2).

The details concerning each of the last 26 patients now under consideration are shown in the accompanying table. In this series of cases the ages varied from 16 months to 15 years. Twelve of the patients were boys and 14 were girls. Fever was present at the onset in all the cases. In each case a stiffened neck and back was noted and a positive Brudzinski sign was obtained. In 2 patients vomiting occurred at the onset. Paralysis or weakness was present in 12 of the 26 patients when first seen. None of these cases who already had paralysis developed any more paralysis after the administration of the thermal antibody; and of the 14 preparalytic cases none developed any weakness or paralysis after treatment with the thermal antibody.

In this series of 26 patients (see Table) 5 either had difficulty in swallowing or could not swallow. This difficulty disappeared within 24 hours in 2 of the patients, in 48 hours in one case, and and in five days in 2 cases, apparently depending inversely on the amount of antibody given.

In the group of 14 preparalytic patients, lost or absent reflexes were noted in 6 patients. Of the remaining 12 cases, 2 had weakness of the right arm and one a weak left leg. In 2 cases both legs were weak. The intercostal muscles and diaphragm were weak in one case. In 2 cases there was weakness of the urinary bladder. Five patients had difficulty in swallowing or were unable to swallow. Head drop was noted in 3 cases and strabismus in one case.

The spinal fluid cell counts varied from 0 to 447. In 10 cases the count was over 100. Eight of these patients were preparalytic, of which 6 had lost reflexes. In 7 patients the cell counts were between 10 and 100, 4 of these had weakness or paralysis, and 3 were preparalytic. Nine patients had cell counts less than 10, 5 of which were preparalytic and 3 were bulbar cases unable to swallow when first seen.

The thermal poliomyelitis antibody was given intramuscularly into the lateral aspect of the thigh in all 26 cases as soon as the diagnosis of acute poliomyelitis was made. The amount given varied from 15 cc. to 110 cc., depending on the severity of the disease, the day of illness, and the age and size of the patient. Twenty patients each received 50 cc. or less, and 6 cases more than 50 cc. each.

---

[1] From the Department of Medicine, Northwestern University Medical School, and the Evanston Hospital. Received for publication. October 30, 1953.

Case No.	Age	Date of Onset	Symptoms and Findings	Spinal Fluid (clear under pressure)	Thermal Antibody: Date & Amount Injected Intramuscularly	
21	11 yrs.	7-15-47	Fever, headache, drowsy, painful neck and back, positive Brudzinski.	Cell count 211 Pandy Positive	7-15-47	40 cc.
22	2 yrs.	8- 1-47	Fever, vomiting, stiff neck & back, positive Brudzinski, head drop.	Cell count 155	8- 3-47	30 cc.
23	4½ yrs.	9-20-47	Fever, headache, vomiting, painful neck and back, positive Brudzinski	Cell count 447	9-20-47	40 cc.
24	3 yrs.	10-21-47	Fever, weakness of legs, headache, stiff neck and back, positive Brudzinski, absent knee reflexes.	Cell count 16	10-21-47	30 cc.
25	14 yrs.	9-18-48	Fever, headache, pain in right lower quadrant, stiff neck and back, positive Brudzinski, weakness of right arm, of both legs and urinary bladder.	Cell count 10	9-21-48	50 cc.
26	10 yrs.	9-19-48	Fever, headache, stiff neck and back, positive Brudzinski, knee reflexes absent.	Cell count 6	9-21-48	30 cc.
27	7 yrs.	9-21-48	Fever, tremors, convulsions, stiff neck and back, positive Brudzinski.	Cell count 133 Ross Jane pos.	9-24-48	25 cc.
28	22 mos.	9-21-48	Fever, convulsions, vomited, lethargic nystagmus, strabismus, stiff neck and back, positive Brudzinski.	Cell count 10	9-22-48	30 cc.
29	7 yrs.	9-24-48	Fever, headache, backache, positive Brudzinski.	Cell count 5	9-26-48	20 cc.
30	5 yrs.	9-30-48	Fever, backache, headache, positive Brudzinski, left knee reflex absent.	Cell count 120	10- 2-48	40 cc.
31	16 mos.	9-30-48	Fever, tongue deviating to right, saliva running out of mouth, when cries shows weakness of right side of mouth, positive Brudzinski, always assumes knee-chest position.	Cell count 0	10- 1-48	15 cc.
32	15 yrs.	11-12-48	Fever, headache, stiff neck and back, positive Brudzinski, positive Kernig, weakness of urinary bladder.	Cell count 1	11-14-48	60 cc.
33	2 yrs.	11-22-48	Fever, weakness of legs, intercostal muscles, diaphragm, difficulty in swallowing, stiff neck and back, positive Brudzinski, head drop.	Cell count 134	11-25-48 11-28-48	60 cc. 20 cc.
34	5 yrs.	11-27-48	Fever, painful neck and back, positive Brudzinski, positive Kernig, absent knee reflexes.	Cell count 17	11-28-48	25 cc.
35	5 yrs.	8- 1-49	Fever, headache, stiff neck and back, positive Brudzinski	Cell count 1	8-11-49	35 cc.
36	3½ yrs.	8- 2-49	Fever, painful to walk, stiff neck and back, positive Brudzinski, positive Kernig.	Cell count 12	8- 2-49	30 cc.
37	8½ yrs.	9- 1-49	Fever, headache, drowsiness, stiff neck and back, positive Brudzinski.	Cell count 101	9- 2-49	50 cc.
38	6 yrs.	9- 6-49	Fever, stiff neck and back, painful legs, positive Brudzinski.	Cell count 227	9- 7-49	50 cc.
39	7 yrs.	9-12-49	Fever, headache, stiff neck and back, could not swallow, positive Brudzinski.	Cell count 0	9-13-49	50 cc.
40	14 yrs.	9-24-49	Fever, backache, throat painful on swallowing, positive Brudzinski.	Cell count 0	9-26-49	30 cc.
41	5 yrs.	11-14-49	Fever, backache, stiff neck and back, painful right leg, positive Brudzinski, head drop, abdominal reflexes absent.	Cell count 32	11-16-49	40 cc.
42	7½ yrs.	6-13-51	Fever, stiff neck and back, could not swallow, positive Brudzinski, knee reflexes absent.	Cell count 4	6-14-51	100 cc.
43	6 yrs.	6-23-51	Fever, headache, backache, stiff neck and back, tremors, positive Brudzinski, head drop, positive Kernig, Right arm and left leg weak.	Cell count 339	6-26 51	110 cc.
44	9 yrs.	7-14-51	Fever, headache, vomiting, stiff neck and back, positive Brudzinski.	Cell count 247	7-15-51	80 cc.
45	5 yrs.	8-18-51	Fever, headache, painful left leg, stiff neck and back, positive Brudzinski	Cell count 0	8-18-51	60 cc.
46	13 yrs.	10-19-51	Fever, backache, positive Brudzinski.	Cell count 10	10-22-51	40 cc.

RAPPAPORT—ACUTE POLIOMYELITIS

Reaction from thermal antibody	Date first improvement noted	Remarks
None	Normal temperature since 7-17-47	8-5-47 Discharged from hospital. No muscular weakness
None	Normal temperature since 8-8-47	8-16-47 Discharged from hospital. No muscular weakness.
None	Normal temperature since 9-24-47	10-5-47 Discharged from hospital. No muscular weakness.
None	Normal temperature since 10-22-47	11-10-47 Discharged from hospital. No muscular weakness.
None	Normal temperature since 9-24-48	10-21-48 Discharged from hospital, urinary bladder normal after 9-26-48. Weakness of right arm and leg gone, right leg weak, but can walk with a cane.
None	Normal temperature since 9-23-48	10-3-48 Discharged from hospital. All reflex present. No muscular weakness.
None	Normal temperature since 9-25-48	10-5-48 Discharged from hospital. No muscular weakness.
None	Normal temperature since 9-25-48	10-6-48 Discharged from hospital. No muscular weakness.
None	Normal temperature since 9-28-48	10-15-48 Discharged from hospital. No muscular weakness.
None	Normal temperature since 10-4-48	10-20-48 Discharged from hospital. No muscular weakness.
None	Normal temperature since 10-1-48	10-20-48 Discharged from hospital. No muscular weakness. Walking around crib. Swallowing saliva normally.
None	Normal temperature since 11-16-48	11-26-48 Discharged from hospital. No muscular weakness.
None	Normal temperature since 11-28-48	2-1-49 Discharged from hospital, with some weakness of right leg. Can walk alone with leg brace. Left leg almost normal, no other weakness remains.
None	Normal temperature since 12-4-48	12-18-48 Discharged from hospital. No muscular weakness. Knee reflexes normal.
None	Normal temperature since 8-14-49	8-29-49 Discharged from hospital. No muscular weakness.
None	Normal temperature since 8-5-49	8-16-49 Discharged from hospital. No muscular weakness.
None	Normal temperature since 9-3-49	9-15-49 Discharged from hospital. No muscular weakness.
Slight local pain	Normal temperature since 9-8-49	9-21-49 Discharged from hospital. No muscular weakness.
Slight local pain	Normal temperature since 9-16-49	10-4-49 Discharged from hospital. No muscular weakness. By 9-17-49 could swallow normally.
None	Normal temperature since 9-27-49	10-7-49 Discharged from hospital. No muscular weakness.
None	Normal temperature since 11-18-49	12-3-49 Discharged from hospital. No muscular weakness. All reflexes normal.
None	Normal temperature since 6-16-51	6-29-51 Discharged from hospital. No muscular weakness. 6-17-51 Could swallow normally. All reflexes normal.
None	Normal temperature since 6-29-51	7-22-51 Discharged from hospital. Left leg slight weakness, but can walk alone.
None	Normal temperature since 7-19-51	7-28-51 Discharged from hospital. No muscular weakness.
None	Normal temperature since 8-20-51	9-1-51 Discharged from hospital. No muscular weakness.
None	Normal temperature since 10-24-51	10-29-51 Discharged from hospital. No muscular weakness.

In only 2 patients a slight local pain developed at the site of the injection, and 24 patients had no reaction or pain.

There were no deaths among these patients treated with the thermal antibody. In all the cases the temperature returned to normal in a shorter period of time than in untreated patients. Muscular pain usually subsided in two or three days after the thermal antibody was given. Although there were 5 cases of the bulbar variety, none of the 26 cases needed, or were placed in, the respirator.

Thirty known contacts exposed by these 26 cases of poliomyelitis were each given 10 cc. of the thermal antibody and none developed poliomyelitis.

CONCLUSIONS

The use of thermal antibody for acute cases of poliomyelitis shortened the acute stage of this disease; prevented the development of weakness or paralysis in preparalytic cases; and in those patients with weakness or paralysis when first seen no additional weakness or paralysis developed after the patients had received the thermal poliomyelitis anti-body. The result was a more rapid return to normal for all the patients as compared to patients with this disease who did not receive the thermal antibody. These results are in accord with those reported by Rosenow in preliminary and control studies in treatment with thermal antibody, in which it was found that circulating streptococcal antigen diminished and antibody increased, shown by cutaneous reactions as clinical improvement occurred (3, 4).

REFERENCES

1. Rappaport, B.: Acute Poliomyelitis Treated with Thermal Antibody, Journal-Lancet, 68: 395, 1948.
2. Rosenow, E. C.: Studies on the Nature of Antibodies Produced in *vitro* from Bacteria with Hydrogen Peroxide and Heat, J. Immunol., 55:219-232, 1947.
3. Rosenow, E. C.: A Study of the 1946 Poliomyelitis Epidemic by New Bacteriologic Methods, Journal-Lancet, 68:265-277, 1948.
4. Rosenow, E. C.: Intradermal Antibody-Antigen and Antigen-Antibody Reactions in Persons having Poliomyelitis, Contacts and Non-contacts in Relation to Poliomyelitis, Federation Proc., (Abstract), 8:410, March, 1949.

APPENDIX D3: *Ohio State Medical Journal*, July 1957, Studies on the
Etiology and Specific Treatment of Multiple Sclerosis [reprinted,
with permission]

Edward C. Rosenow, M.D.

[The Author - Dr. Rosenow, Minneapolis, Minn., was formerly a member
of the staff (Bacteriological Research) at Longview Hospital,
Cincinnati; and is emeritus professor of experimental bacteriology,
Mayo Foundation, Rochester, Minnesota.]

In extended studies on the causation of diverse diseases,
including multiple sclerosis, it was found that specifically
virulent nonhemolytic streptococci could be readily separated from
saprophytic types usually also present in the nasopharynxes of
persons having chronic disease. This was done by making serial
dilution cultures of nasopharyngeal swabbings in tall columns of
destrose-brain broth in test tubes at dilutions of 10^{-2}, 10^{-6}, and 10^{-10},, and making subcultures from the end points of growth of such
cultures.

Streptococci thus isolated and injected intravenously into rabbits
and white mice localized electively in the brains and spinal cords
of the animals.[1-3]   Periods of exacerbation of multiple sclerosis
occurred in varying degrees and incidence in each of the 56 white
persons studied. Twenty-six were males and 30 were females. The
ages ranged from 26 to 72 years. Nystagmus, intention tremor,
ataxia, slurring speech, exaggerated reflexes in involved
extremities, weakness and undue hopefulness characteristic of the
disease were noted in varying degrees and incidence.

METHODS OF STUDY

Diagnostic skin tests for specific circulating streptococcic
antigen were made by injection into the skin of the forearm, 0.05
ml. of thermal antibody solutions in the supernatant of NaCl
solution suspensions containing 20 billion streptococci per
milliliter that had been isolated in studies of multiple sclerosis,
autoclaved for 96 hours and diluted with equal parts of NaCl
solution plus 0.2 per cent phenol. As a control measure,
streptococcic antibody was injected that had been similarly prepared
from streptococci isolated in studies of other diseases.

Skin test for circulating streptococcic antibody were made by
injecting 0.05 ml. of the supernatant of NaCl Solution suspensions
containing 2 billion streptococci per milliliter that had been
heated at 70 degrees C for one hour.[4] Specific streptococcic thermal
antibody for therapeutic use and agglutination studies also was made
from NaCl solution suspensions containing 10 billion streptococci
per milliliter to which 1.5 per cent hydrogen peroxide from a 30 per
cent solution was added, autoclaved for three hours and brought to
pH 7.0. Streptococcic antibody solutions made with and without
hydrogen peroxide were injected subcutaneously in comparable dosage
in treatment. After degree of erythematous reaction had been noted
at the point of injection and the clinical effects of the

administration of varying dosages of both vaccine and thermal antibody solutions had been assessed, the following schedule of skin test and of dosage was used routinely:

One-tenth milliliter of the autogenous or stock vaccine containing 200,000,000 streptococci per milliliter isolated from the nasopharynxes of persons who had multiple sclerosis was injected subcutaneously for the first injection. This dose was increased by 0.1 ml. twice weekly up to the amount of 1 ml. Then 1 ml. was injected each week for an indefinite period, provided local and constitutional reactions were minimal and provided favorable clinical effects occurred.

One-half milliliter of the stock or autogenous [multiple sclerosis] thermal streptococcic antibody from 10 billion streptococci per milliliter was injected separately subcutaneously, but at the same time or more often, if favorable results ensued. This dose was increased to 2 ml. and was given twice weekly or daily, provided local reactions at the point of injection were minimal or negative and provided clinical results were favorable.

Erythematous reaction at the point of injection of vaccine and antibody, and clinical results were used as guides for increments or diminutions of doses. Since such injections were harmless and had to be repeated over long periods, some members of the family of a nurse was instructed to give the injections. Local reactions to repeated injections usually diminished, in respect to both vaccine and antibody, as clinical improvement occurred.

RESULTS

Cutaneous reactions to the intradermal injection of antigen and of thermal antibody in persons who had multiple sclerosis are summarized in Table 1. It will be seen that the immediate erythematous reactions to the intradermal injection of streptococcic antibody (taken to indicate specific circulating streptococcic antigen in patients not receiving antibody or vaccine therapeutically) were far greater (7.31, 8.07, and 9.63 sq. cm.), respectively, than in persons receiving therapeutic injections of antibody and vaccine (3.15 sq. cm.).

Cutaneous erythematous reactions indicating antibody (5.75 and 6.25 sq. cm.) were significantly less in persons not receiving such therapeutic injections than in persons receiving such treatment (7.86 sq.cm.). Erythematous reactions following intradermal injection of control antibody solutions were uniformly minimal, but in each of the three groups having multiple sclerosis reactions were greater to injections of 'neurotropic' (8126) streptococcic thermal antibody than to corresponding injections of "arthrotropic" (8134) antibody prepared respectively from streptococci isolated in studies of diseases of the nervous system and arthritis.

In an additional group of 11 persons who had multiple sclerosis, not included in Table 1, the average erythematous cutaneous reaction indicating specific circulating streptococcic antigen was 9.3 sq. cm. before therapeutic injections of thermal antibody, 5.82 sq. cm. the day after the first therapeutic injections of antibody, and 3.3 sq. cm. the day after the second such treatment. In sharp contrast, cutaneous reactions indicating circulating streptococcic antibody increased in size as follows: 3.78 sq. cm. after the first; 5.83

sq. cm. after the second; and 6.65 sq. cm. after the third
therapeutic injection of antibody. Clinical improvement occurred in
parallel with (1) the diminutions in reactions indicating specific
circulating streptococcic antigen as (2) reactions indicating
circulating antibody inccreased.

Evidence indicating specificity of the streptococcus isolated in
studies of multiple sclerosis is indicated also by the respective
agglutinative titers of thermal antibody solutions prepared from the
streptococcus with and without hydrogen peroxide. Thus, the
agglutination titer of "antibody" perpared by autoclaving NaCl
solution suspensions containing 20 billion streptococci per
milliliter for 96 hours withoug hydrogen peroxide at four tenfold
dilutions of 1-10 to 1-10,000 was 65 percent for the autogenous
streptococci isolated in studies of multiple sclerosis; for
streptococci isolated respectively in studies of respiratory
infection, 0 per cent; schizophrenia, 19 per cent; epilepsy, 19 per
cent; coronary heart disease, 44 per cent; hypertinsion, 50 per
cent; and poliomyelitis, 50 per cent.

Moreover, the agglutinative titer of thermal antibody perpared
from NaCl solution suspensions containing 10 billion streptococci
per milliliter from dense glycerol-saturated NaCl solution of
respective suspensions, autoclaved for but three hours after the
addition of 1.5 per cent hydrogen peroxide, was equally specific.
Thus, the average agglutinative titer of thermal antibody at four
tenfold dilutions of 1-10 to 1-10,000 prepared from a composite
csuspension containing 10 strains of streptococci isolated from the
nasopharynxes of persons having multiple sclerosis was 94 per cent;
for streptococci similarly isolated in studies of lymphatic
leukemia, 38 percent; for carcinoma, 31 per cent; experimental
poliomyelitis, 63 per cent; epidemic poliomyelitis, 56 per cent;
respiratory infection, 38 per cent; schizophrenia, 19 per cent;
epilepsy, 25 per cent; and coronary heart disease, 31 per cent.

Clinical response to the subcutaneous therapeutic injection of
heterologous streptococcic vaccine and thermal antibody solutions,
while favorable, was usually not as great nor as constant as it was
to the autogenous preparations. In both instances there was
diminution in cutaneous reactions in repeat tests indicating
specific circulating streptococcic antigen, and an increase in
reactions indicating circulating antibody as symptoms abated.

In persons who had multiple sclerosis associated with undue pain
indicating an associated neuritis in the affected extremities,
vaccine and thermal antibody prepared from the streptococcus
isolated in studies of multiple sclerosis usually did not suffice to
control the pain and progress ofthe disease, whereas the use of
autogenous vaccine and thermal antibody in such cases usually did
suffice to effect such objectives. Return of symptoms in previously
affected regions and erythematous reactions to repeated intradermal
injections of specific antibody, indicating specific circulating
streptococcic antigen, occurred in three patients several months
after specific treatment with vaccine and antibody had been
discontinued. The symptoms and positive reactions indicating
specific circulating streptococcic antigen in each of the three

patients disappeared when treatment with specific vaccine and thermal antibody was resumed."

SUMMARY AND CONCLUSIONS

Results of a bacteriologic and immunologic study on the causation and specific treatment of multiple sclerosis are reported.

Evidence has been adduced to indicate that this strange, persistent, progressive, chronic disease is caused by a specific type of nonhemolytic neurotropic streptococcic infection or intoxication.

The evidence indicates that such peculiar affinity of the streptococcus in multiple sclerosis for the nervous system is acquired in the nasopharynxes of persons stricken with the disease, and that the disease is not caused by streptococci from extraneous sources, such as milk, water supplies or respired air. Results of specific treatment by means of the subcutaneous injection of specific streptococcic vaccine have been favorable, but the best results have been obtained from the separate injection of both specific streptococcic vaccine and thermal antibody. Such treatment, although specific and effective, needs to be continued indefinitely to prevent recurrence.

In this as in other studies, the ability to isolate specific types of nonhemolytic streptococci from nasopharyngeal swabbings in diverse diseases and from other materials is due (1) to the use of dextrose-brain broth in tall columns in test tubes, which affords a gradient of oxygen tension and other conditions highly favorable for the growth af fastidious organisms, (2) to the selection of pure cultures of the streptococci from the end points of growth of serial dilution cultures in this medium, and (3) to the preservation of viability at 10 degrees C for some months and antigenic specificity for years in dense suspensions of 2 parts of glycerol and 1 part of saturated NaCl solution.

REFERENCES

1. Rosenow, E.C.: Bacteriological Studies of Multiple Sclerosis. Ann. Allergy, 6:271-292, May-June, 1948.

2. Rosenow, E.C.: Streptococci in the Etiology of Diverse Diseases, Including Diseases of the Nervous System. J. Nerv. & Ment. Dis., 117:415-428, May, 1953.

3. Rosenow, E.C.: Experimental and Clinical Studies on the Relation of Streptococci to Various Diseases. Illinois M.J., 75:28-38, January, 1939.

4. Rosenow, E.C.: Diagnostic Cutaneous Reactions to Intradermal Injection of Natural and Artificial Antibody and of Antigen Prepared from Streptococci Isolated in Studies of Diverse Diseases. Ann. Allergy, 6:484-496; 500. September-October, 1948.

Table 1*

Persons who had multiple sclerosis \/	Cases \/	Antibody-indicating antigen \/	Antigen-indicating antibody			
			\/	\/	\/	\/
Type of strain:		Multiple-sclerosis			Neurosis	Arthritis
Stain or case #:		8125	8125	7700	8126	8134
Not receiving vaccine or	23	5.75	7.31	9.63	3.14	1.43
thermal antibody	20	6.25	8.07		5.04	2.15
Receiving antibody and vaccine	13	7.86	3.15		3.85	1.86

*Corrected to conform with narrative, S.H. Shakman, 1996)

From Bacteriological Research, Longview Hospital, Cincininati, Ohio. Submitted July 7, 1956.

APPENDIX D4:   *American Practitioner and Digest of Treatment*
(Philadelphia), 9(5), May 1958, pp. 755-761; reprinted by
permission of *Clinical Pediatrics* (successor publication)

Studies on Specific Prevention and Treatment of Diverse Diseases Shown Due to Specific Types of Nonhemolytic Streptococci

EDWARD C. ROSENOW, M.D.*
Minneapolis Minnesota

This article describes the methods used and reports the results
obtained in bacteriologic and imunologic studies of diseases, the
basic etiology and specific treatment of which are only partially
resolved or are wholly obscure.

Methods

Serial dilution cultures at steps of 10^{-2}, 10^{-6} and 10^{-10} were made of
nasopharyngeal swabbings, with cotton-wrapped aluminum wire swabs,
of the nasopharynx of persons having diverse chronic disease. The
material thus obtained was inoculated into tall (8 to 10 cm.)
columns of 0.2 per cent dextrose broth adjusted to pH 7.0, to which
pieces of fresh calf or beef brain were added, comprising
approximately one part of brain substance to six or seven parts of
broth, and autoclaved at 17 pounds'pressure for 20 minutes.

Cultures were made in this freshly prepared medium directly or
soon after sterilization, but after prolonged storage the test tubes
containing the tall columns of medium were heated in a boiling water
bath for 15 minutes to remove absorbed oxygen.

The streptococci isolated in dextrose-brain broth from
nasopharyngeal swabbings of persons having diverse diseases were
much alike in size, chain formation and staining reactions. All
were gram-positive and none produced zones of clear hemolysis on
blood-agar, but instead, small colonies surrounded by a narrow green
or indifferent zone were formed. The freshly isolated strains from
nasopharyngeal swabbings of persons who had diverse acute or chronic
disease on intravenous injection into mice and rabbits, localized
and produced lesions "electively" in the organ or organs
corresponding to those involved in patients from whom the
streptococci were isolated.[1-6]

The nasopharyngeal swabbings were obtained without touching the
tongue. The material on the swabs was washed off in 2 ml. of NaCl
solution, and then a tube of dextrose-brain broth was inoculated
with the swab, representing an extimated dilution of the material
swabbed of 10^{-2}. Two serial transfers were then made, with a nicrome
wire, the length of the column of dextrose brain-broth sterilized in
a Bunsen flame at each step, representing dilutions of inocula of 10^{-6}
and 10^{-10}, respectively. Growth after incubation at 35° C. for 19
to 24 hours, at a dilution of 10^{-2}, consisted of predominating
numbers of gram-staining, short-chained streptococci and, usually,
of moderate numbers of gram-staining micrococci and sometimes [p.
756:] also gram-negative, gas-producing bacilli. Growth at the
dilution of 10^{-6} usually consisted of a pure culture of short-
chained, alpha-type streptococci. Growths usually did not occur at

dilutions of 10^{-10}, but if positive such growth consisted of a pure culture of streptococci. One mililiter of pure cultures of streptococci from such end points of growth in dextrose-brain broth were inoculated into 200 ml. or gallon lots of 0.2 percent dextrose broth, and the streptococci, thus grown at 35° C. for 18 hours in the smaller lots, were harvested in a cup-type centrifuge. Pure cultures of streptococci in the gallon lots of 0.2 percent dextrose broth were harvested in the revolving bowl of the Sharples super-centrifuge. The sedimented streptococci from the cup-type centrifuge were in turn suspended in dense suspension of an estimated 200 bilion streptococci per milliliter, and those from the larger lots from the bowl of the super centrifuge at 1000 billion per milliliter of two parts of chemically pure glycerol and one part of saturated NaCl solution and stored in the dark in the refrigerator at 10°C. Some of the streptococci in this menstruum remained viable for months. All remained gram-positive and antigenically specific for many months on storage at 10°C. Such storage made it readily possible to maintain serologic and other specific properties of streptococci as isolated in diverse diseases.

Preparation, Diagnostic and Therapeutic Use of Streptococcic Thermal Antibody

The material in the supernatant of NaCl solution suspensions of streptococci and other bacteria, after the application of prolonged heat in the autoclave and the application of heat for a far shorter period on the addition of 1.5 percent of the oxidizing agent, hydrogen peroxide, are designated as "antibody" because (1) the supernatant of respective solutions agglutinated specifically the organisms from which they were prepared, (2) they precipitated specifically the respective dissolved antigens and (3) had curative action in the treatment of diseases in which they were causative, in a manner similar to the action of convalescent serum and the serum of horses hyperimmunized with the streptococcus.

In previous studies it was found that the intradermal injection of 0.05 ml of the euglobulin fraction of the serum of horses that had been immunized with streptococci isolated comparably in studies of diverse diseases elicited immediate erythematous reactions diagnostic of specific circulating streptococcic antigen in persons having the corresponding disease in studies of which the streptococcus was isolated.[7]

It was postulated that the formation of both natural and artificial antibody might be due to oxidation of antigen.[8] Accordingly, suspensions of streptococci in NaCl solution were subjected to the oxidative action of prolonged heat (96 hours) without hydrogen peroxide and for but three hours on adding 1.5 per cent hydrogen peroxide in the autoclave. As this was done specific agglutinins and other antibodies developed which had respective curative action on subcutaneous injection in therapeutic dosage in respective persons ill. Moreover, the intradermal injection of thermal antibody solutions prepared without hydrogen peroxide in persons who had a corresponding streptococcal infection elicited immediate erythematous reactions indicating circulating antibody.[8] Hence, skin tests and therapeutic injections were made with streptococcal thermal antibody and with antigen prepared from streptococci isolated in studies of diverse diseases. Thermal antibody solutions, of which 0.05 ml. was injected intradermally in skin tests, were prepared by autoclaving the respective specific and control NaCl solution suspensions containing 20 billion streptococci per milliliter for 96 hours and diluting the supernatant of such autoclaved suspensions with an equal volume of NaCl solution and adding 0.2 per cent phenol as a preservative.

Immediate erythematous reactions similar to reactions which followed the intradermal injection of the euglobulin fraction of the serum of immunized horses at the point of intradermal injection occurred. This was taken to indicate the presence of specific circulating streptococcic antigen. The maximal reaction was outlined with pen and ink and the size of the reaction was determined in square centimeters by superimposing circles of predetermined size on a transparent cellophane sheet 4 by 6 inches.

The maximal size in square centimeters of the immediate erythematous reaction to the intradermal injection of thermal antibody solutions prepared from specific and nonspecific or control alpha streptococci as isolated from the nasopharynx of 13 groups of persons having different diseases, comprising a total of 480 ill persons and 90 well control persons, are summarized in Table 1. The number of specific strains of streptococci from which thermal antibody solutions were prepared, as used in cutaneous testings in the 13 different disease groups and in well persons ranged respectively from four to ten, and antibody prepared from strains of streptococci isolated similarly from well persons ranged from five to six. The average [p. 757:] size of immediate erythematous reactions to the intradermal injection of two respective specific streptococcal thermal antibody solutions A and B, representing antibody from 10 billion streptococci per milliliter of NaCl solution autoclaved for 96 hours, indicating specific circulating streptococcic antigen, varied considerably, but were invariably far larger in each of the 13 groups of persons ill than were reactions to injection of control antibody solutions similarly prepared, from streptococci isolated in studies of well persons (Table 1). The reactions in question also were significantly greater than reactions to antibody prepared from streptococci isolated in studies of related diseases -- epilipsy and neurosis -- and far greater than reactions in unrelated diseases, such as respiratory infections, arthritis and alcoholism.

The reliability of erythematous reactions to the intradermal injection of thermal antibody indicating specific circulating streptococcic antigen is especially well shown in the 11 cases of alcoholism plus schizophrenia by the large reactions to specific antibody solutions A and B (9.25 and 8.25 sq. cm.) and to "schizophrenic" streptococcic antibody (7.85 sq. cm.), respectively. Specificity is also indicated by results obtained in patients having carcinoma and schizophrenia to antibody solutions A and B (6.90 and 10.90 sq. cm.), and to "schizophrenic" antibody (6.06 sq. cm.)

Specificity of Streptococci as Revealed by Agglutinative Titers of Thermal Antibody Solutions

In order readily to make comparisons of the agglutinative titers

of diverse thermal antibody solutions at four tenfold dilutions of
1-10 to 1-10,000, the degrees of agglutination at each of the four
dilutions was recorded in percentages. Thus, a 4 + agglutination at
each of the four dilutions or 16/16 = 100 per cent, and a total of
four pluses in the four dilutions, or 4/16 = 25 per cent. The
agglutinations in per cent, by thermal antibody solutions prepared
by autoclaving respective NaCl solution suspension of streptococci,
each containing 20 billion streptococci per ml. for 96 hours was
uniformly far greater for homologous than for heterologous nonhemolytic streptococci similarly isolated in studies of 174 persons
having respectively 16 diverse disease entities (Table 2). Of the
16 diseases studied, only two, [p. 758:] respiratory infection and
rheumatic fever, are currently considered to be due to infective
agents while the remaining 14 diseases are currently attributed to
causes other than infection.

The agglutination titer for the respective homologous streptococci
isolated similarly in the different disease groups by the homologous
thermal antibody solutions were uniformly significantly greater than
for heterologous streptococci. This is taken to indicate causal
[corrected] relationship of the respective nonhemolytic streptococci
in each of the 16 disease entities studied.

Nonhemolytic streptococci similarly isolated from well persons and
beta-hemolytic streptococci and staphylococci not shown in Table 2
were not agglutinated or were agglutinated in far lower titer than
streptococci isolated in studies of the diseases in question.

The agglutinative titers (Taable 3a) of the supernatants of
comparable NaCl solution suspensions containing respectively 10
billion streptococci per milliliter to which 1.5 per cent hydrogen
peroxide had been added and which had been autoclaved respectively
for 1,3, and 21 hours for suspensions containing 1, 10 and 100
billion streptococci per milliliter of NaCl solution were, with but
few exceptions, directly proportional to the duration of autoclaving
[p. 759] and to the number of streptococci per milliliter as
isolated in studies of schizophrenia, chronic encephalitis,
respiratory infection and persons in normal health. The total
titers of agglutinations, however, were far greater for the ʼ
homologous streptococci isolated in studies of schizophrenia than
for heterologous streptococci isolated in studies of chronic
encephalitis and respiratory infection. Agglutination of
streptococci isolated from well persons was negligible.

In keeping with the concept generally held that leukemia is
"cancer" of the blood are the high fairly comparable crosswise
agglutinative titers for the respective streptococci by thermal
antibody prepared from streptococci isolated in leukemia (69 and 63
per cent) and carcinoma (50 and 81 per cent) respectively. In
attempts perhaps to determine the mechanism involved, as regards the
acquisition of respective specificities of streptococci isolated
from the nasopharynx of persons having, respectively, schizophrenia
or normal health, they were grown crosswise in the serum of persons
having schizophrenia and in the serum of well persons. The effects
on the streptococci thus grown in the first, second and fourth-
culture generations are summarized in Table 4.

It will be seen that the agglutinative titer for "schizophrenic"
streptococci diminished strikingly after growth of the streptococci
in normal serum in each of the three culture generations, and that

the agglutinative titer of "normal" streptococci grown in "schizophrenic" serum caused them to be agglutinated by "schizophrenic" serum in far higher titer than when grown comparably in normal serum.

Similar results were obtained in other experiments not shown in Table 4, indicating that diverse specifities of alpha-type streptococci constantly present in the nasopharynx of human beings acquire specifities characteristic of respective hereditary traits of the host.

Since erythematous reactions to intradermal injection of thermal streptococcic antibody were found to [p. 760:] indicate circulating antigen and comparable injections of antigen were found to indicate circulating antibody in persons having diverse diseases, such skin tests were made in groups of persons having diverse diseases while not receiving and while receiving therapeutic injections of specific streptococcic vaccines and/or thermal antibody. The results obtained are summarized in Table 5. Cutaneous reactions indicating specific circulating streptococcic antigen were far greater in each of the five groups not receiving vaccine nor thermal antibody treatment than reactions indicating antibody (lateral and multiple sclerosis, muscular dystrophy, epilipsy and chorioretinitis). Moreover, reactions indicating circulating antigen were far greater than reactions indicating antibody in each of three groups (multiple sclerosis, schizophrenia and respiratory infections) before vaccine and antibody treatment was given. After such treatment, reactions in square centimeters indicating circulating antigen diminished, and reactions indicating circulating antibody increased comparable to the antibody titer in persons having migraine and poliomyelitis, respectively, who were receiving specific vaccine and antibody treatments.

The clinical results obtained from the combined subcutaneous use of respective specific streptococcic vaccine and thermal antibody solutions in the treatment of diverse diseases shown to be due to respective specific types of nonhemolytic streptococci are sumarized in Table 6. The results were highly favorable in each of six groups comprising a total of 182 persons having, respectively, respiratory infection, arthritis, schizophrenia, epilepsy, multiple sclerosis and migraine. Of the 182 cases thus treated, favorable results were obtained in 150. In the remaining 32 cases, results were indeterminate. Favorable results were also obtained, not shown in Table 6, in each of three cases of chorioretinitis, in both of two cases os sporadic poliomyelitis and in one case each of bronchiectasis, lupus erythematosus, coronary heart disease and myasthenia gravis. No apparent effects were obtained in one case each of muscular dystrophy and spasmodic torticollis.

Comments and Conclusions

Nonhemolytic or alpha-type streptococci culturally and morphologically indistinguishable as isolated from the nasopharynx of althgether, 480 persons (Table 1) having, respectively, 16 widely different or related diseases localized "electively" in the organ or organs of mice or rabbits corresponding to the organ or organs affected in the spontaneously occurring disease in persons from whom the streptococci were isolated (3).

Thermal antibody solutions prepared in the autoclave, without hydrogen peroxide, from NaCl solution suspensions of the streptococci isolated from nasopharyngeal swabbings of persons having respectively widely different diseases elicited immediate erythematous cutaneous reactions similar to reactions obtained following injection of the euglobulin fraction of the serum of horses that had been immunized with the respective streptococci. Such reactions are considered diagnostic of specific circulating streptococcic antigen. Moreover, the thermal antibody solution agglutinated specifically the streptococci isolated from the nasopharynx of persons having diverse diseases (Table 2).

The agglutinative titer of thermal antibody prepared from streptococci by autoclaving for three hours NaCl solution suspensions containing 10 billion streptococci per ml. to which 1.5 per cent hydrogen peroxide had been added was greater than, and as specific as, the titer of antibody prepared from suspensions without hydrogen peroxide autoclaved for 96 hours (Tables 3, 4).

Evidence from the use of the special methods has been obtained which indicates that the diverse specificities of nonhemolytic streptococci as isolated from the nasopharynx of persons having widely different chronic disease is acquired in the respective hosts rather than being due to streptococci from diverse extraneous sources, such as from milk and other foods from air or water supplies (Table 4). In this, as in other studies, the ability to isolate specific types of nonhemolytic streptococci from nasopharyngeal swabbings of persons having diverse diseases and from other sources is due (1) to the use of dextrose-brain broth in tall columns in test tubes which affords a a gradient of oxygen tension and other conditions highly favorable for growth of specific types of alpha streptococci, (2) to the selection of pure cultures of streptococci from the end point of growth of serial dilution cultures in dextrose-brain broth, and (3) to the preservation of viability at 10° C. for weeks and antigenic specificity for years by means of partial dehydration of the streptococci in dense suspensions of glycerol, two parts and of saturated NaCl solution, one part. Beneficial effects from the use of specific streptococcal vaccine and thermal antibody in treatment of the diverse diseases were clinically evident and strikingly indicated by the reduction in cutaneous reaction to intradermal injection of streptococcal thermal antibody indicating circulating streptococcal antigen and an increase in reactions indicating circulating antibody on intradermal injection of streptococcal antigen (Table 5). Similar favorable clinical results from the use of streptococcal vaccine and antibody in treatment of diverse diseases are summarized in Table 6. Thus of 182 persons so treated, favorable results were obtained in 150 persons, or 82 per cent.

*Emeritus member of the staff of the Mayo Foundation, Rochester Minnesota, 3701 Bryant Avenue South, Minneapolis, Minnesota.

References

1. Rosenow, E.C.: Elective localization of streptococci. *J.A.M.A.*,

65:1687, 1916.

2. Rosenow, E.C.: Elective localization of bacteria in diseases of the nervous system. *J.A.M.A.*, 67:662, 1916.

3. Rosenow, E.C. and A.C. Nickel: Results in various diseases from the elimination of foci of infection and of the vaccines prepared from streptococci having elective localizing power. *J. Lab. and Clin. Med.*, 14:504, 1929.

4. Jensen, L.B. and E.C. Rosenow: Cataphoretic mobility and elective localization of arthritic and neurotropic streptococci. *Proc. Staff Meetings, Mayo Clinic*, 5:49, 1930.

5. Sheard, Cleaves, C.B. Pratt, and E.C. Rosenow: Symposium on cataphoresis and localization of streptococci: the high frequency field as an agent in changing the cataphoretic velocity and localization of streptococci. *Proc. Staff Meetings, Mayo Clinic*, 8:496, 1933.

6. Rosenow, E.C. and F.R. Heilman. Newer methods of study and treatment of chronic streptococcal disease. *Proc. Staff Meetings, Mayo Clinic*, 12:252, 1937.

7. Rosenow, E.C.: Diagnostic cutaneous reactions to intradermal injection of natural and artificial antibody and of antigen prepared from streptococci isolated in studies of diverse diseases. *Annals of Allergy*, 6:485, 1948.

8. Rosenow, E.C.: Production in vitro of substances resembling antibodies from bacteria. *J. Inf. Dis.*, 76:163, 1945.

Table 1. [p. 757] *Diagnostic Erythematous Cutaneous Reactions to Intradermal Injection of Streptococcic Thermal Antibody Indicating Specific Circulating Streptococcic Antigen in Diverse Diseases*

Erythematous Cutaneous Reactions (Sq. Cm.) to Intradermal Injection of Streptococcic Thermal Antibody Indicating Circulating Streptococcic Antigen

Diseases Studied	Cases	Specific		Nonspecific					
		A	B	Schi	Epil	Neur	Resp	Arth	Alco
Schizophrenia	27	9.76	9.93			4.55	2.81	2.77	
	28	9.30	11.30		4.91	4.13	2.17	1.85	3.21
	83	10.12	9.20					2.60	
	78	10.25	9.10					2.13	
Multiple Sclerosis	21	9.20	6.87		5.25	4.25	2.90	2.66	2.66
Migraine	17	13.56	10.76			6.61	4.02	1.13	
Epilepsy	19	13.00	15.50					1.40	
	20	14.52	12.80					1.83	
Respiratory Infect	20	14.90	11.73					2.15	
	34	12.80	7.58					2.50	
Epidemic Polio.	19	11.60	10.79			3.16	2.0	2.19	
Arthritis	15	11.26	7.55						
Coronary Heart Dis	11	9.35	11.04	0.83				2.17	
Alcoholism & Schiz	11	9.25	8.25	7.85				1.26	
Lymphatic leukemia	5	8.48	8.76					1.64	
Chorioretinitis	5	8.10	9.70					4.50	
Carcinom	21	7.46	7.80	1.57				0.71	
Carcinoma & Schiz	26	6.90	10.90	6.06				1.92	
Control Well Pers.	90	0.71	0.49			0.18	0.14	0.63	

Total Cases   480
Total Controls   90

Table 2. [p. 758]. *Agglutination of Nonhemolytic Streptococci Isolated from the Nasopharyngeal Swabbing of Persons Having Diverse Diseases*

Suspensions of Nonhemolytic Streptococci Isolated from Nasopharyngeal Swabbings of Persons Having Respectively	Cases	Average Agglutination Titers in Per Cent at Four Tenfold Dilutions of 1-10 to 1-10,000 by the Respective Thermal Antibody Solutions for Suspension of Nonhemolytic Streptococci	
		Specific	Nonspecific
Respiratory infection	19	59	32
Coronary heart disease	14	75	26
Rheumatic fever	4	56	27
Sydenham's chorea	4	69	20
Myasthenia gravis	7	63	32
Hypertension	5	56	27
Schizophrenia	25	61	31
Epilepsy	18	65	38
Multiple Sclerosis	16	78	33
Epidemic Poliomyelitis	20	72	26
Experimental poliomyelitis	11	63	26
Infertility	63	81	30
Alcoholism	8	81	32
Diabetes	4	69	27
Leukemia	8	66	22
Carcinoma	8	65	23
Diseases 16; Cases	174	64	23

Table 3. [p. 758] *Agglutinative Titer for Streptococci Isolated from the Nasopharynx of Persons Having Schizophrenia, Chronic Encephalitis, Respiratory Infection or Normal Health, Respectively, by Thermal Antibody Prepared from Streptococci Isolated in Studies of Schizophrenia*

Suspension of Streptococci in Isotonic NaCl Solution	Agglutinative Titers (Per Cent) of the Supernatant of Comparable NaCl Solution Suspensions of Streptococci Containing 10 Billion per Ml. + 1.5 Per Cent H_2O_2, Autoclaved for 3 Hours, Isolated in Studies of Schizophrenia and Autoclaved respectively for:								
	1 hour			3 hours			21 hours		
Billions per ml.:	1	10	100	1	10	100	1	10	100
Isolated from nasopharynxes of persons having:									
Schizophrenia	25	63	75	50	63	81	75	81	88
Chronic Encephalitis	19	31	38	6	38	44	13	38	44
Respiratory Infection	10	38	44	6	19	44	13	38	44
Normal Health	6	0	0	13	0	0	13	0	0

Table 4. [p. 759] *Induction of "Normal" Agglutinative Properties in "Schizophrenic" Streptococci on Growth in Normal Serum and of "Schizophrenic" Agglutinative Properties in "Normal" Streptococci on Growth in "Schizophrenic" Serum*

Agglutination of Streptococci in Percentages, of Four Tenfold Dilutions of 1-10, 1-10,000 After Growth Respectively in "Schizophrenia" and "Normal" Serums

Material Studied:	Grown in:	Culture Generations		
		First	Second	Fourth
754 "schizophrenic"}	"Schizophrenic serum	44	63	69
streptococci }	"Normal" serum	25	19	25
756 "normal" }	"Schizophrenic" serum	31	63	69
streptococci }	"Normal" serum	13	19	25

Table 5. [p. 758] *Erythematous Cutaneous Reactions to Intradermal Injection of Specific Streptococcic Antigen and Antibody in Diverse Diseases and Specific Diminution in Reactions Indicating Antigen and an Increase in Reaction Indicating Antibody in Persons Ill Receiving Vaccine and Antibody Treatment*

Diseases Studied	Streptococcic Vaccine and Antibody Treatment	Cases	Antigen	Homologous Strains of Streptococci	Antibody
Multiple sclerosis	+	9	3.82		9.30
	+	17	4.32	8463	10.11
	0	17	10.52		4.85
Lateral sclerosis	0	1	19.64	8125	4.99
Schizophrenia	0	9	10.95	8130	6.80
	+	7	4.91		10.17
Migraine	+	7	7.84	8126	10.31
Epidemic poliomyelitis	0	4	11.50	8122	9.92
Muscular dystrophy	0	1	12.57	8140	4.62
Epilepsy	0	1	19.64	8129	4.99
Chorioretinitis	0	1	7.87	8128	3.14
Respiratory Infection	0	12	8.73	8131	4.10
	+	8	5.41		8.68

Table 6. [p. 760] *Clinical Results from the Use of Specific Streptococcal Vaccine and Antibody Treatment of Diverse Diseases*

Persons Having:	Cases	Results	
		Favorable	Indeterminate
Respiratory Infection	55	48	7
Arthritis	15	12	3
Schizophrenia	26	20	6
Epilepsy	22	18	4
Multiple sclerosis	52	43	9
Migraine	12	9	3
Total	182	150	32

APPENDIX D5: *DENTAL CENTENARY CELEBRATION* –1940, reprinted by permission of *The Maryland State Dental Association*:

Rosenow, E.C., Focal infection and elective localization in relation to systemic disease; review and results of further studies, Proceedings, Dental Centenary Celebration, Maryland State Dental Association, 1940, pp. 261-282, 1940.

****

ORAL DIAGNOSIS AND BACTERIOLOGY

Tuesday Afternoon, March 19

2:00–5:00 P.M.

(Fifth Regiment Armory—Room A, Basement Floor)

OFFICERS OF THE SECTION

Weston A. Price, D.D.S., M.S., *Honorary Chairman*, Cleveland, Ohio
Edgar A. Coolidge, B.S., M.S., D.D.S., *Honorary Vice-Chairman*, Chicago, Ill.
Harold Goldstein, D.D.S., *Secretary*, Baltimore, Md.

****

FOCAL INFECTION AND ELECTIVE LOCALIZATION IN RELATION TO SYSTEMIC DISEASE: A REVIEW AND RESULTS OF FURTHER STUDIES

By EDWARD C. ROSENOW, M.D.

(Rochester, Minn.)

(M.D., Rush Medical College, 1902. Professor of Experimental Bacteriology, The Mayo Foundation, Rochester, Minn.)

It is the purpose of this paper to review the clinical and experimental studies which have been made on focal infection and elective localization in relation to systemic disease. The literature on this subject in the field of medicine and dentistry is so enormous that detailed descriptions of results and complete references are beyond the scope of this report. Only the more important recent clinical and experimental results of my own work and that of others with references to the original communications will be given. For a more complete bibliography the reader is referred to previously published articles by myself (1-3) and by others (4-8).

The deleterious effects of bacterial infection on the host wherever found are both general and specific in varying degrees. As a rule, the more virulent the infecting microörganism the greater the general harmful effects, at the same time the greater the antibody response; and the more nonvirulent the infective agent, the less the general effects and antibody response and the more important the factors of specificity and focus. The former conditions usually prevail in acute diseases which often are self-limiting; the latter conditions usually prevail in chronic diseases which are often progressive.

CLINICAL CONSIDERATIONS

The importance of acute symptom-producing localized infections as a source of systemic disease has for years been generally recognized, but despite the large amount of evidence that has been adduced since Billings first showed that chronic, often symptomless, foci of infection may also be a source of disease in remote tissue this fact is still not sufficiently understood. The reasons for the lack of appreciation of the importance of this basic principle are manifold. The principle applies in a wide range of conditions and diseases. Its proper application is often difficult and calls for revision of well established procedures and the coöperation of the general practitioner, internist and widely different specialists including dentists and bacteriologists.

Symptomless foci are prone not to be suspected. They are not easily detected and may be situated in inaccessible regions. The resulting systemic diseases from such foci as a rule are mild in character and hence are usually not recognized in the early stages –the very time when elimination of foci does the most good.

Recurring inflammation in foci is still too often considered necessary to indicate causal relationship of focus to systemic disease. The bacteria isolated from symptomless foci, while having high specific virulence, usually have only a low general virulence and hence are incapable of causing acute symptoms at the primary focus. This is in accord with the fact that exacerbations of existing systemic disease or the first appearance of systemic disease following acute tonsillitis, pulpitis, prostatitis or respiratory infections usually occur not at the time of the acute attack but in from one to two or more weeks as the symptoms at the primary site subside or have disappeared.

Methods for elimination of foci by surgical or other means may be faulty. Removal of tonsils in the presence of focal infection in and about teeth is illogical and may do more harm than good. Statistical studies on the remote effects of removal of foci made by some authors who have had little or no clinical experience in this field have usually erred in not considering sufficiently the question of faulty methods, the presence of other foci, and, most of all, the development of new foci following the removal of certain types of foci such as infected tonsils and infected teeth. Conditions following removal of tonsils, if improperly done, may be worse than before (8–10). Quantitative bacteriologic studies made by Caylor and Dick (11) have shown that remnants of tonsils are more heavily infected than tonsillar tissue removed the first time. Moreover they showed that tonsillar tissue with a high bacterial count was more often associated with arthritis, neuritis and heart disease than that with a low bacterial count. Tonsillar tags, scar tissue covering partially removed tonsils, residual regions of infection in the jaw, with or without root tips, following removal of infected teeth, especially those which contain large areas of rarefaction, have been shown to be infected (table 1) and to predispose to disease in contiguous structures, such as maxillary sinusitis, and to systemic disease, and to prevent recovery from systemic diseases present at the time the primary foci were dealt with. The proper elimination of these infected structures has frequently been followed by enduring improvement or recovery, especially if done early in the course of the systemic disease (7, 12–15).

Roentgenographically positive teeth are usually, but not always, infected teeth. Hence their removal should not always be expected to produce beneficial effects and roentgenographically negative teeth are still nearly always considered sterile and harmless and are allowed to remain despite the fact that they have been shown by special methods to be infected by streptococci having elective localizing power in most instances (table 1) in which patients are suffering from mild or severe systemic disease. One cannot see bacteria at the apexes of these teeth in the roentgenogram. The infection here may or may not cause absorption of bone. Streptococci isolated from roentgenographically negative pulpless teeth in my experience have been more specifically virulent than those isolated from roentgenographically positive teeth.

Clinical studies on the effect of elimination of foci without regard to the organisms present in the focus or in the disease in question, as is commonly done, do not always suffice to establish cause and effect. Improvement, often permanent, following removal of foci from which the causative streptococci were isolated in my experiences has occurred with such regularity that I have come to consider lack of improvement as evidence that the removal was faulty, that the focus did not contain the causative micro-organism or that other foci were overlooked (11). Recurrence of the former symp-

tunity for the early application of a method such as this are especially great.

In general it may be said that the appreciation of the importance of the principle of focal infection by clinicians is in direct proportion to the thoroughness with which it has been applied. Purely theoretical considerations do not suffice. The lack of appreciation of this principle by some clinicians who admit that it applies in some instances and with whom I have had opportunity to examine patients is well illustrated by the conditions found in one large European clinic. The evidence of focal infection in relation to systemic disease had been entirely overlooked by its chief. Infection in foci was actually

TABLE 1
Results of Cultures from Dental Foci of Infection Obtained by Different Investigators

MATERIAL CULTURED	SPECIMENS CULTURED	POSITIVE IN LIQUID MEDIUMS, CHIEFLY DEXTROSE BRAIN BROTH		POSITIVE, 50 COLONIES OR MORE IN SOFT DEXTROSE BRAIN AGAR	
		Number	Per Cent	Number	Per Cent
Pulpless teeth:					
Apex, roentgenogram positive	728	600	82	290	40
Apex, roentgenogram negative	565	447	79	154	27
Root canal	89	67	75		
Total	1382	1114	81	444	32
Vital teeth:					
Normal pulp; roentgenogram negative; no fillings or periodontoclasia	548	210	38	4	0.7
Normal pulp; roentgenogram negative, with or without degenerating pulp or periodontoclasia	459	291	63		
Granulomas	86	78	91		
Residual regions following extraction of infected teeth	285	241	84	27 of 75	36
Root fragments	105	85	81	43 of 75	57

toms or the occurrence of new ones long after relief resulting from removal of a focus is taken to indicate the development of a new focus or activation of dormant foci.

The lack of striking clinical results from elimination of focal infection is often attributable to the fact that even now the attempts are too often made after the disease process has continued for a long time and secondary foci such as those in and about arthritic joints have become thoroughly established. It is a curious fact that the best clinical results usually are not obtained in large medical centers or hospitals, where advanced conditions are chiefly dealt with, but by physicians and dentists in out of the way places, where inclination, need and oppor-

demonstrated in five patients during my short visit. One of these had had recurring attacks of cholecystitis, two had suffered from rheumatic fever for about two months and two had had acute iritis. A history of an attack of acute tonsillitis shortly before the onset of systemic disease was elicited in each of these cases and large amounts of liquid pus were expressed from the tonsils of each patient by the method I use. Acute pulpitis with death of the pulp and draining dental sinuses occurred shortly before the attack in the two cases of acute iritis, and finally, the chief himself had been ill in bed suffering from an unexplained fever for some time prior to my visit. It was clearly evident that his condition was an example of the very problem under discussion. His teeth were literally floating in pockets of pus arising from pyorrhea and his breath was malodorous. He died several years later, long before he should have died, from cardiac disease.

I recall other tragic occurrences which indicate the importance of unrecognized focal infections in men of note who had had little or no experience in this field, who refused to permit removal of symptomless, pulpless teeth which were normal in the roentgenogram and who died of cardiac disease or other diseases or in whom disabling systemic disease developed not long subsequently, long before it should have developed.

These and many other examples which have come to my attention illustrate how far from accurate purely clinical observations may be concerning the etiologic importance of symptomless foci, especially pulpless teeth which are normal in the roentgenogram, most of them with fillings in the canals of the roots. The patient is not aware of their presence. Dentists and physicians generally consider such teeth to be sterile or harmless; roentgenograms are of little help even if they are repeatedly made, and the pathologist who performs the necropsy has not been schooled to consider them as in any way contributory to the cause of death. Experimental evidence that such foci are of importance is not lacking. Barnes and Giordano (16) have isolated from such foci, after death of the patients, streptococci with which they reproduced in animals the disease from which the patient died. I have had similar results. The findings in a most unusual type of case will serve to illustrate. A patient who had undergone an operation for congenital dislocation of the hip, although recovering satisfactorily, died suddenly from pulmonary embolism one month after the surgical procedure. Cultures by my methods from the embolus after surface sterilization yielded the usual green-producing Streptococci found constantly in instances of pulmonary embolism (17). A pulpless tooth normal in the roentgenogram was extracted after thorough disinfection of the site. Cultures from the apical end of this tooth yielded the same type of green-producing Streptococci as the streptococci obtained from the embolus. Pulmonary embolism was reproduced in rabbits and dogs following inoculation of the streptococcus from both the embolus and tooth, and the streptococcus was demonstrated in and isolated from the experimentally produced thrombi and emboli.

Failures to achieve clinical results have repeatedly been traced to inadequate or improper application of this principle. Nickel and Hufford (18), in a study of a series of patients in whom the symptoms of ulcer of the stomach or duodenum were not relieved following gastro-enterostomy or other operative intervention and after it was thought that all foci had been removed and after some had received autogenous streptococcal vaccines without effect, found evident foci from which causative streptococci were isolated. These foci had been overlooked and after removal of them and further administration of vaccines, relief from symptoms and healing occurred. In my own experience it is still common to find one or more evident foci in patients who have had every attention known to medical science, including the removal of foci of infection without relief, and whose symptoms often disappear following removal, for example, of one or more pulpless teeth which in the roentgenogram appear to be normal, or tonsillar tags or tonsils that were considered to be normal but from the upper pole of which liquid pus was expressed, or an abscess ruptured by the method we use in examining tonsils and from which foci the causative streptococci were isolated.

Simple though the question of the relationship of focal infection to systemic disease seems, the proper application and interpretation of all the factors concerned require diagnostic skill of the highest order. The occasional occurrence of exacerbations or extension of systemic diseases following removal or attempts at removal of various foci, especially infected teeth, emphasized by Reimann and Havens (6), deplorable as this is, should not prevent the application of this principle and should be interpreted as proof that a potential or active focus has been dealt with, but by inadequate methods. Such foci would with reasonable certainty do far more harm if retained indefinitely than is entailed occasionally by their removal even by the methods now employed.

In spite of the inherent difficulties which I have mentioned, favorable results from the application of this principle by critical clinical observers in the various branches of the healing art, including dentistry, have been reported in such great numbers and in so many different diseases, that any impartial reviewer must admit that they lend the fullest support to this basic concept. In a critical review of the case of the oral focal infection idea, McCluskie (19) stated:

There are peculiar difficulties due to the limitations of almost every type of evidence and the varying reactions of the individual. But on considering the vast amount of clinical and experimental observations which have been accumulated in recent years, one is driven to conclude that oral focal sepsis is more than mere theory, and though imperfectly understood, is founded on fact. From the practical point of view the rational remedy is early recognition of oral sepsis, an appreciation of its importance, and closer coöperation in treatment between the doctor and dentist.

EXPERIMENTAL STUDIES

Results of experimental studies support the clinical evidence regarding the importance of this principle. Of the different foci, those in the tonsils and in or surrounding the apexes of pulpless teeth are perhaps the most important primary foci chiefly for mechanical reasons, as we shall see. The crypts of tonsils dilated by scar tissue formed as a result of attacks of tonsillitis or of other causes, teeming with microorganisms, in well or sick persons, may be considered as veritable test tubes with permeable walls and as an ideal experiment in focal infection. Atrophy of lymphoid tissue after middle life of the patient, when systemic disease most often occurs or tends to progress, and the almost constant presence of fibrosis and pus, in extirpated tonsils (20), and of erosion or ulceration of the epithelial lining in their crypts afford especially favorable conditions for ready entrance into lymph or blood channels of the bacteria and their toxic and sensitizing products and for maintenance or acquirement of peculiar virulence of the streptococci. The apical ends of pulpless teeth, from the microscopic and bacteriologic standpoint, represent a cancellous, cavernous structure especially favorable for localization and continued growth of bacteria, and for forming a nidus for the dissemination of bacteria and their toxic products. In this circumstance, as in chronic infections in ulcerated crypts of tonsils, healing of an infective process is for mechanical reasons almost impossible. The routine, complete filling of the foramina at

the apex with impervious material through the root canal or any other means is microscopically and mechanically well-nigh impossible. Antiseptic agents placed into the root canal, although they may sterilize the root, cannot always reach or prevent the recurrence of infection at the apex. The filling in of bone after the antiseptic treatment of the root canal of teeth which are not normal in the roentgenogram does not mean that infection has disappeared (4). Cultures by my methods from the apexes of such pulpless teeth, obtained in a sterile manner for me by Professor Hess of Zurich with a trephine, after he reflected the mucous membrane opposite the apex of the tooth and sterilized the field of operation, yielded the usual green-producing streptococci.

It is mainly for these mechanical reasons that these two types of foci are more or less continously heavily infected and hence are especially prone to cause systemic disease. Absence of symptoms in these foci should not be interpreted as indicating freedom from infection, but rather as evidence of adequate drainage into the lymph or bloodstream of the bacteria and their toxic products. The bacteria contained in the granulation tissue at the apexes of pulpless teeth usually are not encapsulated by fibrous tissue, as is commonly taught; rather, since they are the incitants they are present in greatest numbers at the very periphery in which new blood vessels are being formed and in which inflammatory reaction is most in evidence, precisely where absorption channels are especially abundant. Mechanical removal, for the reasons mentioned, of such foci seems the only safe therapeutic method to employ. Experiments are not lacking which demonstrate why foci in tonsils or pulpless teeth are more important from the standpoint of systemic disease than infections in other tissues, such as those of lungs in bronchiectasis, cervix, prostate gland and the nonpocketed lymphoid tissue of nasopharynx and the normally functioning intestinal tract.

Injection of bacteria into soft tissues does not suffice to produce a chronic focus from which bacteria and their products are more or less continuously disseminated. Prompt healing with destruction of microörganisms, unless the microörganisms are highly virulent, usually occurs, whereas the implantation of infected nonabsorbable or porous material such as agar

(21–23), infected pieces of bone (24), suspensions or emulsions or aleuronat (25) and pledgets of cotton (26), does suffice to produce such a chronic focus. It has been shown that the infection in the nidus thus formed continues almost indefinitely, that it is associated with recurring cellular reactions (25), and that it is the cause of systemic effects, especially allergic states (21–23) similar to those attributable to foci, especially in tonsils and teeth. We have shown that it is usually impossible to desensitize or relieve symptoms of various diseases by means of specific vaccines in the face of active foci. Following removal of the responsible focus or foci, this often becomes possible.

The importance of chronic focal infection was well shown by Reith and Squier (27), who made blood cultures in large quantities of dextrose-brain broth in 293 apparently well persons. Positive cultures, chiefly streptococci, were obtained in fifty-three, or 27 per cent, of 194 persons who had chronic focal infection, whereas positive cultures were obtained from only 12 per cent of ninety-nine persons who had no demonstrable focus of infection. Of twenty-four persons harboring foci and having pain in joints or muscles, including chronic infectious arthritis, streptococci or diplococci were isolated from the blood of ten, or 42 per cent. Moreover, Reith and Squier found that the seasonal incidence of positive blood cultures in persons harboring foci of infection was consistently two to three times higher than it was in persons not harboring foci of infection, and in both groups the incidence of positive blood cultures was lowest during summer.

BACTERIOLOGIC ASPECTS OF FOCI OF INFECTION

Ordinary cultural methods usually do not suffice for the isolation of causative streptococci from dental and other foci of infection, or for the demonstration of specific virulence, elective localizing power and other specific properties. It was found very early in my work that microorganisms, especially streptococci in foci and systemic lesions, are highly sensitive to oxygen and other requirements for growth. The addition of pieces of brain to 0.2 per cent dextrose broth and to soft dextrose-brain agar made these mediums highly favorable for the isolation and maintenance of specific properties and of streptococci from the blood, from foci of infection

(especially those at the apexes of pulpless teeth), from prostatic fluid in prostatitis, from the exudate from the cervix in cases of endocervicitis and from metastatic or systemic lesions. The successful use of these or similar methods by others no longer leaves any doubt of their value.

Slight contamination of teeth may occur during extraction, despite every precaution which may in part be the source of the higher incidence of isolations of bacteria in liquid mediums than in the soft agar. Cultures made from apexes of pulpless teeth resected under sterile precautions have been shown by Precht, Rickert (28) and others to be infected. The much higher incidence of isolations from pulpless than from vital teeth simply cannot be referable to the aforementioned source of contamination. The chances for contamination are precisely the same in the removal of the two types of teeth. Moreover, we have found in our studies that the streptococci obtained from saliva and from pyorrheal pockets and gingiva grow readily on the surface of blood agar plates, whereas those obtained from apexes of pulpless teeth are highly sensitive to oxygen and usually do not grow on blood agar plates. We have used this fact to control our cultures, in addition to the swabbing of the gingivae just before extraction of teeth. Heavy growth in our mediums (dextrose-brain broth and dextrose-brain agar, which afford a gradient of oxygen tension and other favorable conditions) and no growth on blood agar, and a negative control swab culture, are considered proof that the organisms which grew were from the apex of the tooth and were not contaminants.

Austin and Cook (29) found by the use of these methods that anterior pulpless teeth quite without regard as to whether they were normal or abnormal in the roentgenogram, were not only more often infected but were also more heavily infected than vital teeth. Thus, 89 per cent of 100 pulpless teeth and 4 per cent of 100 vital teeth yielded streptococci in dextrose-brain broth; 75 per cent of 100 pulpless teeth yielded a heavy growth in dextrose-brain broth and none of the vital teeth yielded a growth. Differential quantitative cultures were also made by Rhoads and Dick (30) who found that the number of colonies obtained from the apexes of pulpless teeth was from 700 to 1000 times greater than the number obtained from vital teeth drawn and cultured in identical manner. Swanson and

Van Kirk (31) cultured the midportion and the apical ends of roots of extracted teeth after surface sterilization with alcohol and burning. Ninety-six per cent of 1220 root-filled pulpless teeth and 98 per cent of 582 non root-filled pulpless teeth yielded a growth, chiefly green-producing streptococci.

By means of a serial dilution method utilizing soft dextrose-brain agar, we have found that the number of viable streptococci at the apexes of pulpless teeth of persons having systemic

reported on the use of this method in culturing pulpless teeth with similar results.

In order that the reader may visualize the bacteriologic aspects, as now recorded in the literature, of infected teeth, granulomas, residual portions and root tips, I have summarized the results of cultures which have been made by different investigators by what we considered as adequate methods. The results of eight different studies made by fourteen different investigators (4, 33-41) are summarized in

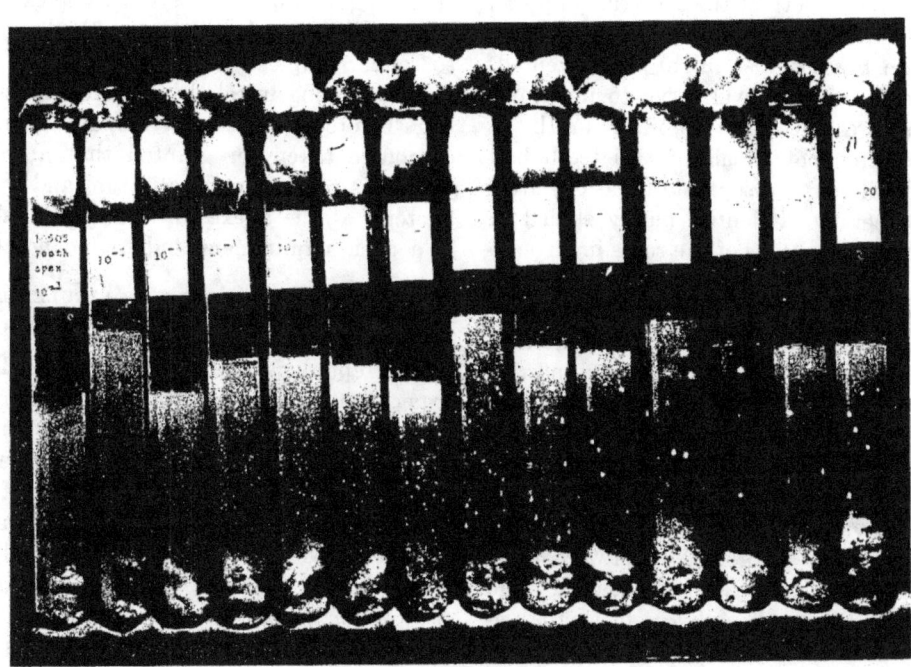

FIG. 1. Serial dilution culture of the washings of the apex of an extracted tooth appearing normal in the roentgenogram, in soft (0.2 per cent) dextrose brain agar. Note the diffuse growth in the first two dilutions, innumerable colonies in the next two dilutions and a progressive diminution in the number of colonies of streptococci, with six colonies in the 10^{-20} dilution ($\times \frac{1}{3}$).

disease, or the ability of these viable streptococci to grow as dilutions are being made, is far greater than the number or ability to grow of viable streptococci at the apexes of vital teeth. The results of growth obtained from pulpless teeth are well shown in figure 1. Washings obtained from the apex of the pulpless tooth yielded six colonies of streptococci at 10^{-20} or a dilution of one billion trillions of the material inoculated, whereas those from nonvirulent streptococci, such as isolated from vital teeth, yielded growth only to a dilution of 10^{-5} or, one hundred thousand. Thomas and Hubbell (32) have

table 1. It will be seen that there was a much higher incidence of growth of chiefly green-producing streptococci in cultures obtained from pulpless teeth, quite irrespective of whether the teeth were normal or abnormal in the roentgenogram, than in cultures obtained from vital teeth. The number of viable streptococci as indicated by the number of colonies that grew was from fifty to seventy times higher in the case of washings from the apexes of pulpless teeth than from the apexes of normal vital teeth without fillings or periodontoclasia. Nearly all granulomas, residual regions following extractions of infected teeth and root tips were found to be infected, and many were heavily infected.

The question of the value of different methods used in the filling of root canals calculated to prevent pulpless teeth from becoming infected has been studied in patients by myself and by Meisser and Brock (42) in dogs. At one time I, with many others, felt that if fillings of the canals of roots of teeth were made first after the material scraped from the canals had been proved to be sterile or in sterile teeth at the time the pulp was removed, then subsequently the infection from blood stream or otherwise might be prevented. The results in one case will serve to illustrate.

After cultures in dextrose-brain broth of scrapings of the root canals of two teeth had remained sterile on two separate occasions after root canal therapy, a dentist highly skilled in this work filled the canals of the roots in a sterile manner, controlling the placement of the fillings in the canals of the roots with the roentgenogram. The patient, of middle age, was well at the time. The teeth remained symptomless and normal in the roentgenogram, but the subject several years later began to suffer from severe progressive myositis and arthritis associated with exhaustion. Rest, fresh air and the best of care proved of no avail. The tonsils had been cleanly removed some years before. No foci were found other than the two teeth whose root canals had been filled, and the only pulpless teeth the patient had. These were drawn in a sterile manner. Cultures from the apexes yielded innumerable colonies of streptococci in dextrose-brain agar and a heavy growth in pure culture of short-chained streptococci in dextrose-brain broth. Intravenous injection in rabbits of the streptococci isolated was followed by extreme myositis and arthritis. The streptococcus was isolated from the experimentally induced lesions in muscles and joints. The patient made a prompt, complete and permanent recovery.

The experiments of Meisser (42) performed on dogs on the question of resistance to infection of teeth from which pulps were amputated or removed in a sterile manner and of which the root canals were filled by methods then in common use in human beings showed (1) that that amputated pulps invariably degenerated, (2) that all teeth from which the pulps were removed and in which the canal had been filled

in a sterile manner became infected in from two to eighteen months, (3) that staphylococci and streptococci having elective localizing power injected intravenously could be isolated more often and in larger numbers and for a much longer time from the pulpless teeth with fillings of the canals of the roots than from vital teeth and (4) that the pulps of vital teeth either remained sterile or rapidly became sterile at about the same time as the kidney, liver and blood, following these intravenous injections of bacteria. It is suggested on the basis of these experiments and many other facts that methods calculated to render pulpless teeth sterile and to prevent their becoming infected be proved efficacious in dogs before being used in human beings. It is of course taken for granted that any method that fails to prevent localization and growth of bacteria at the apexes of such teeth falls short of a basic requirement and should not be used.

THE INFECTING POWER OR VIRULENCE OF STREPTOCOCCI ISOLATED FROM FOCI

The reproduction or simulation of a disease in experimental animals is still the best evidence we have to show the etiologic relationship of an inciting agent to a particular disease entity. The results from intravenous injection of streptococci isolated from foci in a large number of diseases have been reported previously (1-3). I have summarized the results of experiments of my own in seven diseases also studied with my or similar methods by my co-workers and by others. The incidence of localization in the different organs obtained by the different investigators is summarized in tables 2 (1-3), 3 (43-51), and 4 (52-65). In each of the seven diseases, namely, ulcer of the stomach or duodenum, arthritis, iritis and other diseases of the eye, myocarditis, myositis, pyelonephritis and ulcerative colitis, the incidence of grossly visible lesions was consistently higher and usually much higher in each of the three series of experiments in the very organs or tissues affected in the patient from whom the respective strains were isolated (elective localization). Aside from a relatively high incidence of lesions of joints, greatest in the series studied by other investigators, there was no high point of lesions in the different organs following injection alike of nonspecific strains and strains from patients not suffering from systemic disease, a point overlooked by Valentine and Van

Meter (61). The incidence of specific lesions, although it is striking, does not adequately express how very specific these strains usually are on isolation as observed at necropsy.

The technic used by me in experiments on animals is described in detail in the original communications. Although in most instances the in dextrose-brain broth were made in previously warmed dextrose-brain broth in rapid succession (four to six or eight times a day), and single colonies from young (usually six to eighteen-hour) dilution cultures in dextrose-brain agar were transferred to dextrose-brain broth for injection. It is a curious fact that the streptococci from foci

TABLE 2
Elective Localization of Streptococci Obtained in Experiments by Rosenow in Diseases Also Studied by Other Investigators

SOURCE OF STREPTOCOCCI: DENTAL AND OTHER FOCI OF INFECTION IN PERSONS HAVING:	CASES OR STRAINS	ANIMALS THAT RECEIVED INTRA-VENOUS INJECTIONS	PER CENT OF ANIMALS SHOWING LESIONS IN:								
			Stomach or Duodenum	Joints	Eyes	Myocardium	Muscles	Kidneys	Colon	Endocardium	Gallbladder
Ulcer of stomach or duodenum	354	1539	65	9	1	1	2	5	3	5	7
Arthritis	723	1447	8	53	0	1	12	8	1	6	2
Iritis or other diseases of the eye	87	272	2	5	42	0	3	3	0	3	1
Myocarditis	7	36	6	6	0	61	19	3	0	50	0
Myositis	192	891	14	30	1	15	72	9	1	10	2
Pyelonephritis	50	168	7	12	0	4	10	73	3	5	2
Ulcerative colitis	206	527	1	1	0	0	1	1	58	1	1
No systemic disease (control group)	534	1329	14	18	8	6	3	9	5	11	5

TABLE 3
Elective Localization of Streptococci Obtained in Experiments by Co-workers of Rosenow

SOURCE OF STREPTOCOCCI: DENTAL AND OTHER FOCI OF INFECTION IN PERSONS HAVING:	NUMBER OF INVESTI-GATORS	CASES OR STRAINS	ANIMALS THAT RECEIVED INTRA-VENOUS INJEC-TIONS	PER CENT OF ANIMALS SHOWING LESIONS IN:								
				Stomach or Duodenum	Joints	Eye	Myocardium	Muscles	Kidneys	Colon	Endocardium	Gallbladder
Ulcer of stomach or duodenum	6	439	1231	52	6	1	13	16	3	0	2	1
Arthritis	8	511	1225	7	58	1	3	11	6	0	0	2
Iritis or other diseases of the eye	2	107	328	1	4	43	2	2	3	0	0	1
Myocarditis	1	11	39	0	18	3	38	5	5	0	0	3
Myositis	2	19	50	4	22	0	6	58	4	0	2	4
Pyelonephritis	3	21	96	5	17	0	6	12	83	0	6	8
Ulcerative colitis	1	15	60	7	5	0	0	8	3	60	0	0
No systemic disease (control group)	8	278	665	7	11	0	3	7	7	0	0	3

primary cultures (usually pure or nearly pure streptococci) were injected, it must not be supposed that elective localization following intravenous injection was not also obtained following injection of pure single-colony cultures or of pure cultures otherwise far removed from their original source. In order to not destroy the property on which elective localization depends, subcultures at the end point of growth in the serial dilution method in dextrose-brain agar and dextrose-brain broth, often representing an almost unbelievably high dilution, have especially high elective localizing power and other specific properties. One or two platings on the surface of blood agar usually sufficed to destroy this property.

The inoculated streptococci were isolated

routinely from, and often demonstrated in, the experimentally produced lesions and proved to be absent in healthy tissues. On reinjection they again caused the lesions characteristic of the disease in question. Reinjections in dosages small enough for the animals to live for a long time commonly produced a disease picture and microscopic lesions resembling those at hand in patients.

The inability of Lehmann (66) to obtain evidence of elective localization is clearly referable to variation from our technic. He injected from

Nickel and Judd (49) not only produced acute but also chronic cholecystitis and gallstones with streptococci obtained from patients who had cholecystitis. Nickel and Stuhler (67) produced chronic villous and deforming arthritis in rabbits with streptococci obtained from the prostate gland of patients who had rheumatoid arthritis.

The results of experiments by Illingsworth (68) and A. L. Wilkie (69) were particularly striking. D. P. D. Wilkie (70) stated that Illingsworth, working in his clinic, was able to show that, using Rosenow's special medium, streptococci could be

TABLE 4
Elective Localization of Streptococci Obtained in Experiments by Other Investigators

SOURCE OF STREPTOCOCCI: DENTAL AND OTHER FOCI OF INFECTION IN PERSONS HAVING:	NUMBER OF INVESTIGATORS	CASES OR STRAINS	ANIMALS THAT RECEIVED INTRAVENOUS INJECTIONS	PER CENT OF ANIMALS SHOWING LESIONS IN:								
				Stomach or Duodenum	Joints	Eye	Myocardium	Muscles	Kidneys	Colon	Endocardium	Gallbladder
Ulcer of stomach or duodenum	2	101	280	60	39	2	5	13	6		5	2
Arthritis	7	More than 75	415		59	0	13	9	13	0	12	0
Iritis or other lesions of eye	3	67	186	5	45	53	11	17	34	1	11	3
Myocarditis	3	More than 27	94	9	43	3	59	21	32	0	38	2
Myositis	1	14	86	10	44	1	13	56	18	0	13	4
Pyelonephritis	2	More than 10	96	3	45	2	13	16	58		7	
Ulcerative colitis	3	More than 20	119		20		13	3	8	42	12	
No systemic disease (control group)	7	141	300	7	31	2	17	13	19	0	1	6

1 to 2 cc. of broth cultures of streptococci obtained from single colonies, presumably from blood agar, and he killed surviving animals one week or longer after injection. We injected from 5 to 10 cc. of the primary culture of streptococci in dextrose-brain broth and killed animals to search for lesions one to three days following injection. Despite Lehmann's different technic, he did produce endocarditis with Streptococcus viridans in sixteen animals, and by the use of dextrose-brain broth, succeeded in isolating streptococci from 164 or 167 granulomas, results which are in accord with our results and with those of others.

grown from the wall of the gallbladder in quite a large number of cases in which the bile was sterile. He further showed that organisms of the *coli* group are relatively infrequent except in acute suppurative cases. This work has been carried a step further by A. L. Wilkie (69), who has shown that cholecystitis is almost invariably an intramural streptococcal infection, and Rosenow's contention of a selective affinity of this organism for the gallbladder in experimental animals is strikingly true. A. L. Wilkie concluded, after his experimental studies, that (*a*) cholecystitis would appear to be a blood-borne streptococcic intramural infection; (*b*) late changes including formation of gallstones following repeated injection of the streptococcus emphasized the intramural path; (c) the intramural pathologic changes produced experimentally resemble in every detail the changes seen in the human gall-bladder in cholecystitis.

Jarlov and Brinch (8) produced chronic arthritis, and concluded from their long series of experiments that certain strains of streptococci especially those from arthritis produced arthritis more often than others. Cecil and Angevine (71) produced in rabbits, with small doses of streptococci obtained from foci of infection and blood and joint tissues in arthritis, pathologic lesions very similar to those of rheumatoid arthritis in man.

In addition to these aforementioned highly specific effects, there is a close parallelism between the incidence of involvement of various tissues or organs as observed clinically and the incidence of lesions as found in experiments in animals after the intravenous inoculation of organisms recovered from dental and other foci of infection. The lesions most frequently seen in patients referable to focal infection are those of the locomotor system, joints, muscles, tendon sheaths and ligaments. The kidney, skin, heart, stomach, duodenum and eyes are often affected. Less commonly, other organs such as those of the nervous system and blood-building tissues may be involved. Rarely, very unusual localizations of streptococci from dental and other foci of infection such as onychia occurred as shown by Haden and Jordan (72), thyroid disease (especially thyroiditis) as shown by Cantero (73) and lesions of the gasserian ganglion produced electively in experiments of my own in cases of trigeminal neuralgia. The removal of foci in instances of trigeminal neuralgia (and in my experience their presence is constant in this condition) obviously should be done as a preventive measure before central irreversible lesions have occurred, rather than as a curative measure long after the disease has existed. Van Kirk and Swanson (74) produced encephalitis in rabbits by the intravenous injection of streptococci obtained from the pulp-less teeth from patients who had encephalitis, an observation corroborative of our own studies.

Nickel and Mussey (75), Fasting (76), Curtis (77) and Reith (78) have shown that streptococci, isolated from foci of infection in women who had spontaneous abortion not caused by syphilis, had predilection for the uterus and caused abortion in rabbits. Following removal of such foci, pregnancies went to full term. Horton and Dorsey (79) produced vascular lesions with gangrene of the toes in rabbits with material containing streptococci from patients who had thrombo-angiitis obliterans. The intravenous injection of relatively small numbers of streptococci grown not in the test tube but in various foci such as pyorrheal pockets, apexes of pulpless teeth and tonsils, often sufficed to cause lesions referable to streptococci electively in various diseases.

ELECTIVE LOCALIZATION OF STREPTOCOCCI OBTAINED FROM EXPERIMENTALLY INDUCED DENTAL FOCI

Methods other than the intravenous inoculation of freshly isolated living cultures of streptococci have sufficed to show the existence of the property of elective localization. Marked ulceration of the stomach in guinea pigs occurred following the intraperitoneal injection of the streptococcus from a sinus draining an infected tooth of a patient who had acute ulcer of the stomach and recurrent hemorrhage. Cure was prompt and permanent following removal of the infected tooth from which the sinus issued. Suppurative pulpitis and hemorrhagic edema of the periosteum opposite the roots of the teeth of animals followed the intraperitoneal injection of the streptococcus from the pulp of a tooth of a patient who had recurring attacks of pulpitis, dental neuritis and myositis. Squier and Bach (80) produced hypotension in rabbits by injecting the streptococcus isolated from dental and other foci of infection in patients having hypotension into the joints (foci) of rabbits. Moreover, streptococci that manifest elective localizing power have been shown to produce within themselves, and to free in dextrose-brain broth cultures, poisons or toxic products which specifically localize and produce lesions in the same tissues as do the living microörganisms. Specific effects have been produced by the intravenous or intracerebral injection, respectively, of the living streptococci, the dead bacteria or filtrates of active cultures obtained from patients suffering from pyelonephritis, myositis, endocarditis, myocarditis, arthritis, dental neuritis and pulpitis, ulcer of the stomach or duodenum and myasthenia gravis.

Thus, the induction by Meisser and me (81) of

chronic foci in the teeth of dogs with streptococci and staphylococci shown to have elective localizing power was followed by a high incidence of specific localization in the case of strains of streptococci obtained from patients who had nephrolithiasis (7), alkaline phosphatic cystitis, ulcer of the stomach and ulcerative colitis, chorea, encephalitis and epidemic hiccup; and the aforementioned induction was followed by a high incidence of localization in the kidney of staphylococci obtained from the maxillary sinus of a patient who had nephritis.

Jones and Newsom (82), following the production of similar foci in the teeth of dogs with streptococci having affinity for the vascular system, produced symptoms and lesions of the myocardium and endocardium resembling those characteristic of chronic heart disease in human beings. The conditions in the experiments in which elective localization through foci was produced simulated in important respects those at hand in patients. The teeth from which the pulps were removed became discolored. They remained free from pain or tenderness, and at the apexes absorption of bone with formation of granulation tissue in varying degree occurred similar to that observed at the apexes of pulpless teeth in human beings, and as this occurred, specific systemic disease developed in addition to an increased susceptibility to intercurrent infections. At the end of the experiments the streptococci having elective localizing power were isolated from pulp canal and from the granuloma, and were demonstrated microscopically in large numbers in sections. The intravenous inoculation in rabbits of the strains thus isolated revealed the fact that they had retained their elective localizing power for months in the experimentally induced dental foci. The results of these basic experiments were not considered by Holman (83), and Reimann and Havens (6) in their critical reviews. Holman concluded: "However, what Rosenow and his followers particularly showed and what all the other investigators of the problem have definitely demonstrated is that streptococci do localize in various organs and tissues and can produce lesions at least sufficiently suggestive of those found in man so that their potential danger in infected foci cannot be neglected." Reimann and Havens and other critics conceded that the principle of focal infection applies in some cases.

I wish now to discuss other observations which indicate that the streptococci commonly isolated from foci, that is, streptococci that have elective localizing power, have etiologic significance.

RELATIONSHIP OF FOCI OF INFECTION TO HYPERSENSITIVENESS AND ALLERGY

Although I have studied chiefly the specific localizing and necrotizing power of the bacteria isolated from foci and their products, the question of the effect of these and of the focus on the host, aside from the induction of specific disease, has also been considered. Symptoms resembling those of anaphylaxis were produced in guinea pigs, rabbits and dogs by primary intravenous injections of autolysates and of leukocytic digests of pneumococci, streptococci and other bacteria. The appearance, and later disappearance, of these highly toxic properties were associated with proteolysis. Hypersensitiveness to extracts and autolysates of pneumococci and streptococci was also obtained, a point reported on more recently, and with similar results, by Zinsser and Grinnell (84). Leukocytosis and destruction of organisms following the intraperitoneal injection of the corresponding antigen or bacteria in the hypersensitive animals were greater and more rapid than in normal animals. The hypersensitive animals exhibited decreased resistance to the intraperitoneal injection of large numbers of virulent pneumococci, but exhibited increased resistance or immunity following the inoculation of small numbers. The induced hypersensitiveness or allergy in guinea pigs to pneumococcic extracts disappeared on repeated inoculations of dead pneumococci or pneumococcic extracts and autolysates and after recovery of the animals from pneumococcic infections.

The difference in the behavior of normal and sensitized guinea pigs toward unautolyzed and autolyzed extracts of pneumococci was especially illuminating in these early studies. The unautolyzed extracts were nontoxic to normal animals and very toxic to the sensitized animals. Partially autolyzed extracts were very toxic to normal animals, and only slightly toxic, or not at all, to sensitized animals, whereas more completely autolyzed extracts were nontoxic to both. These results and those of Zinsser and Grinnell (84) indicate that a parenteral digestion of bacteria and bacterial antigens into highly toxic cleavage products occurs more rapidly, and, it would seem, in greater amount, in experimental or spontaneous hypersensitiveness, or in the presence of allergy, than in normal animals. Zinsser and Grinnell (84) assert that in the autolysis of various bacteria there are set free substances which stimulate the allergic state and that such autolysates are the best reagents with which to test hypersensitiveness.

Patients who have foci of infection, especially those who have chronic infectious arthritis or myositis and neuromyositis, often were found to be exceedingly sensitive to streptococcic vaccines. The dogs in which we successfully produced chronic foci about the teeth, in addition to exhibiting lesions specific for the strains of streptococci inoculated, lost weight and hair, and became more susceptible to intercurrent infection. A diet sufficient to keep the control animals well was inadequate for the dogs who had chronic foci of infection.

Derick, Hitchcock and Swift (85), and Clawson (22) have shown that focal infection resulting from the inoculation of nonhemolytic streptococci may be followed by a state of hypersensitiveness and they have emphasized the relationship of allergy to streptococci in rheumatic fever. Swift, Derick and Hitchcock (21) induced a hyperergic state in rabbits by the production of focal lesions; this state was maintained for months by making an agar focus infected with allergizing green-producing streptococci. Clawson (22) and Birkhaug (23) obtained similar results. Moon and Stewart (86) produced lesions in rabbits and dogs essentially like those of rheumatic fever by establishing foci of infection in the subcutaneous tissues with pledgets of cotton soaked in cultures of streptococcus viridans obtained from persons who had rheumatic fever. Harkary (87), in a memorial volume to Dr. Emanuel Libman, stressed the importance of focal infection in bacterial allergy in asthma and arthritis. Cook, in his paper at the Dental Centenary Celebration at Baltimore stressed the importance of focal infection in relation to allergic states. Weisberger (88) showed that dissemination of bacteria from foci established at the apexes of teeth in rabbits was far greater following injection of horse serum into sensitized animals than it was following injection of the same serum into nonsensitized animals.

Patients whom I have found to be extremely sensitive and whose condition improved following removal of foci and guarded use of vaccines became less sensitive to the vaccine as improvement occurred. The mechanism of bacterial and protein hypersensitiveness has been shown to be the same. Hence, a focus, in addition to affording conditions favorable for the production of specific systemic disease, may have more general deleterious effects, the nature of which may be determined in part by the bacterial antigens absorbed from chronic bacterial foci, and in part by the peculiar reactivity of the host.

Streptococci which had specific elective localizing power and characteristic cataphoretic velocity repeatedly have been demonstrated to be present in various foci of infection and elsewhere (carrier state) for a period of years, and long after the onset of symptoms among patients suffering from certain chronic diseases, such as arthritis and encephalitis. This is believed to be of fundamental significance, for it indicates that the patient's tissues or tissue juices afford the conditions favorable for streptococci to acquire and maintain particular elective localizing power and cataphoretic velocity, peculiar to the disease from which the patient is suffering.

May not this be a reason why so many chronic diseases tend to persist, recur and run a progressive course with so few localizations elsewhere, and why they are so difficult to cure? Might not the inherited rheumatic diathesis, the neuropathic or the allergic constitution and other "diatheses" and "constitutional predispositions" be expressions in part of a peculiar interaction between host and invading organism, and not expressions merely of an inherited "weakness" of joint, brain or other organ, as is usually assumed? The focus furnishes a ready source of infecting organisms and bacterial antigens to which the host reacts variously, depending, among other factors, on inherited or acquired constitutional peculiarities. If of allergic tendency, local and general hypersensitiveness are prone to develop; if of normal constitution, increased resistance or immunity is probable. The particular tissue in which local hypersensitiveness develops and in which allergic manifestations are especially marked is determined, it would seem, by the specific or elective localizing power of either or both the bacteria and their antigens or toxins.

ELECTROPHORETIC MOBILITY OR VELOCITY AND ELECTIVE LOCALIZATION OF STREPTOCOCCI

To obviate the use of animals and to determine, if possible, more precisely wherein lie the reasons for elective localization, Jensen and I (89) have studied cataphoretically streptococci that have elective localizing power, and Sheard, Pratt and I (90) have studied the effects of exposing streptococci having elective localizing power and characteristic cataphoretic time and velocity to the high frequency field. Among other interesting facts, it has been discovered that there is a close parallelism between elective localization and cataphoretic time and velocity of streptococci. The details of the technic are described in pub-

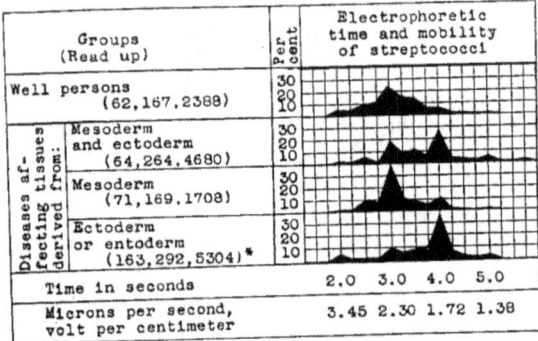

Groups (Read up)	Per cent	Electrophoretic time and mobility of streptococci
Well persons (62,167,2388)	30 20 10	
Diseases affecting tissues derived from: Mesoderm and ectoderm (64,264,4680)	30 20 10	
Mesoderm (71,169,1708)	30 20 10	
Ectoderm or entoderm (163,292,5304)*	30 20 10	
Time in seconds		2.0 3.0 4.0 5.0
Microns per second, volt per centimeter		3.45 2.30 1.72 1.38

*The figures in parenthesis indicate, respectively, the number of strains, cultures and streptococci timed in each group studied.

FIG. 2. Distribution curves of cataphoretic time and velocity of streptococci isolated from dental and other foci of infection, according to the embryologic origin of the tissues chiefly affected.

lished reports. It is sufficient to state herein that the migration rate, under constant voltage in an electrical field, of the different streptococci is determined in the cataphoretic cell of the Northrop-Kunitz-Mudd apparatus. Since under these conditions migration rate is directly proportional to surface charge, it follows that the greater the charge, the faster the streptococci move. For example, streptococci from atria of infection of patients who have chronic infectious arthritis and other diseases involving tissues derived from the mesoderm and which have respective elective localizing power, have, by our measurements, chiefly a cataphoretic time of 3.0 seconds and velocity of 2.22 microns per second, volt per centimeter, whereas streptococci from similar sources, among patients who have encephalitis and certain other diseases of the nervous system

and which tend to localize electively, have a cataphoretic time and velocity of chiefly 4.0 seconds and 1.67 microns per second, volt per centimeter.

In figure 2 are given the average distribution curves of cataphoretic time and velocity of streptococci isolated from infected teeth and other foci of infection of persons having streptococcic diseases affecting tissues derived from ectoderm or endoderm, mesoderm, and mesoderm and ectoderm and of well persons. The higher the column at a given time or velocity, the larger the number of streptococci that traversed the unit distance (50 microns) at that particular time or velocity. The cataphoretic time and velocity of streptococci isolated from the depths of the jaws and from apexes of pulpless teeth of persons having various diseases during epidemics of influenza, although characteristic of each disease when influenza was not at hand, were, as in the case of streptococci isolated from the nasopharynx, also more like those of streptococci from influenza.

Exposure to the high-frequency field caused marked changes in the cataphoretic time and velocity of streptococci and, concomitantly, in their elective localizing power. Thus, in a series of experiments in which animals were injected with unknown cultures of streptococci, it was found that when the cataphoretic time and velocity of streptococci isolated from instances of chronic infectious arthritis (which streptococci, when untreated, manifested marked affinity for joints) had become cataphoretically like those of streptococci isolated from instances of encephalitis, the streptococci had lost affinity for joints, and concomitantly, had acquired affinity for the nervous system. Conversely, when streptococci isolated from instances of encephalitis (which streptococci on isolation had marked affinity for the nervous system) had become cataphoretically like those isolated from instances of arthritis, they had lost affinity for the nervous system and had acquired affinity for joints of animals that had received intravenous injections.

The work on cataphoresis has proved of importance in still other respects. I could often predict before injection of a given culture whether or not localization would be specific by determining the distribution curve of cataphoretic time and velocity of the streptococci. This has made clear an otherwise puzzling fact, often observed in elective localization work; namely, the sudden disappearance of elective or all localizing power, or the appearance of new affinities following successive animal passage and repeated transfers in cultures. It has yielded information which makes more explicable certain discrepancies of some workers in this field, for consideration of the inherent property of changeability of streptococci, is basic in studies on focal infection and elective localization. A lack of appreciation of this fact and lack of sufficient attention to technical details have led to misinterpretations and failures to repeat some of these results.

Of great importance is the fact that the medium dextrose-brain broth with which I have obtained the best results in experiments on elective localization, is by far the best medium for preserving characteristic cataphoretic time and velocity of streptococci of any mediums that we have tested. Several transplants in other mediums, such as plain broth, dextrose-beef broth, veal infusion broth, heart muscle infusion broth, yeast broth and even the same dextrose-brain broth minus the brain, often sufficed to convert a strain in which originally most organisms had characteristic cataphoretic velocity and which had elective localizing power, into one of very different velocity with changed localizing power or without this faculty.

As has been pointed out, the antibody content of the serum of patients suffering from the different diseases studied was not uniformly high enough to obtain consistent results by the usual methods of agglutination and precipitation to prove causal relationship. The work on cataphoresis has furnished a method whereby consistent results have been obtained. The serum obtained from patients suffering from various diseases in which elective localization has been demonstrated has specific slowing (charge-reducing) action on the respective streptococci having characteristic distribution curves of cataphoretic time and velocity and elective localizing power. Among the diseases in which this has been demonstrated are acute and chronic arthritis and encephalitis, epidemic hiccup, persistent postoperative hiccup, epidemic vertigo, acute and chronic poliomyelitis, and multiple sclerosis and chorea.

SEROLOGIC PROOF OF SPECIFICITY OF STREPTOCOCCI

Because of the great variability of streptococci as isolated from infected teeth and other foci

of infection in various diseases, the prompt loss of specific properties on artificial cultivation, their tendency to agglutinate spontaneously as grown on the usual mediums, and the use of inadequate methods of agglutination with the serums of patients, little evidence has been obtained with which to indicate the causal relationship of streptococci to chronic disease. In a large measure, these difficulties have been overcome by the use of dextrose-brain broth for the primary isolation, by growing the streptococci for purposes of agglutination in this medium or in dextrose broth for one culture generation and by preserving the centrifuged streptococci in dense suspension in glycerol (two parts) and 25 per cent solution of sodium chloride (one part). One cubic centimeter of this menstruum was made to contain the growth of from 50 to 500 cc. of the culture. The antigens for agglutination were prepared by diluting the suspension in glycerol-sodium chloride solution to the density of a broth culture with salt solution to which 0.2 per cent phenol had been added. The patient's serum was likewise diluted in sodium chloride solution to which 0.2 per cent phenol had been added, to one-half the desired dilution and then 0.2 per cent of suspension and serum dilutions were mixed and placed at 50°C. (122°F.) for from eighteen to twenty-four hours, at the end of which time readings were made. Highly specific results were obtained with many, but not all, of the serums obtained from patients who had chronic disease.

The streptococci isolated, grown and preserved in the manner indicated were found to be highly satisfactory also for the preparation of hyperimmune serums in horses and for agglutination experiments with these antiserums. Moreover, the antiserums prepared in this way caused precipitation (antibody-antigen reaction), often specific, when overlaid in small precipitation tubes with cleared washings in sodium chloride solution of nasopharyngeal swabbings or with the serum of patients. The results summarized in table 5 show how very specific this reaction was with the serums obtained from the respective patients. The demonstration by the precipitation test of the common presence of streptococcic antigen in the serums of patients who had chronic disease that was antigenically related to the streptococcus with which the reacting serum was prepared is new, and, from the

TABLE 5
Precipitation Reaction with the Serum of Patients and the Serum of Horses Hyperimmunized with Streptococci

SOURCE OF SERUMS (ANTIGENS)	CASES STUDIED	PERCENTAGE OF POSITIVE REACTIONS WITH						
		Antiserums Prepared with Streptococci from:					Control Serums	
		Encephalitis	Poliomyelitis	Chronic Ulcerative Colitis	Myasthenia Gravis	Chronic infectious Arthritis	Pneumococcus I, II, III	Normal Horse
Encephalitis	55	78	31	40	45	64	0	0
Spasmodic torticollis	12	75	41	41	25	58	0	13
Chronic poliomyelitis	20	50	60	30	25	35	0	5
Acute poliomyelitis:								
Human beings	28	46	64	4	17	18	0	7
Monkeys	9	55	89	44	33	33	0	0
Neuritis, herpes, hiccup	12	92	8	33	17	42	0	0
Epidemic gastro-enteritis	51	67	33	90	60	45	0	0
Myasthenia gravis	8	63	25	38	88	75	0	13
Neurofibromyositis	24	63	29	41	33	83	0	13
Asthmatic bronchitis	16	68	25	37	31	37	0	0
Chronic infectious arthritis	12	50	8	8	8	67	0	0
Iritis	11	27	9	9	0	45	0	0
Normal controls	48	8	0	6	2	10	0	0

TABLE 6
Erythematous Reactions to Intradermal Injection of the Euglobulin Fraction of Antistreptococcic Serums

SOURCE OF SERUMS (ANTIGENS)	PERSONS TESTED	AVERAGE REACTIONS (SQ. CM.) TO:											
		Euglobulins Prepared with Streptococci from:										Control Serums	
		Encephalitis Chronic	Acute*	Poliomyelitis Typical	Los Angeles	Chronic Ulcerative Colitis	Ulcer of Stomach or Duodenum	Myasthenia Gravis	Chronic Infectious Arthritis	Iritis	Pyelonephritis	Pneumococcus I, II, III	Normal Horse
Encephalitis	92	6	5	3	3	3		2	3		0	1	0
Spasmodic torticollis	30	5	4	4	4	1	2	4	5			1	1
Hiccup	10	10	8	4		1		1	2			1	1
Amyotrophic lateral sclerosis	19	4	5	5	8			5	1				0
Chronic poliomyelitis	27	3	2	8	8	6		3	2			1	0
Optic or peripheral neuritis	17	8	7	7				3	4			1	0
Chronic ulcerative colitis	13	5			3	10	4		5		2	1	1
Epidemic gastro-enteritis	69	3				12	3	2	5		1	2	1
Ulcer of stomach	39	5	3	4	5	10	11		4		2	0	0
Neuromyositis and fibrositis	35	5	5	6	5	4	2	3	9	3	3	0	0
Rheumatic arthritis, neuromyositis and carditis	28	5	5	5		4			9	1		2	0
Myasthenia gravis	19	4	2	2		1		11	3			1	1
Chronic infectious arthritis	42	3	3	0	3	3	3	1	8		2	2	0
Osteitis deformans	10	3	2		1			1	8				0
Iritis	12	6		1		5			14	11		4	1
Pyelonephritis	19	1	8	1		5	2		3		9	3	0
Diseases not due to streptococci	33	0	0	1		1	0	0	1		1	0	0
Well persons	32	1		1		1	1	0	1			1	1

* St. Louis type.

standpoint of pathogenesis and specific therapy, is considered to be of great importance.

It was also found that intradermal injections of the euglobulin fraction of the antiserum prepared in horses, in the manner indicated, elicited an immediate (ten minutes) erythematous-edematous reaction in patients suffering from a streptococcic disease identical to, or closely related to, the one in studies of which the immunizing strain of streptococcus was isolated. This test is an application to streptococcic diseases of the Foshay antigen-antibody reaction, first noted in relation to tularemia. It serves to determine whether or not a patient is suffering from a streptococcic infection, and if so, of what particular type and what antiserum or stock vaccine had best be used therapeutically. The results recorded in table 6 well illustrate how specific the test is as applied to patients having different diseases.

COMMENT AND SUMMARY

A review and results of further studies of clinical, bacteriologic and experimental observations on focal infection and elective localization are reported.

Despite the lack of clinical improvement or cure following the elimination of foci of infection in many cases and in certain diseases, alleviation of symptoms occurs so often and in so many diseases that this principle should be applied not so much as a form of therapy unrelated to other conditions but as one of other well-established procedures in diagnosis, prognosis and treatment.

Bacteriologic studies conducted by adequate methods no longer leave any doubt that chronic, often symptomless, foci, especially those of tonsils and teeth, are infected, usually heavily infected, and chiefly by green-producing streptococci. The results of earlier experimental studies have been corroborated sufficiently often by myself, my co-workers and other investigators to indicate conclusively that the bacteria (especially the green-producing streptococci found in the presence of chronic focal infection) are not only virulent but are usually specifically virulent. Their probable or undoubted causal relationship to a number of diseases has been shown by intravenous and other methods of injection in animals, by the induction with streptococci of chronic foci especially at the apexes of teeth in dogs, by cataphoretic studies, by diagnostic cutaneous tests made with the euglobulin fraction of the serum of horses hyper-immunized with the respective freshly isolated strains, by the precipitation reaction with the respective undiluted antistreptococcic serums of horses and the blood serum of patients and by agglutination tests made by special methods.

The property or tendency of these streptococci to localize and to produce lesions electively has been shown to be referable to a toxic substance or substances elaborated by the organisms within themselves and free in the medium in which they grow. Filtrates of actively growing cultures of the respective streptococci, the dead bacteria and the live culture, all tend to localize and produce symptoms and lesions specifically or electively in the tissues or organs characteristic of the disease the patient had and from whose foci the streptococci were isolated. The specificity of the streptococcus on isolation from dental and other foci is often so marked that the clinical and pathologic pictures of certain diseases have been reproduced by the induction of chronic foci of infection at the apexes of pulpless teeth in dogs, and these pictures simulate in all essential respects those commonly at hand in human beings. The streptococci in chronic foci maintain their specific infecting and other properties for many months, whereas artificial cultivation (especially on aerobic mediums) destroys specificity promptly, especially the property on which elective localization depends.

The focus affords ready entrance of bacteria and their toxic products which may, depending on inherited or acquired predispositions or other factors, cause infection in remote tissues, general ill effects, hypersensitiveness or allergy or a combination of some or all of these in the same persons, or perhaps at times increased resistance and immunity.

The localizing and necrotizing power peculiar to these organisms (usually streptococci) determines largely the site or tissues to be affected. The sooner foci are eliminated, after the onset of a disease, or preferably even before systemic symptoms have occurred, the better should be the immediate and end results. The common practice of waiting until the disease is far advanced or until a serious condition, such as a hemorrhage in ulcer or a cardiac attack in heart disease, has developed, or until advanced age has occurred, before evident foci, especially pulpless teeth, are removed, is most deplorable.

Since streptococci appear to be a cause of so many diseases, since immunity is of short duration, and since mechanical factors play so large a part in maintaining infection in structures so commonly the seat of foci, mechanical correction or removal, so far as possible, probably always will be necessary, even if highly effective specific or other remedial agents are discovered. Recurrence of the previous condition or new localization is prone to occur unless the predisposing cause, the focus, is eliminated. Likewise, operation probably always will be indicated in many of the chronic systemic lesions, such as chronic indurated ulcer, cholecystitis with gallstones and appendicitis with fecal stones or a constricted lumen resulting from previous attacks.

The removal of pulps of teeth and the filling of the roots of teeth calculated to prevent subsequent infection and root canal therapy are so difficult, so expensive and the results so uncertain, as to preclude their routine adoption. Many who formerly skillfully practiced the art find it no longer necessary, and consider it safer to remove pulpless teeth and to attach restorations in a way harmless to vital teeth. It is to be hoped that efficient methods may be found that will not only sterilize pulpless teeth and periapical tissues that have become infected, but will also prevent subsequent infection, especially of the periapical tissues. Considering the mechanical difficulties, the fulfilment of the latter requirement seems almost unattainable, and until this has been accomplished, it would seem wiser to remove teeth that have become infected or that require extirpation of the pulp, rather than to retain them at the risk of having them become the source of an insidious, incapacitating and perhaps fatal infection. Vital teeth free from pyorrhea and fillings should never be extracted except as it becomes necessary for restorative work, but the extraction of pulpless teeth seems to me to be indicated, wholly regardless of the appearance of the roentgenograms. Not too much should be expected or promised from the removal of a given focus, especially in chronic conditions, because a similar condition may be present in inaccessible foci and in foci too small to be detected. The source may not be a focus at all. Moreover, recovery may be made difficult by local tissue sensitivity or unusual mechanical conditions, and living bacteria in a metastatic lesion may continue the process independently of the focal source.

Elective localization of streptococci isolated from pyorrheal pockets occurred commonly following intravenous injection, emphasizing the importance of recognizing periodontoclasia as a focus of infection. Steps to prevent and correct this most common of evils should continue.

Teeth, especially multirooted teeth, with deep fillings or caries, which manifest evidence of infection of the pulp, with or without pulp stones, and even symptomless teeth which react positively to vitality tests and that have deep fillings, may be the source of systemic effects and may need to be removed. However, this should be done only after due consideration has been given to other sources of infection. I have repeatedly seen marked benefit following the removal of such teeth when all other efforts had failed, especially teeth in which pulps had died and were found to be heavily infected. Direct injection of the material containing the bacteria in such teeth often was followed by extremely specific effects.

The importance of good hygiene, proper living and inheritance as factors in preventing infective diseases from any source is granted. But why jeopardize or break down these barriers of nature through foci of infection, provided the latter can be prevented or eliminated? The fact that some persons may harbor foci of infection for a long time without apparent harm or systemic disease should not be interpreted as proof of the harmlessness of such foci, any more than polluted water was considered blameless in the days of water-borne typhoid because only a few of the many who drank the contaminated water contracted typhoid fever.

It must not be supposed that other regions, not foci in a mechanical sense, may not also harbor the streptococcus or other bacteria with which the disease from which the patient is suffering may be reproduced. I have isolated streptococci in some instances, not only from foci, but also from the more nearly normal mucous membrane of the upper part of the respiratory tract and from the stool. This may be a reason why the condition of some patients does not improve following removal of one focus or more. It also serves to show that the concept of the principles embodied in focal infection must not place too much emphasis on mechanical factors. The bacteria that gain entrance through foci must overcome the same inherent resistance of the host to produce diseases as those that gain entrance elsewhere. The factors determining localization are the same in both instances.

The clinical, bacteriologic and experimental studies now extant no longer leave any doubt of the basic fact that localized or pocketed infections or foci in the dental and other regions predispose to systemic disease, that prevention and removal of foci at the proper time and by proper methods are indicated and that mere elimination of foci does not always suffice to cope successfully with the many diseases which still beset human beings. More than removal of foci is necessary; this much seems established; these are matters on which all can agree. How often foci are responsible for the occurrence and for the progressive course of systemic diseases and how often preventive and curative effects may be expected from the elimination of primary or secondary foci in different diseases are still unsettled questions and call for further study.

REFERENCES

(1) ROSENOW, E. C.: Studies on elective localization; focal infection with special reference to oral sepsis. Dental Research, September, 1919, **1**: 205–249.

(2) ROSENOW, E. C.: Focal infection and elective localization. Internat. Clin., June, 1930, **2**: 29-64.

(3) ROSENOW, E. C.: Studies on focal infection, elective localization and cataphoretic velocity of streptococci. Dental Cosmos, July, 1937, **76**: 721–744.

(4) HADEN, R. L.: Dental Infection and Systemic Disease. Philadelphia, Lea & Febiger, 1928, 165 pp.

(5) BIERRING, W. L.: Focal infection: quarter century survey. (Frank Billing's lecture.) J. A. M. A., October 29, 1938, **111**: 1623–1627.

(6) REIMANN, H. A., AND HAVENS, W. P.: Focal infection and systemic disease; a critical appraisal; the case against indiscriminate removal of teeth and tonsils. J. A. M. A., January 6, 1940, **114**: 1-6.

(7) VON ALBERTINI, A., AND GRUMBACH, A.: Die experimentelle Streptokokkeninfektion des Kaninchens in ihren Beziehungen zur Herdinfektion. Ergebn. d. allg. Path. u. path. Anat., 1937, **33**: 314-423.

(8) JARLØV, E., AND BRINCH, O.: Focal infection, especially stomatogenic: experimental studies on chronic joint diseases produced by infection with streptococci of medium virulence. Hospitalstid., January 18, 1938, **81**: 80–85.

(9) RHOADS, P. S., AND DICK, G. F.: Efficacy of tonsillectomy for the removal of focal infection. J. A. M. A., October 20, 1928, **91**: 1149–1154.

(10) BORDA, JULIO M.: Dermatologia e Infeccion Focal. Thesis for Doctorate of Medicine, Buenos Aires, 1939.

(11) CAYLOR, H. D., AND DICK, G. F.: Quantitative bacteriology of the tonsils. J. A. M. A., February 25, 1922, **78**: 570–571.

(12) KAISER, A. D.: Incidence of rheumatism, chorea and heart disease in tonsillectomized children; a control study. J. A. M. A., December 31, 1927, **89**: 2239–2245.

(13) ANDREWS, G. C., AND MACHACEK, G. F.: Pustular bacterids of hands and feet. Arch. Dermat. & Syph., December, 1935, **32**: 837–847.

(14) GOLDBERG, H. G.: Ten years' research of dental infections and their relations to systemic disease. Am. J. Orthodontics, March, 1938, **24**: 272–280.

(15) IRONS, E. E.: Some less frequently considered portals of infection in arthritis and iritis. J. A. M. A., June 30, 1923, **80**: 1899-1902.

(16) BARNES, A. R., AND GIORDANO, A. S.: Bacteria recovered postmortem with special reference to selective localization and focal infection; preliminary report. J. Indiana M. A., January 15, 1922, **15**: 1-7.

(17) ROSENOW, E. C.: A bacteriologic study of pulmonary embolism. J. Infect. Dis., 1927, **40**: 389–398.

(18) NICKEL, A. C., AND HUFFORD, A. R.: Elective localization of streptococci isolated from cases of peptic ulcer. Arch. Int. Med., February, 1928, **41**: 210-230.

(19) McCLUSKIE, J. A. W.: Focal sepsis. Tr. Roy. Med.-Chir. Soc. Glasgow, pp. 13-17, 1936-1937; in Glasgow M. J., December, 1936.

(20) WILKINSON, H. F.: Pathologic changes in tonsils: a study of ten thousand pairs of tonsils, with special reference to the presence of cartilage, bone, tuberculosis and bodies suggestive of actinomycosis. Arch. Otolaryng., August, 1929, **10**: 127–151.

(21) SWIFT, H. F., DERICK, C. L., AND HITCHCOCK, C. H.: Bacterial allergy (hyperergy) to nonhemolytic streptococci: in its relation to rheumatic fever. J. A. M. A., March 24, 1928, **90**: 906–908.

(22) CLAWSON, B. J.: Experiments relative to a possible basis for vaccine therapy in acute rheumatic fever. J. Infect. Dis., July, 1931, **49**: 90–97.

(23) BIRKHAUG, K. E.: Rheumatic fever; bacteriologic studies of non-methemoglobin-forming streptococcus with especial reference to its soluble toxin production. J. Infect. Dis., May, 1927, **40**: 549-569.

(24) RHODES, G. B., AND APFELBACH, C. W.: Chronic localized streptococcus infections in dogs; experimental focal infection. J. Infect. Dis., September, 1928, **43**: 215-217.

(25) RÖSSLE, R.: Experimenteller Beitrag zum Verständnis der Herdinfektion. Virchows Arch. f. path. Anat., 1939, **304**: 1-18.

(26) MOON, V. H., AND KONZELMANN, F. W.: A method of producing chronic focal infections. Arch. Path., October, 1930, **10**: 587-588.

(27) REITH, A. F., AND SQUIER, T. L.: Blood cultures of apparently healthy persons. J. Infect. Dis., 1932, **51**: 336-343.

(28) RICKERT, U. G.: Significance of passive bacteremias. Oral Health, March, 1931, **21**: 162-171.

(29) AUSTIN, L. T., AND COOK, T. J.: Bacteriologic study of normal vital teeth. J. A. D. A., May, 1929, **16**: 894-896.

(30) RHOADS, P. S., AND DICK, G. F.: Roentgenographically negative pulpless teeth as foci of infection; results of quantitative cultures. J. A. D. A., November, 1932, **19**: 1884-1893.

(31) SWANSON, W. F., AND VAN KIRK, L. E.: Results of culturing 1800 pulpless teeth. J. Dent. Research, September, 1936, **15**: 315.

(32) THOMAS, B. O. A., AND HUBBELL, A. O.: New culture method for dental bacteriology. J. A. D. A., December, 1939, **26**: 2024-2029.

(33) HENRICI, A. T., AND HARTZELL, T. B.: Bacteriology of vital pulps. J. Dent. Research, December, 1919, **1**: 419-422.

(34) NICHOLS, ANNA C.: The virulence and classification of streptococci isolated from apical infections; a preliminary report. J. A. D. A., September, 1926, **13**: 1218-1231.

(35) LUCAS, C. D.: Periapical infection. Dental Cosmos, June, 1929, **71**: 555-562.

(36) CRAMER, H. C., AND REITH, A. F.: Quantitative bacteriologic study of pulpless teeth correlated with dental roentgenograms. J. A. D. A., June, 1932, **19**: 976-982.

(37) TOPLEY, W. W. C., AND WILSON, G. S.: The Principles of Bacteriology and Immunity. New York. William Wood & Company, 1929, vol. I, pp. 357-367.

(38) CANBY, C. P.: Incidence of pulpal infection in periodontoclasia. J. A. D. A., October, 1936, **23**: 1871-1880.

(39) FUENDELING, M. J., AND CARTNEY, T. L.: Roentgenographic diagnosis of vital pulp infection confirmed by bacteriological examination. Am. J. Roentgenol., September, 1938, **40**: 386-391.

(40) ELLIOTT, S. D.: Bacteriaemia and oral sepsis. Proc. Roy. Soc. Med., May, 1939, **32**: 747-754.

(41) RHOADS, P. S., AND DICK, G. F.: Roentgenographically negative pulpless teeth as foci of infection; results of quantitative cultures. J. A. D. A., November, 1932, **19**: 1884-1893.

(42) MEISSER, J. G., AND BROCK, SAM: A clinical and experimental study in chronic arthritis. J. A. D. A., December, 1923, **10**: 1100-1110.

(43) BROWN, R. O.: A study on the etiology of cholecystitis and its production by the injection of streptococci. Arch. Int. Med., February, 1919, **23**: 185-189.

(44) BUMPUS, H. C., JR., AND MEISSER, J. G.: Focal infection and selective localization of streptococci in pyelonephritis; study I. Arch. Int. Med., March, 1921, **27**: 326-337.

(45) BUMPUS, H. C., JR., AND MEISSER, J. G.: Foci of infections in cases of pyelonephritis; study II. J. A. M. A., November 5, 1921, **77**: 1475-1479.

(46) MEISSER, J. G., AND GARDNER, B. S.: Elective localization of bacteria isolated from infected teeth. J. Nat. Dent. A., 1922, **19**: 578-592.

(47) MARGOLIS, H. M., AND DORSEY, ANNA H. E.: Chronic arthritis; bacteriology of affected tissues. Arch. Int. Med., July, 1930, **46**: 121-136.

(48) MOENCH, LAURA M.: The relationship of chronic endocervicitis to focal infection with special reference to chronic arthritis. J. Lab. and Clin. Med., February, 1924, **9**: 289-309.

(49) NICKEL, A. C., AND JUDD, E. S.: Cholecystitis; bacteriologic and experimental study of 300 surgically resected gallbladders. Surg., Gynec. and Obst., April, 1930, **50**: 655-662.

(50) COOK, T. J.: Focal infection of the teeth and elective localization in the experimental production of ulcerative colitis. J. A. D. A., December, 1931, **18**: 2290-2301.

(51) BERNHARDT, HERMANN: Zur Frage der Fokalinfektion und der "elektiven Lokalisation." Ztschr. f. klin. Med., 1931, **117**: 158-174.

(52) ROTHSCHILD, M. A., AND THOLHIMER, WILLIAM: Experimental arthritis in the rabbit, produced with Streptococcus mitis. J. Exper. Med., May 1, 1914, **19**: 444-449.

(53) IRONS, E. E., BROWN, E. V. L., AND NADLER, W. H.: The localization of streptococci in the eye; a study of experimental iridocyclitis in rabbits. J. Infect. Dis., March, 1916, **18**: 315-334.

(54) KELLY, T. H.: The results of animal inoculations with material obtained from the tonsils of cases of acute rheumatic fever. Ohio State M. J., April 1, 1918, **14**: 221-223.

(55) TOPLEY, W. W. C., AND WEIR, H. B.: The lesions produced in rabbits by the inoculation of streptococci isolated from rheumatic and other lesions in the human subject. J. Path. and Bact., 1921, **24**: 333–346.

(56) PRICE, W. A.: Dental Infections; Oral and Systemic. Cleveland, Ohio, The Penton Publishing Company, vol. 1, 1923, p. 287.

(57) THOMPSON, MURIEL J.: An experimental study of the streptococci found in pyorrhea alveolaris. Edinburgh M. J., December, 1925, **32**: 781–806.

(58) SMALL, J. C.: The bacterium causing rheumatic fever and a preliminary account of the therapeutic action of its specific antiserum. Am. J. M. Sc., January, 1927, **173**: 101–129.

(59) HADEN, R. L.: The pulpless tooth from a bacteriologic and experimental standpoint. J. A. D. A., August, 1925, **12**: 918–934.

(60) PRECHT, EDWARD: Fokalinfektion. Deutsche med. Wchnschr., June 21, 1929, **55**: 1035–1037.

(61) VALENTINE, E., AND VAN METER, M.: Localization of streptococci in tissues of rabbits. J. Infect. Dis., July, 1930, **47**: 56–82.

(62) CLAWSON, B. J.: Experimental streptococcic inflammation in normal, immune and hypersensitive animals. Arch. Path., June, 1930, **9**: 1141–1153.

(63) STEINFELD, FRITZ: Untersuchungen über elektive Lokalisation. Ztschr. f. d. ges. exper. Med., 1931, **80**: 472–486.

(64) LUSENA, M., AND CHINI, V.: Le infezioni focali. Riforma med., October 14, 1933, **49**: 1533–1535.

(65) VON ALBERTINI, A., AND GRUMBACH, A.: Ergebnisse experimenteller Forschung zur Frage der Herdinfektion. Schweiz. med. Wchnschr., December 3, 1938, **68**: 1309–1315.

(66) LEHMANN, WALTHER: Zur Herdinfektion. Deutsche Gesell. f. inn. Med., 1930, **42**: 482–486.

(67) NICKEL, A. C., AND STUHLER, L. G.: The prostate gland as a focus of infection in arthritis. M. Clin. North America, May, 1930, **13**: 1519–1527.

(68) ILLINGSWORTH, C. F. W.: Types of gallbladder infection; study of 100 operated cases. Brit. J. Surg., October, 1927, **15**: 221–228.

(69) WILKIE, A. L.: The bacteriology of cholecystitis; a clinical and experimental study. Brit. J. Surg., January, 1928, **15**: 450–565.

(70) WILKIE, D. P. D.: An address on some aspects of gall-bladder disease. Brit. M. J., March 24, 1928, **1**: 481–484.

(71) CECIL, R. L., AND ANGEVINE, D. M.: Experimental streptococcus arthritis in rabbits. Tr. A. Am. Physicians, 1938, **53**: 310–317.

(72) HADEN, R. L., AND JORDON, W. H.: Multiple onychia as a manifestation of focal infection; experimental production of onychia in rabbits. Arch. Dermat. and Syph., July, 1923, **8**: 31–36.

(73) CANTERO, ANTONIO: Bacteriology of the thyroid gland in goiter. Surg., Gynec. and Obst., January, 1926, **42**: 61–63.

(74) VAN KIRK, L. E., AND SWANSON, W. F.: Experimental encephalitis in rabbits; intravenous injection of streptococci from pulpless teeth in human encephalitis. J. Dent. Research, September, 1936, **15**: 315–316.

(75) NICKEL, A. C., AND MUSSEY, R. D.: Experiments on the relations of focal infection to abortion. M. J. and Rec., April 6, 1927, **125**: 467–470.

(76) FASTING, G. F. C.: Focal infection and elective localization: evaluation of bacteriological procedures and biological factors. Am. Dent. Soc. of Europe, Nice, France, April 21, 1930, pp. 122–138.

(77) CURTIS, A. H.: Streptococcus infection as a cause of spontaneous abortion. J. A. M. A., December 9, 1916, **67**: 1739–1741.

(78) REITH, A. F.: Streptococci as a cause of spontaneous abortion. J. Infect. Dis., 1927, **41**: 423–427.

(79) HORTON, B. T., AND DORSEY, ANNA H. E.: Experimental thrombo-angiitis obliterans: bacteriologic and pathologic studies. Arch. Path., June, 1932, **13**: 910–925.

(80) SQUIER, T. L., AND BACH, CATHERINE T.: Experimental hypotension in rabbits. Arch. Int. Med., July, 1928, **42**: 56–63.

(81) ROSENOW, E. C., AND MEISSER, J. G.: The production of urinary calculi by the devitalization and infection of teeth in dogs with streptococci from cases of nephrolithiasis. Arch. Int. Med., 1923, **31**: 807–829.

(82) JONES, N. W., AND NEWSOM, S. J.: Experimentally produced focal (dental) infection in relation to cardiac structure. Arch. Path., March, 1932, **13**: 392–414.

(83) HOLMAN, W. L.: Focal infection and "elective localization:" critical review. Arch. Path. and Lab. Med., January, 1928, **5**: 68–136.

(84) ZINSSER, H., AND GRINNELL, F. B.: Further studies on bacterial allergy; antigen involved in pneumococcus allergy. J. Bact., November, 1927, **14**: 301–315.

(85) DERICK, C. L., HITCHCOCK, C. H., AND SWIFT, H. F.: Reactions of rabbits to nonhemolytic streptococci: study of modes of sensitization. J. Exper. Med., July, 1930, **52**: 1–22.

(86) MOON, V. H., AND STEWART, H. L.: Experimental rheumatic lesions in dogs and in rabbits. Arch. Path., February, 1931, **11**: 190–206.

(87) Harkary, Joseph: Focal Infections and Bacterial Allergy in Asthma and Arthritis. In: Libman Anniversary Volume, New York, The International Press, 1932, vol. 2, pp. 551–559.

(88) Weisberger, D.: Relation of hypersensitivity to localization in and dissemination of Streptococcus viridans from incisor teeth of rabbits. Yale J. Biol. and Med., May, 1937, **9**: 417–427.

(89) Rosenow, E. C., and Jensen, L. B.: Elective localization and cataphoretic potential of streptococci. Proc. Soc. Exper. Biol. and Med., February, 1930, **27**: 442–444.

(90) Sheard, Charles, Pratt, C. B., and Rosenow, E. C.: Symposium on cataphoresis and localization of streptococci; the high frequency field as an agent in changing the cataphoretic velocity and the localization of streptococci. Proc. Staff Meet., Mayo Clin., August 16, 1933, **8**: 496–504.